Drug Design Using Machine Learning

Scrivener Publishing
100 Cummings Center, Suite 541J
Beverly, MA 01915-6106

Publishers at Scrivener
Martin Scrivener (martin@scrivenerpublishing.com)
Phillip Carmical (pcarmical@scrivenerpublishing.com)

Drug Design Using Machine Learning

Edited by
Inamuddin
Tariq Altalhi
Jorddy N. Cruz
and
Moamen Salah El-Deen Refat

Scrivener Publishing

WILEY

This edition first published 2022 by John Wiley & Sons, Inc., 111 River Street, Hoboken, NJ 07030, USA and Scrivener Publishing LLC, 100 Cummings Center, Suite 541J, Beverly, MA 01915, USA

For more information about Scrivener publications please visit www.scrivenerpublishing.com.

Wiley Global Headquarters
111 River Street, Hoboken, NJ 07030, USA

For details of our global editorial offices, customer services, and more information about Wiley products visit us at www.wiley.com.

Library of Congress Cataloging-in-Publication Data

ISBN 9781394166282

Cover image: Pixabay.Com
Cover design by Russell Richardson

Set in size of 11pt and Minion Pro by Manila Typesetting Company, Makati, Philippines

Printed in the USA

10 9 8 7 6 5 4 3 2 1

Contents

Preface

Traditionally, the design of new drugs has been a long process that requires an investment of billions of dollars. In the last decades, molecular modeling techniques have been used in the pharmaceutical industry and large laboratories to accelerate this process in order to reduce the amount of money that needs to be invested. More recently, machine learning approaches to drug discovery have aroused great interest in the scientific community. This has occurred, among other reasons, due to advances in high-performance computing and the availability of an abundance of biological and chemical information on thousands of compounds. Through machine learning and artificial intelligence approaches, this information can be filtered quickly and at a low cost. From this, algorithms can be trained to be used in the different stages of drug design.

The objective of this book is to bring together several chapters that function as an overview of the use of machine learning and artificial intelligence applied to drug development. The initial chapters discuss drug-target interactions through machine learning for improving drug delivery, healthcare, and medical systems. Further chapters also provide topics on drug repurposing through machine learning, drug designing, and ultimately discuss drug combinations prescribed for patients with multiple or complex ailments. This book should be useful for information technology professionals, pharmaceutical industry workers, engineers, university students and faculty members, medical practitioners, researchers and laboratory workers who have a keen interest in the area of machine learning and artificial intelligence approaches applied to drug advancements. A chapter-by-chapter summary of the work reported in the 12 chapters of this book follows.

- Chapter 1 describes the use of molecular recognition for drug development through various mathematical models. Molecular docking of the main elements is discussed in detail to consider which elements are important for obtaining a reliable prediction of protein-ligand complexes. The role of machine learning in molecular recognition models is also analyzed.

- Chapter 2 reviews classical and machine learning-based approaches to study target-drug interactions in the field of drug discovery, from target identification to the optimization of the lead compound. In addition, a special section discusses peptide-based drugs.
- Chapter 3 gives a brief overview of the various machine learning techniques that underpin artificial intelligence, poly-pharmacology, and drug repurposing to improve healthcare services. The way in which machine learning is used throughout the drug development process to help increase its efficacy and robustness, resulting in a significant reduction of the time and cost of bringing new drugs to market, is discussed in detail.
- Chapter 4 elaborates on the advancements in artificial intelligence technologies along with their applications, enumerates the challenges faced by these technologies that retard their full-scale implementation, and also provides an overview of their social, legal, and economic aspects. All these are discussed for various applications such as drug delivery, healthcare, and medical systems.
- Chapter 5 details the various machine learning approaches for drug repurposing. The network-based approach, text mining-based approach, and semantics-based approach are discussed in fair detail. Furthermore, case studies of drugs repurposed through machine learning programs are also discussed.
- Chapter 6 summarizes the recent developments in the machine learning-mediated drug discovery process within industrial and academic contexts. More precisely, machine learning algorithms used for drug discovery, bioactivity prediction using machine learning, and application of machine learning in chemo-informatics are reviewed. Furthermore, an in-depth analysis of the challenges and suggestions are provided.
- Chapter 7 details the basic principles underlying supercritical fluid technology and its main techniques. Furthermore, the more representative biodegradable polymers impregnated with supercritical fluid technology are described. Finally, the state of the art of supercritical fluid technology for improving drug absorption in biopolymer and the delivery processes are thoroughly reviewed.
- Chapter 8 details the different *in vivo, in vitro* and *in silico* techniques applied to study the protein-protein interactions through the active sites. The role of the active sites of protein is also discussed. Moreover, databases and algorithms are mentioned along with their uses and advantages.
- Chapter 9 describes various machine-learning methods involved in protein redesign and engineering along with strategies ranging from designing the model to predicting hot spots. The chapter also focuses on additional

support vector machines, nearest neighbor, decision trees, neural networks, Bayesian networks, ensemble learning, and deep learning.

– Chapter 10 describes computational methods used for the selection of bioactive compounds. In this context, various approaches based on transcriptomics and artificial intelligence are discussed. Additionally, methods and applications of de novo synthesis are also addressed along with its future endeavors in drug designing.

– Chapter 11 discusses the application of computer-aided techniques for the prediction of drug effectiveness and toxicity, including artificial intelligence, artificial neural networks, and machine learning. A hierarchical method for drug design is followed as drug discovery, drug design through new techniques and application, machine learning methods, deep learning, applications, and problems.

– Chapter 12 details the use of artificial intelligence in assessing the side effects to drugs. Practicing artificial intelligence necessitates the skills and awareness for data-intensive analysis, knowledge-based management, and definite challenges. A smarter future can be envisaged using artificial intelligence-guided new scientific accomplishments in the field of pharmacovigilance.

The Editors
Inamuddin
Tariq Altalhi
Jorddy N. Cruz
Moamen Salah El-Deen Refat
July 2022

1

Molecular Recognition and Machine Learning to Predict Protein-Ligand Interactions

A. Reyes Chaparro[2], J.A. Moreno-Melendres[1], A.L. Ramos-Jacques[3] and A.R. Hernandez-Martinez[2]*

[1]PCeIM-UNAM, Centro de Física Aplicada y Tecnología Avanzada (CFATA), Universidad Nacional Autónoma de México (UNAM), Querétaro, México

[2]Centro de Física Aplicada y Tecnología Avanzada (CFATA), Universidad Nacional Autónoma de México (UNAM), Querétaro, México

[3]Edit Academy, México, Querétaro, México

Abstract

Molecular recognition is part of several chemical-biological processes, and is the interaction between macromolecules (such as proteins and ligands) through noncovalent bonds. This phenomenon has been extensively studied for developing new drugs. Molecular modeling is an affordable method (compared with laboratory experiments) for predicting which macromolecules may interact and, through molecular docking, which will form a stable complex. Molecular docking has two main components: (1) search algorithm and (2) scoring function. The search algorithm studies the conformational space of the ligand at the binding site. The scoring function is a mathematical model that evaluates the interaction energy of each complex, and it could be empirical by using databases of ligand-protein complexes. Results of the search algorithm are satisfactory compared with experimental data, but the scoring function still must improve its performance. Due to the complexity of analysis and management of databases, accurate predictions are difficult to obtain. Machine learning can contribute to achieve better results for predicting macromolecular interactions. Computational predictions of the interaction between macromolecules complexes enhance the development of applied technology in medicine.

**Corresponding author*: angel.ramon.hernandez@gmail.com

Inamuddin, Tariq Altalhi, Jorddy N. Cruz and Moamen Salah El-Deen Refat (eds.) Drug Design Using Machine Learning, (1–20) © 2022 Scrivener Publishing LLC

Keywords: Molecular docking, search algorithm, scoring function, mathematical models

1.1 Introduction

Life is based on four main groups of macromolecules: carbohydrates, lipids, proteins, and nucleic acids. Each group of molecules separately cannot create an organism, life and all its functions arise when there is a dynamic and continuous interaction between these macromolecules and small organic and inorganic molecules. Molecular recognition refers to the process in which biological macromolecules interact with each other or with small molecules through noncovalent interactions to form a complex [1]. Molecular recognition is not a physiological process, it is rather a component of many processes, such as cell signaling, genetic regulation, metabolism, immunity, and all those processes in which there is an interaction between macromolecules (or between a macromolecule and a ligand) [2, 3]. For example, in the expression of genes, there must be a molecular recognition between the inducing proteins and the DNA chain to generate the mRNA. Subsequently, there is molecular recognition between the mRNA and the ribosomes, and thus in each of the steps until generating a functional protein, which in turn has molecular recognition according to its function [4]. Another example is the enzymatic reactions that are carried out for the energy metabolism of the carbohydrate and lipid pathways, in addition to the xenobiotic metabolism, which is carried out simultaneously in cells, all the time [5]. The chapter discusses the ligand-protein molecular recognition using data and algorithms for improving mechanisms predictions.

1.1.1 Molecular Recognition

The molecular recognition model has evolved since 1894 when Emil Fischer proposed the "lock key" model in which the ligand and the protein were kept rigid and had a highly specific interaction [6]. Later, in 1958, Koshland [7] proposed that molecules promote a conformational change in proteins and it was called the "induced fit" model. The induced fit model considers that the protein does not always have the same conformation and that different ligands could lead to different induced fit; with these new concepts, phenomena, such as noncompetitive and allosteric inhibition, could be explained [1]. More recently, the idea of conformational selection was raised, in which proteins are found naturally in different conformations and ligands have a different affinity for each conformation [8]. Current interaction models consider that the induced fit and conformational selection phenomena occur in a complementary manner (Figure 1.1) [9].

The phenomenon of molecular recognition has been studied extensively in the development of new drugs. When a new protein involved in a physiological process or disease is described, it is considered as a potential target molecule. New drugs are tested and designed for having an interaction with that target molecule to obtain a potential therapeutic effect [10]. The most widely used experimental tool for finding new molecules with potential biological activity is the high-throughput screening (HTS), which is an automated process to screen large amounts of ligands with a single protein that allows identifying molecules with activity against the target protein [11]. Although HTS is a highly optimized process, the number of

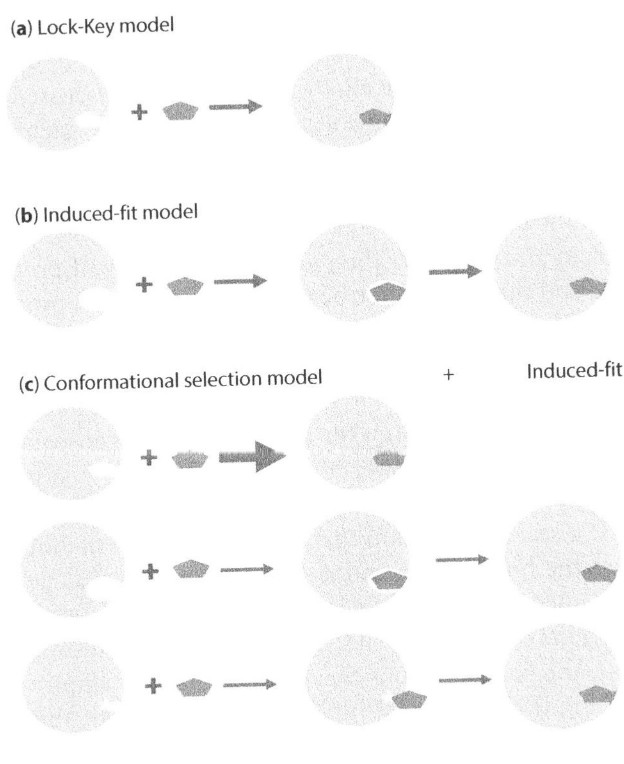

Figure 1.1 Molecular recognition models.

existing molecules currently amounts to millions of compounds, and it is not cost-effective enough to be used as an initial tool for drug discovery screening [12]. For this reason, computational methods are of great interest in the screening of millions of compounds at a reasonable cost. Structure-based virtual screening is one of the most widely used to screen databases of millions of compounds, based on their affinity for the target protein [13]. The only requirement is to have the three-dimensional structure of the target protein to be able to carry out the interaction tests, these are called molecular coupling.

1.2 Molecular Docking

The use of computers for drug development is known as computer-aided drug design (CADD); many different techniques are supported by the pharmaceutical industry and universities to accelerate the development of new drugs. Some of the tools used are quantitative structure-activity relationship (QSAR) models, pharmacophore modeling, lead optimization, molecular dynamics, and molecular coupling [14]. In addition, different machine learning applications, which will be discussed in section 1.3, have complemented the same techniques but with a machine learning algorithm.

Molecular coupling is a computational test that allows studying the interaction at the molecular level between a macromolecule, which is normally a protein and a ligand. The molecular modeling of proteins began in the 1980s, and this allowed the beginning of simulation processes, such as molecular ligand-protein recognition [15]. The results of the coupling made it possible to select a large number of substances according to their energy of interaction with the target protein. Currently, molecular docking is widely used in the search for new drugs, as a consequence of the increase in computational power and the availability of large databases of ligands and proteins [16]. Molecular docking protocols have two main components: a search algorithm that shows the conformational space of the ligand at the binding site and a scoring function that quantitatively evaluates the interaction energy of each of the conformations [17]. Finally, after sampling the conformational space and evaluating the binding energy of each pose, the conformations that present the best affinity energy are obtained. Using these results of molecular docking tests, the best molecules can be proposed to be chemically synthesized by carrying out new experimental tests (Figure 1.2) [18].

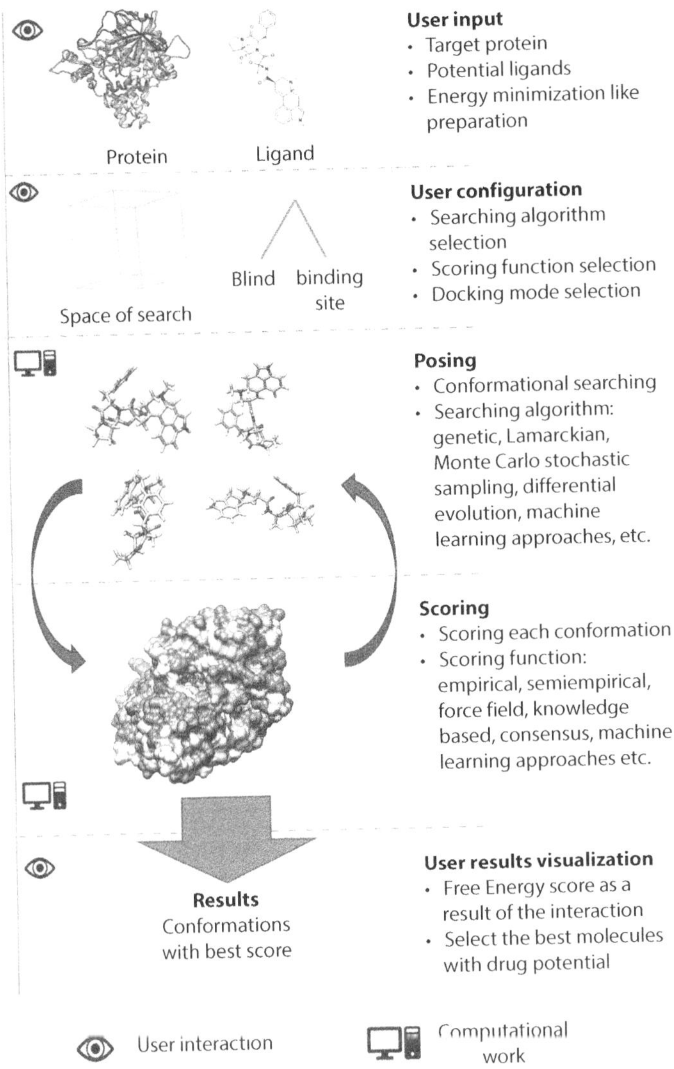

Figure 1.2 General protocol of docking work.

1.2.1 Conformational Search Algorithm

The binding pose refers to the conformation that the ligand has, with respect to the protein; in molecular docking, a large number of binding poses are evaluated trying to cover the entire conformational space of the ligand within the sampling space [19]. Taking into account the sampling space, two types of molecular docking are known: blind docking and binding-site docking. Blind docking includes all the protein within the sampling space, it is used to find out which is the site with the highest affinity energy of the ligand for the protein, this is mainly useful when the binding site of the target protein is unknown. On the other hand, binding-site docking has a sampling space limited to a particular area that is usually the protein-binding site; it can also target an allosteric site or any region of interest [16].

The conformational search stage is about sampling all the possible conformations that the ligand can take in the search space. Conformations are based on the structural parameters, torsion, translation, and the degrees of freedom of torsion (dihedral) of the ligands [20]. The amount of conformations that can be tested increases exponentially as the degrees of freedom increase, that is, the rotatable bonds of the ligand; this phenomenon is known as combinatorial explosion [21]. The aim of the conformational searching is to generate all possible conformations so that they can be evaluated with the score function, and find the conformation in which the ligand has the greatest stability with the protein. In molecular docking, the most stable position that the ligand can take in interaction with the protein is known as the global minimum; there are also local minimums that are stable conformations, but with lower energy than the global minimum (Figure 1.3) [22].

There are two options to perform the conformational search, using stochastic or systematic methods [23, 24]. In systematic methods, different conformations of the same ligand are used, in each one, small conformational changes in the molecules are tested and evaluated by the scoring function. Modifications continue until they converge to the energy minimum after long cycles of conformational search and interaction energy evaluation. The method has computational performance advantages over stochastic, however it is more likely that the results will converge on a local minimum and the global minimum will not be reached, simultaneous searches must be performed from different conformations to increase the probability of reaching a global minimum [22]. For their part, stochastic methods also start from different ligand conformations, but with the stochastic type function the conformational changes are random, obtaining a greater number of different ligand conformations covering a larger sampling area [25]. The stochastic method has a greater probability of reaching a "minimum global" of energy; however, generating random numbers in a system greatly increases the computational cost of the process, so although it is more efficient it also demands more resources [26].

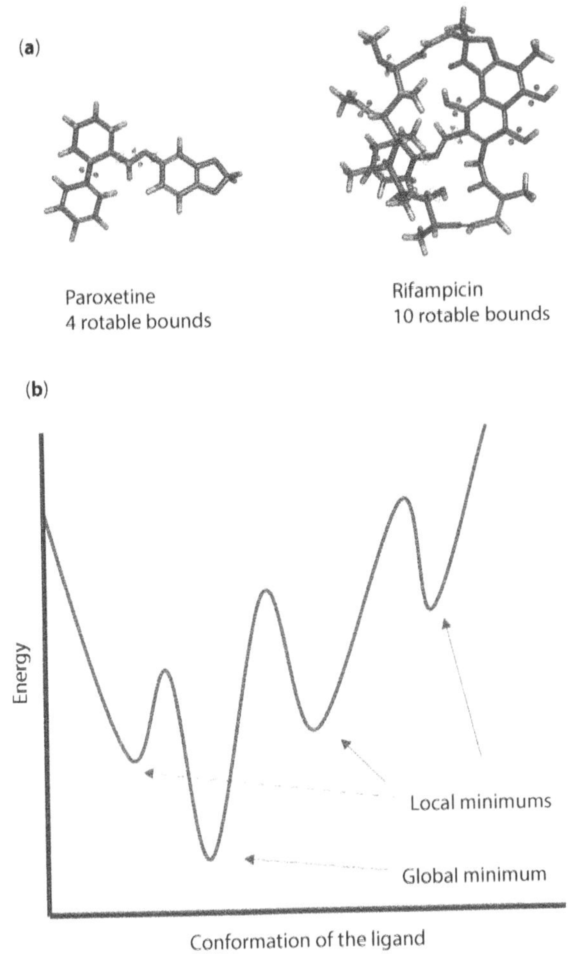

Figure 1.3 Conformational searching. (a) Rotatable bonds of two common drugs. (b) Conformational searching of the best ligand pose (global minimum).

Each conformation generated by any method will be evaluated by the scoring function and the conformations with the best interaction energy will be selected to perform new conformational modifications again by either method.

1.2.2 Scoring Function with Conventional Methods

The scoring function is a mathematical or predictive model that calculates a score that represents the binding free energy of each of the conformations that the software tests [27]. Conventional calculation methods for the score function are based on the physical calculation of the atomic interactions between the ligand and the protein; the set of equations involved in the calculation is called the force field. Force fields are based on five terms: potential energy, torsion terms, bond geometry, electrostatic terms, and Lennard-Jones potential [28]. When the scoring function of a software uses a force field, it is known as a force field-based score function. However, there are also empirical and knowledge-based score functions. The empirical scoring function has a different calculation system, the energy resulting from the calculations is composed of weighted energy terms; the terms describe a chemically intuitive interaction, these include hydrogen bonding, desolvation effect, van der Waals interactions, hydrophobicity, and entropy [29]. The reference data for the empirical score function also have an experimental origin that is adjusted to calibrate the different coefficients using linear regressions [30]. On another hand, knowledge-based scoring functions are based on large databases of ligand-protein complexes that are studied using statistical approaches. Thus, rules and models are obtained and then used to calculate the affinity energy of the new ligand-receptor complexes [31]. In comparison, the conformational search function has achieved a good reproducibility rate with respect to the experimental crystallography data; however, the scoring function has presented poor performance compared to the experimental data [32].

The validation of the molecular docking protocols is performed through comparisons of the results obtained with the docking test and the results of the cocrystallized ligand-receptor complexes. This comparison is made using the root mean square deviation (RMSD), which is a measure of the variation between the position of the same molecule, but with the conformation that was obtained by docking test and that was obtained by crystallography (Equation 1.1) [33]. The RMSD tests allow the selection of the best search protocol for the trials that are planned to be performed. The DockBench platform has been developed to facilitate the task of selecting docking protocols, in this platform, autocoupling routines are performed to reproduce the cocrystallized complexes; thus measuring the capacity of each protocol to replicate the crystallographic pose, using the RMSD as a reference measure. A more comprehensive evaluation of the protocols uses the lowest, the highest, and the average RMSD values ($RMSD_{min}$, $RMSD_{max}$, and $RMSD_{ave}$, respectively), as well as the largest number of conformations with a lower RMSD than the corresponding crystal at x-ray resolution (R) RMSD value (RMSD <R) [33].

$$RMSD = \sqrt{\frac{1}{N}\sum_{i=1}^{N}(X_{ci} - x_{di})^2 + (y_{ci} - y_{di})^2 + (z_{ci} - z_{di})^2} \quad (1.1)$$

Equation 1.1. Root mean squared deviation for two sets of N atoms on c and d coordinates, in x, y, z axis.

Currently, there are diverse software available to perform molecular docking assays, this allows for approximations using different conformational search algorithms and combinations of scoring functions. Torres *et al.* [27] made a compilation of the different software available, also showing a brief description of his algorithm for conformational search and scoring. The most recommended currently is to use different scoring functions to validate the docking results, this is known as consensus docking. Each scoring function has different scopes and details, they can complement each other but their comparison and combination is not recommended [34]. Combining three or four scoring functions is considered optimal to improve results, although sufficient predictive power has not yet been achieved, especially in the case of highly flexible ligands [16, 35]. That is why new approaches are emerging using machine learning, to achieve a better score function.

1.3 Machine Learning

Advances in computational science have made it possible to generate better molecular recognition simulations, leading to a wide use in developing new drugs. Machine learning (ML) has found acceptance in all fields of science and technology, pushing the frontiers of knowledge, since there are now large databases that work to train algorithms. The first computer-aided techniques began in the 1950s; however, the large databases that are available today were not yet available. Machine learning relies on data science, and through the development of mathematical and statistical models, predictive models can be built in computer-aided drug development. Currently, machine learning models are also widely used in autonomous car development, speech recognition, search engines, cybersecurity, etc. [36]. Machine learning algorithms have been incorporated into all steps of the drug discovery process, such as prediction of interactions with target molecules (molecular docking), prediction of physical and chemical properties of drugs, biomarker analysis, optimization of biomolecules, and prediction of properties, pharmacokinetics, and pharmacodynamics [37, 38].

However, all the machine learning algorithms developed so far can be grouped into two categories; supervised and unsupervised. Algorithms developed from supervised learning, learn from training samples with known labels and are then tested to determine the labels of new samples. On the other hand, the algorithms that are developed under an unsupervised scheme recognize patterns of a set of samples generally without labels. To recognize high-dimensional patterns, the data are transformed into a lower dimension, which is useful since in reduced dimensions, unsupervised learning is more efficient, and the recognized patterns can be more easily interpreted [14]. When a combination of both types of learning is used, it is called semi-supervised and reinforcement learning [39].

The databases available for the development, evolution, and feasibility of machine learning algorithms are essential at every step of the process. Currently, there are various databases on proteins, ligands, interactions, biological activities, etc., that have made it possible to develop models with greater predictive power. With the development of omics sciences, the amount of data that can be obtained have grown exponentially in recent years. The increase in the capacity to handle and process large amounts of data has allowed a greater number of variables that can be used to train a machine-learning algorithm. Because of the large amount of data and increasingly efficient algorithms, a new search has recently emerged to arrive at precision and personalized medicine. In the same form, personalized medicine was already a discipline and machine learning enhances many aspects of its application, also molecular docking has benefited from algorithms developed with machine learning to have greater predictive power on ligand-receptor interactions.

1.3.1 Machine Learning in Molecular Docking

As mentioned before, machine learning is not a molecular docking technique, it is a set of tools and techniques based on a wide range of algorithms, collectively known as "Computational Intelligence," designed to interpret and obtain knowledge from databases. ML can be widely used to improve some of the steps in the molecular docking process. The main use of ML applications for molecular docking is for improving the scoring function, which has not reached high precision with conventional methods [32]. However, there are several recent efforts to predict ligand-receptor interactions using ML techniques throughout the molecular docking process, mainly focused on the design of new drugs, using different approaches, such as Random Forest, Naive Bayesian Classification (NBC), multiple linear regression (MLR), Logistic Regression (LR), linear discriminant analysis (LDA), probabilistic neural networks (PNN), multi-layer perceptron (MLP), support vector machine (SVM), which are some of the most used algorithms in machine learning [40–42].

Semisupervised training techniques have been effective in addressing the use of incomplete databases, where the lack of labels or null data in some items can be overcome with the use of previously established criteria. However, with complete and properly labeled databases, better results will be obtained. In addition, with the semisupervised techniques that have integrated the chemical structure, the data of the drug-protein interaction network and the data of the genome sequence, the results obtained have been much more successful [42–44]. On the other hand, training techniques based on deep learning have shown promising potential in molecular docking, due to their great ability to recognize hidden patterns in extremely large data sets (Big data). Deep learning approaches have been investigated to replace classical scoring functions, showing still a moderate success for their potential. An advantage of the deep learning approach is its multi-layered function-based techniques for automatically extracting information from available initialized databases. While the functions are designed to extract information from databases, in traditional machine learning models they are done manually [40, 41, 45–50].

1.3.2 Machine Learning Challenges in Molecular Docking

Conformal scoring is the most challenging aspect of molecular docking; the same scoring function represents a limitation in virtual screening as it serves to score and classify molecules. Classic scoring functions simplify the function to maintain computational efficiency [16]. Conventional score functions assume a parametric system with nonbinding interactions as input variables; these variables were established by reference values of available systems [51]. Rigid systems of input variables prevent the algorithm from adapting to different situations, this section is where they have had the greatest impact on machine learning approaches [52]. There are several success stories on the use of machine learning in molecular docking, for example, in native pose prediction and virtual binder screening [53–55].

The most recent applications of machine learning require even greater optimizations to achieve adequate performance, it is required to train the algorithms with large databases that increase their versatility to have a greater field of application [56]. On the other hand, if the algorithm

Table 1.1 Developments using machine learning (ML) algorithms in molecular docking. Modified from: Torres *et al.* 2019 [27].

SF name and reference	ML algorithm	Training database	Best performance	Generic or family specific	Type of docking study
RF-Score [51]	RF[a]	PDBbind	Rp[b] = 0.776	Generic	BAP[c]
B2BScore [59]	RF	PDBbind	Rp = 0.746	Generic	BAP
SFCScore^{RF} [57]	RF	PDBbind	Rp = 0.779	Generic	BAP
PostDOCK [55]	RF	Constructed from PDB	92% accuracy	Generic	VS[d]
- [54]	SVM[e]	DUD	-	Both	VS
ID-Score [58]	SVR[f]	PDBbinf	Rp = 0.85	Generic	BAP
NNScore [60]	NN[g]	PDB;MOAD; PDBbind-CN	Ef = 10.3	Generic	VS
CScore [61]	NN	PDBbind	RPgen = 0.7668 Rpfam = 0.8237	Both	BAP
- [62]	Deep NN	CSAR, DUD-E	ROCAUC = 0.868	Generic	VS

(Continued)

Table 1.1 Developments using machine learning (ML) algorithms in molecular docking. Modified from: Torres *et al.* 2019 [27]. (*Continued*)

SF name and reference	ML algorithm	Training database	Best performance	Generic or family specific	Type of docking study
- [56]	Deep NN	DUD-E	ROCAUC = 0.92	Both	VS
DLScore [63]	Deep NN	PDBbind	Rp = 0.82	Generic	BAP
DeepVS [64]	Deep NN	DUD	ROCAUC = 0.81	Generic	VS
Kdeep [65]	Deep NN	PDBbind	Rp = 0.82	Generic	BAP

[a]Random Forest; [b]Pearson's Correlation Coefficient; [c]Binding Affinity Prediction; [d]Virtual Screening; e Support Vector Machine; [f]Support Vector Regression; [g]Neural Network.

becomes too complex it will have problems being interpreted and having a relationship with the structure. Coupling machine learning studies focus on improving predictive powers and there are few applications in drug discovery, most algorithms have not been implemented in available software. Torres *et al.* [27] study the machine learning applications and the predictive power that was achieved, Table 1.1 summarizes that information. Some algorithms are designed specifically for a group of molecules, this causes specific algorithms to improve the predictive power for a group of compounds of interest. On the other hand, generic algorithms can be applied to any type of molecule, but the predictive power can vary between groups of molecules. Machine learning allows having nonparametric predictions, which provokes more versatile predictions. The implementation of machine learning algorithms in analysis software is the next step for its implementation in the research and pharmaceutical industry [57, 58].

The recent advances that ML tools represent great opportunities in molecular docking, but they also pose relatively new challenges. These challenges are related with the database availability; e.g., the widely used ZINC library showed a growth between 2005 and 2019 of 1000 times the molecules stored in itself; and went from 700,000 entries to more than 1,300 million molecules [66–68]. There is a lack of experience in; *(i)* the selection of libraries and data sets; *(ii)* how to coupling databases with smaller data collections; *(iii)* assigning appropriate labels to ultra-large chemical libraries for diverse users with diverse interests [68–75]. There are also challenges, apparently less complicated to solve, related to the approaches in using the technology; *(i)* conformational flexibility of the ligand, *(ii)* conformational flexibility of the receptor, *(iii)* sampling of binding sites and binding poses more efficiently, and *(iv)* scoring different binding modes with greater precision. However, these challenges are addressed in different efforts, each time with better results [76–80].

1.4 Conclusions

Advances in computational science enabled better molecular recognition simulations. The progress in molecular docking is related with the scoring function improvement. This requires the analysis and processing of large quantities of data, which complicates the reliable prediction of stable protein-ligand complexes. Machine learning can contribute to achieve better results for predicting macromolecular interactions. Machine learning algorithms available can be trained by existing databases, but this process must include labeling those databases for increasing algorithm efficiency;

semi-supervised training techniques are recommended. This process can be incorporated in the development of new drugs, for the prediction of interactions with target molecules (molecular docking), physicochemical drugs properties, biomarker analysis, pharmacokinetics, and pharmacodynamics features. Computational predictions of the interaction between macromolecules complexes enhance the development of applied technology in medicine and could aid in the establishment of personalized medicine.

References

1. Demchenko, A.P., Recognition between flexible protein molecules: Induced and assisted folding. *J. Mol. Recognit.*, *14*, 42, 2001.
2. Kavraki, L.E. and Docking, Protein-ligand, including flexible receptor-flexible ligand docking, in: *Geometric Methods in Structural Computational Biology, L.E*, Kavraki, (Ed.), 2009.
3. Du, X., Li, Y., Xia, Y.L., Ai, S.M., Liang, J., Sang, P., Ji, X.L., Liu, S.Q., Insights into protein–ligand interactions: Mechanisms, models, and methods. *Int. J. Mol. Sci. 17*, 2, 144, 2016.
4. Mitsis, T., Efthimiadou, A., Bacopoulou, F., Vlachakis, D., Chrousos, G.P., Eliopoulos, E., Transcription factors and evolution: An integral part of gene expression (Review). *World Acad. Sci. J.*, *2*, 3, 2020.
5. Strogatz, S.H., Exploring complex networks. *Nature*, *410*, 268, 2001.
6. Böhm, H.J. and Schneider, G., *Protein-ligand interactions: From molecular recognition to drug design*, pp. 3–20, Weinheim, Germany, Wiley-VCH Verlag, 2003.
7. Koshland, D.E., Application of a theory of enzyme specificity to protein synthesis. *Proc. Natl. Acad. Sci.*, *44*, 98, 1958.
8. Vogt, A.D., Pozzi, N., Chen, Z., Di Cera, E., Essential role of conformational selection in ligand binding. *Biophys. Chem.*, *186*, 13, 2014.
9. Paul, F. and Weikl, T.R., How to distinguish conformational selection and induced fit based on chemical relaxation Rates. *PloS Comput. Biol.*, *12*, e1005067, 2016.
10. Ammar, O., *In silico* pharmacodynamics, toxicity profile and biological activities of the saharan medicinal plant limoniastrum Feei. *Braz. J. Pharm. Sci.*, *53*, 1, 2017.
11. Inglese, J., Johnson, R.L., Simeonov, A., Xia, M., Zheng, W., Austin, C.P., Auld, D.S., High-throughput screening assays for the identification of chemical probes. *Nat. Chem. Biol.*, *3*, 466, 2007.
12. Lyne, P.D., Structure-based virtual screening: An overview. *Drug Discovery Today*, *7*, 1047, 2002.

13. Marrone, T.J., Briggs, J.M., McCammon, J.A., Structure-based drug design: Computational advances. *Annu. Rev. Pharmacol. Toxicol.*, *37*, 71, 1997.
14. Patel, L., Shukla, T., Huang, X., Ussery, D.W., Wang, S., Machine learning methods in drug discovery. *Mol. Basel Switz.*, *25*, 22, 5277, 2020.
15. Naqvi, A.A.T. and Hassan, Md., II, Methods for docking and drug designing, in: *Methods and Algorithms for Molecular Docking-Based Drug Design and Discovery*, S. Dastmalchi, M. Hamzeh-Mivehroud, B. Sokouti (Eds.), pp. 39–53, Hershey, P, IGI Global, 2016.
16. Kitchen, D.B., Decornez, H., Furr, J.R., Bajorath, J., Docking and scoring in virtual screening for drug discovery: Methods and applications. *Nat. Rev. Drug Discovery*, *311*, 935, 2004.
17. Pagadala, N.S., Syed, K., Tuszynski, J., Software for molecular docking: A review. *Biophys. Rev.*, *9*, 91, 2017.
18. Sousa, S.F., Fernandes, P.A., Ramos, M.J., Protein-ligand docking: Current status and future challenges. *Proteins Struct. Funct. Genet.*, *65*, 15, 2006.
19. Rarey, M., Kramer, B., Lengauer, T., Klebe, G., A fast flexible docking method using an incremental construction algorithm. *J. Mol. Biol.*, *261*, 470, 1996.
20. Ferreira, L.G., Dos Santos, R.N., Oliva, G., Andricopulo, A.D., Molecular docking and structure-based drug design strategies. *Molecules*, *20*, 13384, 2015.
21. Dias, R. and de Azevedo Jr., W., Molecular docking algorithms. *Curr. Drug Targets*, *9*, 1040, 2008.
22. Zsoldos, Z., Reid, D., Simon, A., Sadjad, S.B., Johnson, A.P., EHiTS: A new fast, exhaustive flexible ligand docking system. *J. Mol. Graph. Model.*, *26*, 198, 2007.
23. Agrafiotis, D.K., Gibbs, A.C., Zhu, F., Izrailev, S., Martin, E., Conformational sampling of bioactive molecules: A comparative study. *J. Chem. Inf. Model.*, *47*, 1067, 2007.
24. Yuriev, E., Agostino, M., Ramsland, P.A., Challenges and advances in computational docking: 2009 in review. *J. Mol. Recognit.*, *24*, 149, 2011.
25. Gorelik, B. and Goldblum, A., high quality binding modes in docking ligands to proteins. *Proteins Struct. Funct. Genet.*, *71*, 1373, 2008.
26. McGann, M., FRED and HYBRID docking performance on standardized datasets. *J. Comput. Aided Mol. Des.*, *26*, 897, 2012.
27. Torres, P.H.M., Sodero, A.C.R., Jofily, P., Silva-Jr, F.P., Key topics in molecular docking for drug design. *Int. J. Mol. Sci.*, *20*, 1, 2019.
28. Monticelli, L. and Tieleman, D.P., Force fields for classical molecular dynamics. *Methods Mol. Biol.*, *924*, 197, 2013.
29. Korb, O., Stützle, T., Exner, T.E., Empirical scoring functions for advanced protein-ligand docking with plants. *J. Chem. Inf. Model.*, *49*, 84, 2009.
30. Hans-Joachim, B., The Development of a simple empirical scoring function to estimate the binding constant for a protein-ligand complex of known three-dimensional structure. *J. Comput. Aided Mol. Des.*, *8*, 243, 1994.

31. Rimac, H., Grishina, M., Potemkin, V., Use of the complementarity principle in docking procedures: A new approach for evaluating the correctness of binding poses. *J. Chem. Inf. Model.*, *61*, 4, 1801, 2021.
32. Chaput, L. and Mouawad, L., Efficient conformational sampling and weak scoring in docking programs? Strategy of the wisdom of crowds. *J. Cheminformatics*. *9*, 1, 37, 1–18, 2017.
33. Ciancetta, A., Cuzzolin, A., Moro, S., Alternative quality assessment strategy to compare performances of GPCR-ligand docking protocols: The human adenosine A2A receptor as a case study. *J. Chem. Inf. Model.*, *54*, 2243, 2014.
34. Huang, S.Y., Grinter, S.Z., Zou, X., Scoring functions and their evaluation methods for protein-ligand docking: Recent advances and future directions. *Phys. Chem. Chem. Phys.*, *12*, 12899, 2010.
35. Wang, R. and Wang, S., How does consensus scoring work for virtual library screening? An idealized computer experiment. *J. Chem. Inf. Comput. Sci. 41*, 1422–1426, 2001.
36. Kimber, T.B., Chen, Y., Volkamer, A., Deep learning in virtual screening: Recent applications and developments. *Int. J. Mol. Sci.*, *22*, 443, 2021.
37. Gertrudes, J.C., Maltarollo, V.G., Silva, R.A., Oliveira, P.R., Honorio, K.M., da Silva, A.B.F., Machine learning techniques and drug design. *Curr. Med. Chem.*, *19*, 4289, 2012.
38. Lo, Y.C., Rensi, S.E., Torng, W., Altman, R.B., Machine learning in chemo-informatics and drug discovery. *Drug Discovery Today*, *23*, 1538, 2018.
39. Rifaioglu, A.S., Atas, H., Martin, M.J., Cetin-Atalay, R., Atalay, V., Doğan, T., Recent applications of deep learning and machine intelligence on *in silico* drug discovery: Methods, tools and databases. *Brief. Bioinform.*, *20*, 1878, 2019.
40. Li, H., Hou, J., Adhikari, B., Lyu, Q., Cheng, J., Deep learning methods for protein torsion angle prediction. *BMC Bioinf.*, *18*, 417, 2017.
41. Spencer, M., Eickholt, J., Cheng, J., A Deep learning network approach to *ab initio* protein secondary structure prediction. *IEEE/ACM Trans. Comput. Biol. Bioinform.*, *12*, 103, 2015.
42. Xia, Z., Wu, L.-Y., Zhou, X., Wong, S.T., Semi-supervised drug-protein interaction prediction from heterogeneous biological spaces. *BMC Syst. Biol.*, *4*, S6, 2010.
43. Wang, C. and Kurgan, L., Survey of similarity-based prediction of drug-protein interactions. *Curr. Med. Chem.*, *27*, 5856, 2020.
44. Dara, S., Dhamercherla, S., Jadav, S.S., Babu, C.M., Ahsan, M.J., Machine learning in drug discovery: A review. *Artif. Intell. Rev.*, *54*, 1–53, 2021.
45. Lavecchia, A. and Giovanni, C., Virtual screening strategies in drug discovery: A critical review. *Curr. Med. Chem.*, *20*, 2839, 2013.
46. Schmidhuber, J., Deep learning in neural networks: An overview. *Neural Netw.*, *61*, 85–117, 2015.

47. Angermueller, C., Pärnamaa, T., Parts, L., Stegle, O., Deep learning for computational biology. *Mol. Syst. Biol.*, *12*, 878, 2016.
48. LeCun, Y., Bengio, Y., Hinton, G., Deep learning. *Nature*, *521*, 436, 2015.
49. Jiménez-Luna, J., Cuzzolin, A., Bolcato, G., Sturlese, M., Moro, S., A deep-learning approach toward rational molecular docking protocol selection. *Molecules*, *25*2020, 2487, 2020.
50. Gentile, F., Agrawal, V., Hsing, M., Ton, A.-T., Ban, F., Norinder, U., Gleave, M.E., Cherkasov, A., Deep Docking: A deep learning platform for augmentation of structure based drug discovery. *ACS Cent. Sci.*, *6*, 939, 2020.
51. Ballester, P.J. and Mitchell, J.B.O., A Machine learning approach to predicting protein-ligand binding affinity with applications to molecular docking. *Bioinformatics*, *26*, 1169, 2010.
52. Bharadwaj, Prakash, K.B. and Kanagachidambaresan, G.R., Pattern recognition and machine learning, in: *Programming with TensorFlow, ruting*, pp. 105–144, Ghent, Belgium, Springer, 2021.
53. Cândida, G.S., Carlos, J.V.S., Pedro, C., Rui, M.M.B., Enhancing scoring performance of docking-based virtual screening through machine learning. *Curr. Bioinforma.*, *11*, 408, 2016.
54. Kinnings, S.L., Liu, N., Tonge, P.J., Jackson, R.M., Xie, L., Bourne, P.E., A machine learning-based method to improve docking scoring functions and its application to drug repurposing. *J. Chem. Inf. Model.*, *51*, 408, 2011.
55. Springer, C., Adalsteinsson, H., Young, M.M., Kegelmeyer, P.W., Roe, D.C., PostDOCK: A structural, empirical approach to scoring protein ligand complexes. *J. Med. Chem.*, *48*, 6821, 2005.
56. Imrie, F., Bradley, A.R., Van Der Schaar, M., Deane, C.M., Protein family-specific models using deep neural networks and transfer learning improve virtual screening and highlight the need for more data. *J. Chem. Inf. Model.*, *58*, 2319, 2018.
57. Zilian, D. and Sotriffer, C.A., SFCscoreRF: A random forest-based scoring function for improved affinity prediction of protein-ligand complexes. *J. Chem. Inf. Model.*, *53*, 1923, 2013.
58. Li, H., Li, C., Gui, C., Luo, X., Chen, K., Shen, J., Wang, X., Jiang, H., GAsDock: A new approach for rapid flexible docking based on an improved multi-population genetic algorithm. *Bioorg. Med. Chem. Lett.*, *14*, 4671, 2004.
59. Liu, Q., Kwoh, C.K., Li, J., Binding affinity prediction for protein-ligand complexes based on β contacts and B factor. *J. Chem. Inf. Model.*, *53*, 3076, 2013.
60. Durrant, J.D. and McCammon, J.A., NNScore: A neural-network-based scoring function for the characterization of protein-ligand complexes. *J. Chem. Inf. Model.*, *50*, 1865, 2010.
61. Ouyang, X., Handoko, S.D., Kwoh, C.K., CScore:A Simple yet effective scoring function for protein ligand binding affinity prediction using modified Cmac learning architecture. *J. Bioinform. Comput. Biol.*, *9*, 1, 2011.

62. Ragoza, M., Hochuli, J., Idrobo, E., Sunseri, J., Koes, D.R., Protein-ligand scoring with convolutional neural networks. *J. Chem. Inf. Model.*, *57*, 942, 2017.
63. Hassan, M.M., Mogollón, D.C., Fuentes, O., Sirimulla, S., *DLSCORE: A deep learning model for predicting protein-ligand binding affinities*, ChemRxiv, Cambridge, Massachusetts, USA: Cambridge Open Engage, 2018.
64. Pereira, J.C., Caffarena, E.R., Dos Santos, C.N., Boosting docking-based virtual screening with deep learning. *J. Chem. Inf. Model.*, *56*, 2495, 2016.
65. Jiménez-Luna, J., Cuzzolin, A., Bolcato, G., Sturlese, M., Moro, S., A deep-learning approach toward rational molecular docking protocol selection. *Molecules*, *25*, 1, 2020.
66. Irwin, J.J. and Shoichet, B.K., ZINC – A free database of commercially available compounds for virtual screening. *J. Chem. Inf. Model.*, *45*, 177, 2005.
67. Sterling, T. and Irwin, J.J., ZINC 15 – Ligand discovery for everyone. *J. Chem. Inf. Model.*, *55*, 2324, 2015.
68. Chen, Y., de Bruyn Kops, C., Kirchmair, J., Data resources for the computer-guided discovery of bioactive natural products. *J. Chem. Inf. Model.*, *57*, 2099, 2017.
69. Stumpfe, D., Bajorath, J., Trends, current, overlooked issues, and unmet challenges in virtual screening. *J. Chem. Inf. Model.*, *60*, 4112, 2020.
70. Chen, Y., Garcia-de-Lomana, M., Friedrich, N.-O., Kirchmair, J., Characterization of the chemical space of known and readily obtainable natural products. *J. Chem. Inf. Model.*, *58*, 1518, 2018.
71. Yang, B., Mao, J., Gao, B., Lu, X., Computer-assisted drug virtual screening based on the natural product databases. *Curr. Pharm. Biotechnol.*, *20*, 293, 2019.
72. Yoo, S., Yang, H.C., Lee, S., Shin, J., Min, S., Lee, E., Song, M., Lee, D., A deep learning-based approach for identifying the medicinal uses of plant-derived natural compounds. *Front. Pharmacol.*, *11*, 584875, 2020.
73. Diallo, B.N., Glenister, M., Musyoka, T.M., Lobb, K., Tastan Bishop, Ö., SANCDB: An update on South African natural compounds and their readily available analogs. *J. Cheminformatics*, *13*, 37, 2021.
74. Berenger, F., Kumar, A., Zhang, K.Y.J., Yamanishi, Y., Lean-docking: exploiting ligands' predicted docking scores to accelerate molecular docking. *J. Chem. Inf. Model.*, *61*, 2341, 2021.
75. Joshi, T., Mathpal, S., Sharma, P., Joshi, T., Pundir, H., Maiti, P., Nand, M., Chandra, S., *Molecular docking study of drug molecules from drug bank database against COVID-19 Mpro protein*, OSF Preprints, April 11, 2020.
76. Shen, C., Ding, J., Wang, Z., Cao, D., Ding, X., Hou, T., From machine learning to deep learning: Advances in scoring functions for protein–ligand docking. *Wires Comput. Mol. Sci.*, *10*, e1429, 2020.

77. Ain, Q.U., Aleksandrova, A., Roessler, F.D., Ballester, P.J., Machine-learning scoring functions to improve structure-based binding affinity prediction and virtual screening. *Wires Comput. Mol. Sci.*, *5*, 405, 2015.
78. Harmalkar, A. and Gray, J.J., Advances to tackle backbone flexibility in protein docking. *Curr. Opin. Struct. Biol.*, *67*, 178, 2021.
79. Salsbury, A.M. and Lemkul, J.A., Recent developments in empirical atomistic force fields for nucleic acids and applications to studies of folding and dynamics. *Curr. Opin. Struct. Biol.*, *67*, 9, 2021.
80. Choi, J., Yun, J.S., Song, H., Kim, N.H., Kim, H.S., Yook, J.I., Exploring the chemical space of protein–protein interaction inhibitors through machine learning. *Sci. Rep.*, *11*, 13369, 2021.

2

Machine Learning Approaches to Improve Prediction of Target-Drug Interactions

Balatti, Galo E.[1*], Barletta, Patricio G.[2], Perez, Andres, D.[3], Giudicessi, Silvana L.[4,5] and Martínez-Ceron, María C.[4,6†]

[1]*Departamento de Ciencia y Tecnología, Universidad Nacional de Quilmes, Roquez Sáenz-Peña, Bernal, Argentina*

[2]*International Center for Theoretical Physics, Trieste, Italia*

[3]*IFLP, CONICET - Dpto. de Física, Universidad Nacional de La Plata, La Plata, Argentina*

[4]*Universidad de Buenos Aires, Facultad de Farmacia y Bioquímica, Cátedra de Biotecnología, Buenos Aires, Argentina*

[5]*Universidad de Buenos Aires (UBA) - Consejo Nacional de Investigaciones Científicas y Técnicas (CONICET), Instituto de Nanobiotecnología (NANOBIOTEC), Buenos Aires, Argentina*

[6]*Instituto de Ingeniería Biomédica, Facultad de Ingeniería, Universidad de Buenos Aires, Consejo Nacional de Investigaciones Científicas y Técnicas (CONICET), Buenos Aires, Argentina*

Abstract

From the initial steps of early drug discovery, the traditional techniques, like docking, QSAR, or molecular dynamics, have been used for decades identifying targets, ranking molecule candidates and optimizing the lead compounds chemically to decrease toxicity and improve drug absorption, distribution, metabolism, and excretion (ADME) properties. Nowadays, computational tools are increasingly used not only in the drug discovery process but also in drug development. Information technologies like artificial intelligence (AI) and machine learning (ML) participate in practically every step in the pharma value chain, improving and accelerating the overall drug development and design. Besides the rise of new methodologies, the improvement of relative old computational techniques, like docking, QSAR, or cavity search with new ML-based algorithms like random forest, support vector machines, or neural networks are being developed and

**Corresponding author*: camartinez@ffyb.uba.ar; mc4camila@gmail.com

†*Corresponding author*: balatti@live.com; gbalatti@ffyb.uba.ar

Inamuddin, Tariq Altalhi, Jorddy N. Cruz and Moamen Salah El-Deen Refat (eds.) Drug Design Using Machine Learning, (21–96) © 2022 Scrivener Publishing LLC

promises to reduce time and operational costs mainly in the drug design process. In this chapter, we review some of these approaches, briefly introducing the most used ML techniques in study drug-target interactions. Also, a special section about peptide-based drugs and its advantages over small organic molecules is discussed.

Keywords: Drug design, cavity searching, binding site prediction, scoring functions, docking, support vector machine, random forest, neural networks

2.1 Machine Learning Revolutionizing Drug Discovery

2.1.1 Introduction

In the last years, with the SARS-CoV-2 outbreak, the way drugs are developed and approved changed forever. Traditionally, the development of a new drug involves several steps or phases. 1) A first phase of discovery consists of the identification of a disease causal factor and a drug with the potential to correct it. 2) The preclinical phase is where the pharmacokinetics and pharmacodynamics of the drug are studied, both *in vivo* and *in vitro*. 3) Clinical phases, numbered as Phase I, II and III, and consist of the safety and kinetics of the drug (phase I), its efficacy and interaction with other drugs (phase II) and its performance in comparison with other drugs already approved or placebo are evaluated using volunteer candidates (phase III). 4) Finally, a Phase IV of pharmacovigilance is achieved (Figure 2.1). This whole process can take from 8 to 15 years [1]. Not only it is time-consuming but also expensive, and most drugs do not overcome the different stages [2, 3]. For example, between 2015 and 2020 the United States' Food and Drug Administration (FDA) only approved 14 antiviral drugs [4]. Between 2015 and 2019, FDA authorized only 208 new drugs, 15 of them were peptides or molecules that

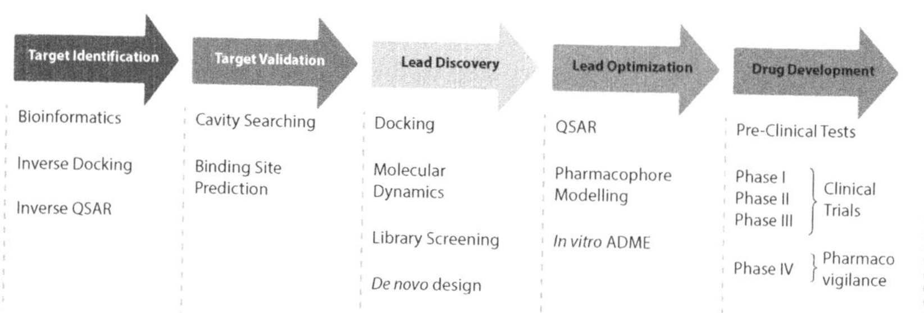

Figure 2.1 The overall process of developing a drug. Target identification and validation as well as lead discovery and optimization belong to the drug design steps, and this chapter is focused on those techniques, since ML participate in all of them.

contained peptides [5]. Wouters *et al.* reported that the cost of bringing a new drug to market was around $985 million 3 years ago [6]. That is why a new way of discovering drugs is needed, based on the knowledge acquired both about the etiology of diseases, as well as the innumerable databases that contain information on toxicity, pharmacodynamics, pharmacokinetics, physical-chemical characteristics, adverse effects, among others [3].

Current COVID-19 pandemic (produced by SARS-CoV-2 virus) has challenged health systems around the world, forcing both to design new drugs or to use already approved drugs with new applications. At the same time, it led to a redesign the approval process for new drugs and vaccines, carrying out several phases at the same time [4, 7–9]. On the other hand, the high costs involved in the approval of new drugs makes rare or orphan disease drug research more complex since the pharmaceutical industry does not see the possibility of economic recovery in the short term [10].

Computational techniques, such as QSAR or docking, became an *in silico* approach to adding data to experimental results or vice versa. Several databases (some of them enlist in Table 2.1) provide structural information on proteins bound to different ligands (peptides, small organic molecules,

Table 2.1 Several databases which collected protein structures; approved or next to be approved by FDA drugs; antimicrobial peptides from food, plants, bacteria; among others.

Database	Description
Protein Data Bank [40]	3D shapes of proteins, nucleic acids, and complex assemblies
DrugBank [41]	containing information on drugs and drug targets
BRENDA [42]	collection of enzyme functional
ChEMBL [43]	bioactive molecules with drug-like properties
BindingDB [44]	measured binding affinity interactions of protein to be drug-targets
PDB bind [45]	experimentally measured binding affinity data for complexes

(Continued)

Table 2.1 Several databases which collected protein structures; approved or next to be approved by FDA drugs; antimicrobial peptides from food, plants, bacteria; among others. (*Continued*)

Database	Description
PepBDB [46]	biological complex structures of peptide-mediated protein interactions
Propedia [47]	peptide-protein complexes
PDBsum [48]	Pictorial database of 3D structures in the Protein Data Bank
PRM-DB [49]	Peptide Recognition Modules
Cppsite 2.0 [50]	Experimentally Validated Cell-Penetrating Peptides
CAMP [51]	Collection of Antimicrobial Peptides
THPdb [52]	FDA approved therapeutic peptides and proteins
PepTherDia [53]	Peptide Therapeutics and Diagnostics
BactiBase [54]	collection of bacteriocin
LAMP2 [55]	AMPs collection
DBAASP [56]	AMPs collection
PeptBind [57]	sequence-based method for protein-peptide binding residues prediction
PinaColada [58]	design of peptide inhibitors for protein-protein interactions
FermFooDb [59]	bioactive peptides derived from fermented foods
AHTPDB [60]	antihypertensive peptides, which are majorly from natural resources
FeptideDB [61]	bioactive peptides from food protein
MBPDB Search [62]	milk protein-derived bioactive peptides
StraPep [63]	structure database of bioactive peptides
PlantPepDB [64]	plant peptide database
DrumPID [65]	drugs and their protein networks
PDID [66]	Protein-Drug Interaction Database in the structural human proteome

cofactors, etcetera); enzymes participation in a metabolic and pathometabolic pathway; drugs lethal dose or effective dose; drug-cell membrane penetration; among others. But being able to take advantage of all this information is time-consuming when it is manually done and wrong conclusions can be drawn. Artificial intelligence (AI) strategies can offer a faster and more efficient way to discover new drugs based on the ability of computers to "think." Machine learning (ML), a branch of AI, has the ability to learn from input data and "think" like humans do through computer programs. Some data along with a certain algorithm is entered into a computer. This system will be able to learn without being explicitly programmed and then make predictions on any new data set [11, 12]. Machine learning makes it possible to automate repetitive data processing, which could reduce the costs of designing a new drug, lead to the reuse of drugs already approved for the treatment of other diseases, or even find solutions for rare diseases. Perhaps, in the not-too-distant future it will be able to achieve the paradigm of personalized medicine [1] and, in fact, AI is being increasingly used in practically every step of drug discovery and development [13].

On the other hand, the quality of input data, the algorithm used to train the system, the algorithm selection criteria and the interpretability of the result obtained, are some ML drawbacks that make its application limited [12]. However, new techniques and approaches along with the increase in simultaneous and parallel analysis capacity, due to the increase in computing power can provide a solution in this regard.

2.1.2 Virtual Screening and Rational Drug Design

Computational tools to predict drug-target complex formation are especially important in early drug-design stages (small organic molecules, peptides, or biosimilar) because they can significantly reduce development costs [14, 15]. Currently, it depends mainly on the researcher's criteria, but ML can be independent of it since it is able to learn and process data without human intervention in an automatic way, reducing the operator's effect.

Different strategies are implemented to analyze *in silico* the prediction of drug-target complex formation [16], that is governed by hydrogen bonding forces and hydrophobic and electrostatic interactions [17], as well as entropic effects. These strategies are encompassed by the name of virtual screening (VS), in which different tools like docking, molecular dynamic simulations or pharmacophore modeling are used to predict drug-target interactions [18–23]. Virtual screening makes it possible to evaluate the interaction between a target (protein, cell-membrane surface; etcetera) and a drug (small organic molecules or peptides) database to find suitable ligands in a faster and more complete way than a wet laboratory experiment can give [16, 20]. This approach can be based on ligand (ligand-based VS) or structure information (structure-based VS). Ligand-based VS tries to predict binding forces based on known ligand information, residue orientation, residue charges, etcetera, hypothesizing that similar molecules can bind a target protein and produce certain activity. Not prior target structure information is needed. On the other hand, the structure-based approach extracts information from a given three-dimensional compound structure, since it considers that two molecules union occurs according to their atom orientation. Since structure-based models need target structure and to precisely know the pockets that bind the ligands [9, 24], the development of ligand-based models based on Machine learning techniques (MLT) are increasingly used in VS [25].

However, many structure-based tools like docking are being enhanced by the use of MLT, as well as novel tools for the identification of druggable pockets and to optimize lead compounds by Quantitative structure activity relationship (QSAR). We will see these kinds of ML applications in the present book chapter.

2.1.3 Small Organic Molecules and Peptides as Drugs

For the FDA, drugs are substances used in diagnosis, to cure, for the treatment or prevention of disease. They can affect the structure or any function of the body [26]. The most common type of drugs are also known as small organic molecules. They have low molecular weight (less than 900 daltons) [27, 28], can cross cell membranes and binds specifically biomolecules (proteins, cell-membrane phospholipids, nucleic acids, among others) and generates an effect modifying its function [28]. They also can be administered orally [29]. But spotlights are over peptide-based drugs. Peptides are short chains composed of less than 50 amino acids [30] and linked by peptide bonds. These structures are found in all living beings, fulfilling different vital functions. Many times, these functions are determined by the building blocks that constitute them and their physical-chemical characteristics [31, 32]. Peptides are among small molecules and proteins due to their size, but with biochemical and therapeutic characteristics significantly different from them. Peptides are involved in cell signaling functions, so it is interesting to know their mechanisms of action in order to be able to use them in disease treatment [33]. They are also the first line of defense in all living beings [34–36]. Peptides can be used to targets that were not possible to intervene using more classical drugs [37].

Even though peptides are less stable than small organic molecules and more difficult and expensive to manufacture, they have interesting characteristics such as their specificity, safety and tolerability that make them the future of medicine. They can be applied in the treatment of several diseases, like metabolic, oncologic, infectious ones, etcetera [30, 33, 37–39].

This book chapter is organized as follows: section 2.2 will briefly explain the theoretical basis of most commonly used MLT on Drug Discovery, section 2.3 will introduce classical and ML tools to discover novel druggable sites on drug protein receptors in the Target Validation process, sections 2.4 and 2.5 the classical and ML approaches for receptor and ligand-based virtual screening (Lead Discovery) and the Lead Optimization. All these techniques have been mainly applied for small organic molecules. But peptides have promising applications as drugs that is why section 2.6 will briefly explain the advantages of using them as drugs and how MLT can help to improve peptide-based drugs development.

2.2 A Brief Summary of Machine Learning Models

We briefly summarize some concepts about Machine learning (ML) that are going to be useful for the following discussions. This section can be skipped if the reader is familiarized with the subject.

Artificial intelligence (AI) is a very general field based on the automation of data analysis tasks. As such, AI contains ML as a subset, but also involves approaches that do not include learning. For example, algorithms known as "symbolic AI" require hard-coded rules written by the programmer to perform some task. As expected, increasingly complex problems need an increasing set of explicit rules, and that was the dominant paradigm and effort up to 1990. AI worked very well for well-defined problems, but eventually turned out to be really hard to craft explicit rules for more elaborated problems that include a huge amount of information, such as speech or image recognition.

Then, a new paradigm emerged. In symbolic AI, the programmer would input the rules into a program, and the data would be analyzed with those rules to obtain some answer. On the other hand, with ML instead of crafting the rules, the focus is to automatically find them (or learn them) using the available data and the expected answers as inputs [67]. Afterward, new data can be analyzed with the learned set of rules.

As a consequence, ML algorithms are "trained." A subset of the data is presented as examples to find some structure that allows the system to obtain the desired rules. To do so, usually a ML program needs:

- input data points, often large datasets,
- the expected outputs for the inputs (for supervised learning). It is important to notice that the "right answer" is known beforehand and used as examples to extract a statistical structure,
- a function to measure the algorithm performance. This is done by comparing the current and expected output, and used as feedback to modify the algorithm parameters.

Therefore, ML is the automated search for some useful representation of the input data within a space of possibilities, adjusting its parameters in a series of steps guided by the current performance of the system.

Although a detailed description of ML algorithms is out of the scope of this chapter, next we will briefly discuss some examples. We will also summarize some deep learning algorithms, a specific subfield of machine learning that rose to prominence in the 2010s and is increasingly relevant. Finally, we will comment on some commonly used methods to evaluate the performance of regression and classification methods.

2.2.1 Support Vector Machines (SVM)

Support vector machines (SVM) are supervised learning algorithms part of so-called kernel methods developed in the early 1990s by Vapnik and collaborators [68, 69]. They were initially designed to solve classification problems, although the same concepts can be generalized and applied for regression. The classification task is achieved by finding a decision boundary (hyperplane) between sets of points that belong to two different categories. First, the data is mapped into a new high dimensional space where the classification problem becomes simpler. Then, the decision boundary is computed by a procedure called "maximizing the margin," where the distance between the hyperplane and the closest data points from each class is maximized (see Figure 2.2). In the regression case, the hyperplane is defined optimizing the sum of the distances from the data points to the decision boundary [70].

Mapping data to a high-dimensional space is done with a technique called "kernel trick." Instead of explicitly computing the coordinates of the data points in the new representation, the distance between pairs of points is used. Nonlinear kernel functions map any two points in the original space into the distance between these two points in the representation space, bypassing the computation of the new coordinates. An important property of SVM is that kernel functions are not learned from data, but are

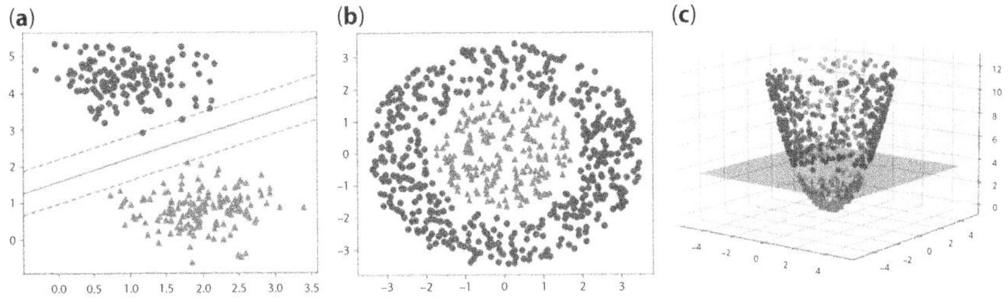

Figure 2.2 SVM classification examples. (a) Linearly separable datasets. The solid line shows the hyperplane found with SVM technique that maximizes the distance to the closest points of each class (margin). The dashed curves delimit the margins. (b) Example where the datasets are not linearly separable. (c) Same datasets as in panel b, mapped into a high-dimensional space with a kernel transformation (z=x2+y2). Now the data is linearly separable by a hyperplane.

required beforehand to construct the algorithm and define the new high dimensional space where the data is going to be analyzed. The hyperplane that separates the data points is learned. Among the different kernel functions that are crafted, four are usually employed in SVM modeling: linear, polynomial, sigmoid, and radial basis function (RBF), of which the latter is the most widely adopted kernel.

SVM can handle high dimensional variables and small datasets, however they are hard to scale and usually do not perform very well in complex scenarios, like image classification, where useful representations are hard to obtain manually.

2.2.2 Random Forests (RF)

Random forest (RF) is a supervised machine learning method constructed from a set of decision tree (DT) algorithms, used to solve both regression and classification problems [71]. A DT is a decision support technique with a tree-like structure, as its name suggests, with two basic components: decision nodes, and leaf nodes (see Figure 2.3a). The training dataset is divided in each decision node, which further segregates into other branches until a leaf node is reached. The decision nodes represent the attributes or conjunctions of features that are used to analyze the data, and the leaves the class labels if we are dealing with a classification problem.

As already mentioned, RFs consist of a large number of individual DTs working as an ensemble (see Figure 2.3b). Especially after the 2000s, RFs are widely used since they can handle large datasets efficiently. The key feature of the RF method is that each tree is trained using different samples

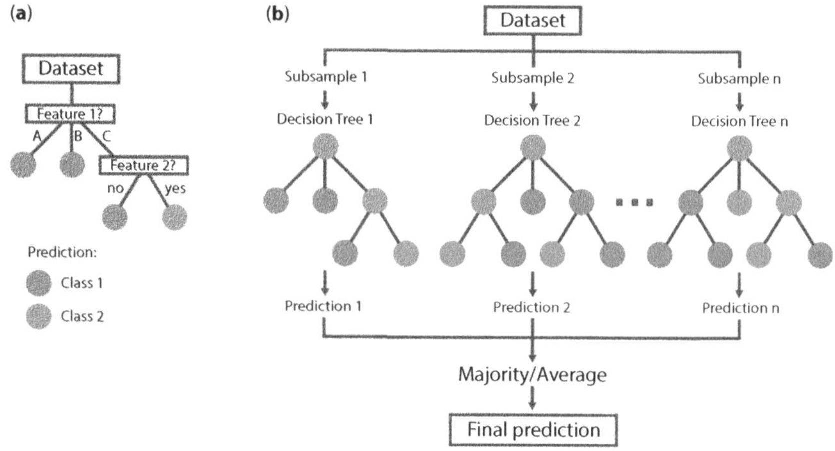

Figure 2.3 (a) Decision tree example. The dataset in each decision node is divided depending on the analyzed feature, until a leaf node is reached determining the final prediction. (b) Random forest example showing its structure. The dataset is divided randomly into n training sets (bootstrap separation) with replacements. For each subsample, an independent decision tree is constructed. Then, the results from all the decision trees are considered to provide the final prediction (bootstrap aggregation) by taking the most predicted class or the mean, for classification or regression.

of data rather than the original sample. This technique called bootstrap or bagging selects a random sample with replacements (for example repeating some data points) and therefore de-correlates the trees by showing them different training sets. In this way, variation among trees is achieved, as each DT considers the features that produce the most separation between the observables in their decision nodes. Then, a large number of relatively uncorrelated trees working as an ensemble produces a better model performance than any of its constituents. While some individual trees may produce a wrong prediction, many others will point towards the correct direction. Finally, the output of the RF is the class selected by most DTs, or the mean of the individual DTs, for classification and regression tasks respectively.

2.2.3 Gradient Boosting Decision Tree

Gradient boosting decision tree (GBDT) is a machine learning method based on ensembling DTs as base learners used to solve both regression and classification problems, popular after 2014 [72–74]. Unlike RF, where the DTs are trained in a parallel way (a technique called "bagging"), GBDT models employ a technique called "boosting," where the base learners are combined in an iterative way.

Each subsequent base learner, or DT, attempts to improve the weak points of its predecessor by adding a new estimator that corrects the errors of the last DT. Although there exist other boosting models, to determine the difference between the predicted and actual target value in each step, GBDT algorithms use a differentiable loss function. This function is optimized though gradient descent, and hence the name gradient boosting. For example, the mean square error and logarithmic loss are usually considered for regression and classification tasks respectively.

Then, the goal of the algorithm is to minimize the loss function by incremental adjustments with subsequent DTs, and the final model aggregates the result of each step. GBDTs usually outperforms RF models. While the addition of new DTs do not cause overfitting issues in the latter, GBDT requires a careful selection of hyperparameters (e.g. number of trees, tree depth, learning rate) to avoid this problem, for which techniques as regularization to slow down learning or subsampling the dataset to reduce correlation are available.

2.2.4 K-Nearest Neighbor (KNN)

K-nearest neighbors (KNN) is a supervised machine learning algorithm used to solve both regression and classification problems [75–77]. One particular feature of these models is that no explicit training step is required. The method assumes that data points with similar characteristics exist in close proximity, and to determine this similarity a notion of distance has to be calculated, that usually depends on the problem. For continuous variables the distance metric can be the Euclidean distance, but for discrete variables other metrics like Hamming distance, where the measure is related to the minimum number of substitutions required to transform one variable into the other, can be employed.

For each new example that the user wants to classify, the distances between the new unlabeled point and the labeled data are calculated and sorted in ascending order. Then the algorithm selects the first K entries (e. g. the K-nearest neighbors) from the sorted collection and returns a predicted output for the current example point as the mode of the K labels. For example, if K=1 the predicted label is simply the class of the nearest data point. In regression, the object property value is taken into account, and the predicted output of the query example is the mean value of the K nearest neighbors.

The determination of the K value that maximizes the performance is usually done manually with an independent validation dataset. Increasing the value of K makes the predictions more stable due to averaging, but eventually also the substructures are averaged hence the number of errors increases. On the other hand, if K is too low, we find a loss of generalization, since local variations become dominant.

The algorithm is versatile, simple and easy to implement in a multidimensional feature space with few parameters. There are common and useful techniques to improve its accuracy, like normalizing the training data, or assigning weights to the contributions of each neighbor. For example, the weight can be equal to $\frac{1}{d}$, with d as the distance, so the nearer points contribute more than the more distant ones. However, the KNN method has the major drawback of becoming significantly slower for increasing datasets and gets usually outperformed by other machine learning methods.

2.2.5 Neural Network and Deep Learning

Neural networks are a set of flexible ML methods represented by an array of interconnected nodes, called "neurons," arranged in a series of layers. Each neuron can have several inputs but produces a single output by applying a nonlinear function, denoted "activation function," over the product of the inputs and parameters called "weights." This output would be the input for one or several neurons of the subsequent layer depending on the connections between the nodes. Since the neurons are arranged in layers, the output of a layer becomes the input of the next one (see Figure 2.4).

The weights of each neuron are adjusted during the training process with the goal of minimizing a loss function that computes a distance score between the overall output with the desired output, in the case of supervised learning. This is done by an "optimizer" algorithm implementing a technique called "backpropagation" [78] a gradient-descendent method in which the networks works backward, from the output to the input units, using the loss function score as feedback signal to modify the weights in the direction that would lower the loss score for the current example.

In this context, artificial neural networks (ANN) usually refers to algorithms with one or two layers of neurons, regarded as "shallow learning," and can suffer from poor generalization for high dimensional data. On the other hand, deep learning methods like deep neural networks (DNN) solve these problems by finding successive and increasingly meaningful representations from data in a multi-stage way with successive layers. Then, the term "deep" refers to the idea of multiple representations through multiple layers.

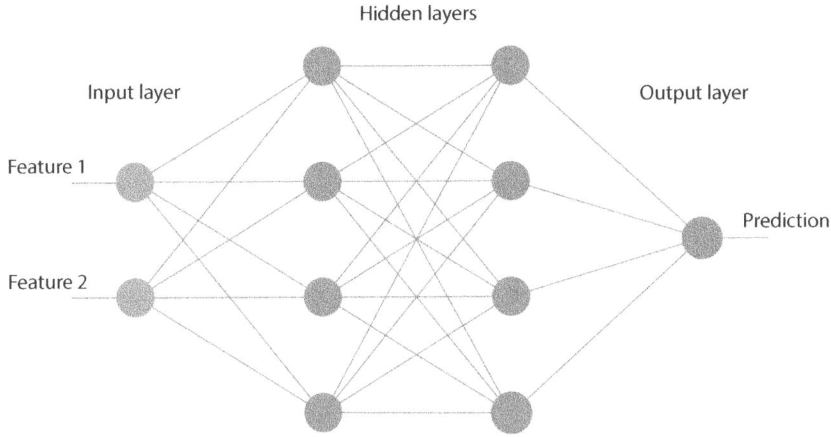

Figure 2.4 Example of a fully connected neural network with one input layer (two neurons, in green), two hidden layers (each with four neurons, in blue), and one output layer (one neuron, in red). This architecture could be used to analyze data points with two features (e.g. solubility, bioavailability or lipophilicity) to obtain a binary classifier, e.g. to distinguish between two classes (e.g. high or low bioavailability).

Another important deep learning method is called convolutional neural networks (CNN), usually used to analyze images. CNNs have three main types of layers: convolutional layers, pooling layers, and fully-connected layers. The first type of layers requires input data in matrix form whose entries would be, for example, the values of the pixels of an image, and a kernel or filter represented by another matrix (a two-dimensional array of weights) with lower number of elements than the input image (usually 2x2 or 3x3). The kernel applies a dot product between the elements of the kernel and the pixels of an area of the image to produce a single output. Then, the process is repeated "moving" the kernel to cover the entire image and to produce an output matrix or convolved image. The objective of each kernel is to extract features from the input image. While lower convolutional layers may identify low-level features (for example edges or color), subsequent layers may extract increasingly high-level concepts. Remarkably, these features are not specified manually, but learned automatically. The values of the kernel's weights are adjusted during training using backpropagation, although it is important to notice that to analyze an example its values are fixed, e. g. the convolution of the entire image is done with a fixed kernel. This provides a translation or space invariant response, meaning that the kernel can identify the desired feature regarding its position within the image.

Pooling layers are used to reduce the size of the convolved images. They are made up of a filter or kernel that moves across the image, but unlike convolutional layers, does not have weights. There are two main types of pooling layers: max pooling and average pooling, which return the maximum value or the average of the elements within the area covered by the filter, respectively. Besides reducing the computational power required to process the data, pooling layers are useful to boost efficiency, avoid overfitting, and to improve space invariance.

Finally, after a set of convolutional and pooling layers, the output is flattened and is analyzed with a set of fully-connected layers: a ANN or DNN network, depending on the number of layers. The main goal of this section is to perform the classification task based on the features extracted by the previous filters.

Although the key ideas of deep learning have been well-known since late 1980, the models can be computationally demanding. Therefore, it rose to prominence after 2012 due to advances in hardware, datasets, and algorithms (e.g. better activation functions and optimization algorithms). Today it is one of the most popular and used machine learning schemes, because in many scenarios it offers better performance that other methods, can handle huge datasets, high dimensional data, can be trained on additional data without having to start from scratch, and unlike shallow methods that require human manual intervention and data preparation to be able to extract a useful representation, in deep learning this process is automated and therefore much simpler.

To summarize, two key characteristics of deep learning are highlighted: a model learns increasingly complex and abstract representations by breaking them down in a series of simpler transformations with each successive layer, and that these incremental representations are learned jointly, e. g. if an internal feature is adjusted all the other features will be automatically modified to adapt the change and minimize the error of the network. The end result is a much more powerful method than stacking shallow models.

2.2.6 Gaussian Process Regression

Gaussian process (GP) is a Bayesian nonparametric approach to solve nonlinear (not constrained to a specific functional form) optimization problems such as regression [79, 80]. It is flexible enough to handle small datasets, uneven sampling, diverse range of dynamic behaviors, and can provide uncertainty measurements on the predictions.

Unlike the previous supervised machine learning methods where the exact values of every parameter in a function is learned, GP infers a probability distribution over all compatible functions that fit the data. It uses Bayes's rule: an input distribution has to be given, called "prior," which is updated based on the training dataset. The resulting distribution, called "posterior," encompasses the information from both the dataset and the prior.

The prediction for a new data point, that for GP is actually a new distribution called "predictive," can be obtained by weighting the possible predictions (integrate over all the possible parameters) by the calculated posterior. To be able to perform the calculation, the prior and likelihood are usually assumed to be Gaussian distributions, and with this choice the predictive turns out to be also Gaussian, and hence the name of the method. Finally, we can consider the predictive mean as the predicted value for our data point, with its variance as uncertainty.

2.2.7 Evaluating Regression Methods

There are several methods to evaluate the results in a regression problem. One useful concept often used is correlation, e. g. how two or more variables are related to each other. Among the many correlation coefficients that measure the degree of correlation, the Pearson correlation coefficient [81], denoted by "r," is widely used. It measures the linear correlation between two datasets dividing the covariance (*cov*) of the two variables by the product of their standard deviations (*var*). For a set of n data points (x_i, y_i) this means:

$$r = \frac{cov(x,y)}{\sqrt{var(x)var(y)}} = \frac{\sum_{i=1}^{n}(xi-\overline{x})(yi-y)}{\sqrt{\sum_{i=1}^{n}(xi-\overline{x})^2}\sqrt{\sum_{i=1}^{n}(yi-\overline{y})^2}},$$

where $\overline{x}$ and $\overline{y}$ represent the mean of x_i and y_i, correspondingly. In practice this quantity tells us how two variables behave as a pair to find the linear relationship between them by measuring how far or close are the points to the fitted regression line. The coefficient "r" can take values from -1 to 1. If r=0, the variables (x_i, y_i) are completely uncorrelated; and a perfect linear relation is obtained when r=-1 or 1, depending on the slope.

It is important to notice that correlation does not imply causation. Also, the Pearson correlation coefficient is not used to determine how well predictions match observation. For example, given a dataset with a value of "r," we could add additional data points that follow the previously found linear relationship without modifying the Pearson coefficient. However, the confidence about the prediction of the fitted line would be different for different sample sizes.

In that regard, the coefficient of determination [82], denoted R^2, is used for judging the goodness of fit in a linear regression model, e. g. a comparison of the observed data with the data expected under the model. Then, R^2 is a measure of how much the variance of the dependent variable can be explained by its relation with the independent variable, in other words, the percentage of correct predictions obtained. It can be calculated as:

$$R^2 = \frac{var(y) - var(y(x))_{fitted}}{var(y)} = 1 - \frac{var(y(x))_{fitted}}{var(y)},$$

where $var\,(y(x))_{fitted}$ denotes the variance of the data with respect to the fitted curve (values predicted by the regression model), and is proportional to the sum of squares of residuals:

$$var\,(y(x))_{fitted} = \frac{1}{n}\sum_{i=1}^{n}(yi - y(xi))^2,$$

R^2 can take values in the range [-∞,1], being 1 a perfect fit. Although in some cases the Pearson correlation coefficient and the coefficient of determination are related, the latter need not be the square of the former.

Another very common metric to evaluate a regression is the root mean squared error (RMSE), defined as:

$$RMSE = \sqrt{var(y(x))fitted} = \sqrt{\frac{1}{n}\sum_{i=1}^{n}(yi - y(xi))^2},$$

e. g. the square root of the sum of the squared errors (differences between the predicted and observed values), normalized by the number of points. RMSE can take values in the range [0,∞]. Values closer to zero point towards a good regression model, and in the limit RMSE=0 represents a perfect fit since in that scenario the errors vanish. However, RMSE is a quantity with units, therefore evaluating if the calculated value is sufficiently small depends on the accuracy needed and the particular problem we are probing.

A similar issue can be found with the metric called mean absolute error (MAE) defined as the average of the absolute value of the errors:

$$MAE = \frac{1}{n}\sum_{i=1}^{n}|y1 - y(xi)|,$$

although its interpretability is easier as the absolute value of the error of each data point contributes linearly. In practice, MAE represents how much the predictions differed from the mean, in average.

2.2.8 Evaluating Classification Methods

Many pharmaceutical questions (e.g. Ligand Binding Site Prediction or Virtual Screening) are binary classification problems. Thus, its evaluation is a simple binary hypothesis testing problem, the prediction is either true or false. Thus, it is convenient to review the metrics employed in the field. The possible outcomes of a prediction are:

- True Positive (TP), the model correctly identifies a positive class sample,
- True Negative (TN), the model correctly identifies a negative class sample,
- False Positive (FP), the model incorrectly identifies a positive class sample,
- False Negative (FN), the model incorrectly identifies a negative class sample.

From the above quantities we can obtain the following metrics:

$$Accuracy = \frac{TP + TN}{TP + TN + FP + FN}.$$

While **Accuracy** is the most intuitive and general metric, other metrics may help model improvement by highlighting weaknesses. For example, we may know the accuracy of our model, but what is our true positive rate? How many of the true samples were we able to detect? **Recall**, also referred to as **Sensitivity**, is the metric that evaluates that:

$$Recall = \frac{TP}{TP + FN}.$$

But optimizing recall alone might lead the model astray. The algorithm may become overeager labelling samples as positive, thus increasing the number of False Positives. So Recall has its counterpart, the true negative rate, called **Specificity**:

$$Specificity = \frac{TN}{TN + FP}.$$

So Recall (or Sensitivity) and Specificity are 2 concepts that go hand in hand and it is often the case that there is a trade-off between them and researches decide which type of error must be minimized, either the False Negatives (by increasing Recall), or the False Positives (by increasing Specificity).

The problem is multifaceted, so other measurements show up too. **Precision** is used to evaluate the performance of a method when the output is a Positive:

$$Precision = \frac{TP}{TP + FP}.$$

Remembering that a high recall indicates that the model is not missing Positives, Precision deals with the certainty of those positives. Thus, Precision also helps to minimize False Positives, but it does so by comparing them to the True Positives, unlike Specificity that compares them to True Negatives.

Slightly more convoluted metrics are also used. When searching for a balance between Recall and Precision, researchers often use the **F1-score**, which performs the harmonic mean of the former two:

$$F_1 = 2\frac{Precision.Recall}{Precision + Recall}.$$

Which ranges from 0 to 1, 1 meaning perfect Recall and Precision.

The bioinformatics field also makes heavy use of the Mattheu's Correlation Coefficient (**MCC**) as an overall indicator:

$$MCC = \frac{(TP.TN) - (FN.FN)}{\sqrt{(TP + FP).(TP + FN).(TN + FP).(TN + FN)}}.$$

As the name implies, the MCC is essentially a correlation parameter between the predicted and the observed classifications and its value ranges from -1 to 1. Although alternative, and perhaps even more appropriate methods have been proposed [83], the MCC score is the most widely used, due to its relative simplicity.

2.3 Target Validation

2.3.1 Ligand Binding Site Prediction (LBS)

Once a target is defined, the next step in drug discovery is the identification of its Ligand Binding Site (LBS), and since interactions have to be established in order to form a stable complex, proteins have developed cavities. They are usually located in the concave surface of the protein but they can also be found in the interior, after traversing a tunnel. Hence, the identification and characterization of protein cavities, pockets, clefts, tunnels, or channels of a protein structure is key in the process of drug discovery.

When approaching an old problem with new methods (ML in this case), the lack of specific domain knowledge is among the main causes of failure. We therefore proceed to make a review of the old, and not so old, approaches. The story of finding a LBS is in great part the story of detecting, delineating, calculating and characterizing these cavities, pockets, clefts, tunnels, or channels. Throughout this chapter we will refer to all of them as "voids."

2.3.2 Classical Approaches

The first steps in this field could be traced back as early as 1975 [84]. These initial approaches did not look for cavities, but mostly tried to find a suitable surface of interaction between protein and ligand. Perhaps influenced by Fischer's lock-key model [85], these methods sampled the protein (the lock) with a probe (the key), trying to find suitable interaction points. These points were not continuous but laid on a discretization of the 3D space, a grid, a construct that will be present in almost all cavity software. These first methods can be named energy probe methods. The last of these methods came out in 1985 [86].

Starting with Cavity Search [87], LBS field took a more modest approach than straight up determining binding sites and started discovering cavities where ligands could, in principle, bind. Since most cavities are in direct contact with the solvent, the Solvent Accessible Surface Area (SASA) definition from Lee & Richards [88], in 1971, was instrumental in cavity search and calculation. The SASA is the surface that the center of a probe (in lieu of a solvent molecule), traces when rolling along the Van der Waals radii of a macromolecule. Later, Shrake & Rupley [89], Connolly [90, 91] and Michel Sanner [92] provided their own alternative methods to calculate the SASA. To this day, newly published cavity detection tools employ one of these methods to delineate protein voids. We will refer to these methods as **rolling probe** methods.

In 1983, the first of Edelsbrunner alpha shapes papers was published, which was followed by more publications that refined Edelsbrunner's algorithms to calculate these alpha shapes [93–95], until Edelsbrunner's own software was published, CAST [96]. These alpha shapes are a set of curves that approximate the shape of a set of points, the same goal the rolling probe methods have but unlike these previous methods, calculation of alpha shapes is done by subdividing the 3D space in tetrahedra, which later aids in the search of voids. Many algorithms have been developed to find these Alpha Shapes and their related constructs such as Convex Hulls, Delaunay Triangulations and Voronoi Diagrams. All of these are fundamentally associated, and we will group them as **tessellation** methods.

New programs keep coming out almost every year, but almost all of them are based on 3 kinds of methods, which we will now briefly describe: grid, rolling probe and tessellation methods.

The grid method is perhaps the most intuitive. Many tools, if not most, incorporate it in some way, especially more modern ones, since the increase of available computational power is necessary in dealing with the elevated running times this method usually implies.

It should be noted that in this section we will refer to pure grid methods. As we said, many programs use grids at some stage, but they serve auxiliary functions.

These methods divide the space using cubic **cells**, sometimes called **voxels**. The size of the cells is defined as the **resolution** of the method and their centers are usually called **points**. After dividing the space into cells, they determine which of them are free and which are occupied by protein atoms. This is done by going through all the cells in the grid and evaluating the following: for each cell, compare the distance from the point (its center) to the nearest atom; if the distance is less than the atoms Van der Waals radius, the cell will be considered occupied; if the distance is greater than the radius, then the cell will be considered free. After evaluating all the cells, the volume of the cavity is obtained from multiplying the volume of the cells (which is defined by the resolution) and the number of free cells.

This way of evaluating cell occupancy poses the first disadvantage of the method: the grid of points is equidistant, so the cells are cubic, but the method to determine if these cells are free uses only the coordinates of the center of the cell and the center of the atom, so we cannot ensure that the entire cell is free, but only its circumscribed sphere, whose center coincides with that of the cell and whose radius is half the size of the cell (the grid resolution). This problem of the difference between the volume of a cubic section and the volume of its circumscribed sphere is often called the sphere packing problem and is illustrated, in 2 dimensions, in Figure 2.5a.

As we said, a decision has to be made as to whether calculating the free volume using the formula of the volume of a cube or that of a sphere. Most grid programs calculate the total free volume, as the sum of the volumes of the circumscribed spheres:

$$V = N\frac{4}{3}\pi\left(\frac{G}{2}\right)^3$$

where N: number of free spheres, G: grid resolution.

Naturally, the solution to the sphere packing problem is to increase the resolution of the grid, but this entails a high computational cost since the complexity of this algorithm in its naive version (without optimizations) is quadratic[97]: $\Theta\ (mn)$, where **m** is the number of cells in the grid and **n** is the number of atoms of the protein. Since all possible combinations must be calculated among all the atoms and all cells.

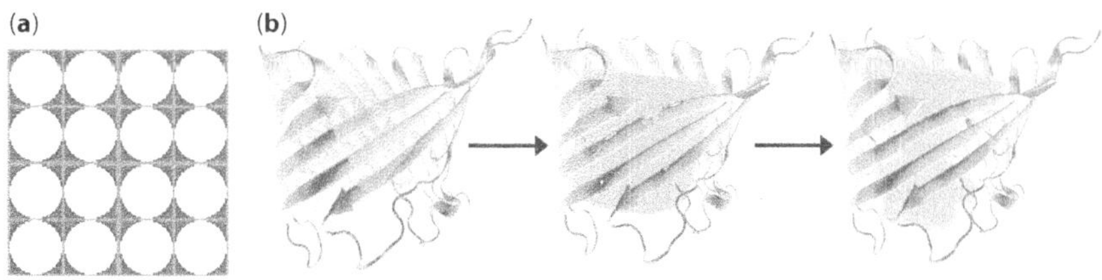

Figure 2.5 (a) The sphere packing problem in 2 dimensions. Grid methods only check for atoms inside the blue circles, but the area is calculated as the sum of the green boxes area, there is no telling if the red surfaces are occupied or not. (b) The steps of a pure grid program, applied on the tunnel of a porin (blue, PDB ID: 1PRN). A green cylinder defines the grid volume, where the cavity will be calculated. Later, the cylinder is filled with the grid voxels (shown in orange). After removing the voxels that overlap with the atoms, the porin tunnel remains.

In addition to the sphere packing problem, grid methods have another disadvantage: the calculated volume depends on the orientation of the molecule. Grid programs, for simplicity, tend to apply the grid on a fixed XYZ reference frame in space; if the protein rotates, the volume obtained will vary. This problem is a consequence of the space discretization. One way to mitigate it is, again, to increase the resolution. Some methods recalculate the volume at different grid angles, others place the grid axes along the protein's moment of inertia axes.

None of the currently available programs based on grid methods count with cavity detection methods, so the user must define manually. This may seem like an inconvenience, but in practical terms, it allows a greater control in the definition of the cavity compared to other methods. The preferred way to define the search area of the cavity is by means of geometric figures such as spheres, prisms or cylinders. For example, if the user decides to use a sphere for the definition of the cavity, they will set its radius and position and the volume covered by this sphere will be divided into grid cells and the process already described in the previous section will be carried out. Only in the volume enclosed by this sphere will voids be detected. Figure 2.5b shows the entire process carried out by the Epock [98] tool.

The second group of methods, the *rolling probes,* are all based on the Solvent Accessible Surface Area (SASA) definition by Lee & Richards [88] and the subsequent algorithms [89–92]. Their method was not developed to study cavities but to define and study the surface of proteins. Consequently, they are usually not the best choice for dealing with occluded pockets or tunnels, but they are very effective at capturing the geometry of more shallow voids such as grooves.

These methods model the protein as a set of spheres centered on the atoms and of radius equal to the Van der Waals radius of their respective atom. They then define 3 surfaces, the first of which is the Van der Waals Surface (VdWS), it corresponds to the boundary of the set of spheres (atoms), that is, it follows the exact line of the perimeter of the spheres exposed to solvent.

To delineate the next 2 surfaces, a spherical probe of a certain radius representing the solvent (1.4 Å for water), will be rolled across the VdWS. This probe traverses the entire VdWS defining on its way the other 2 surfaces: the SASA and the Solvent Excluded Surface Area (SESA). The SASA will be the trace of the center of the probe and the SESA will be the trace of the contact point between the probe and the spheres (the atoms). The trace is defined as the line that describes the path followed by a given point on the probe as it traverses the protein. As already said, if that point is the center of the probe, the trace will describe the SASA; if the point is the point of contact between the probe and the atoms of the protein, the trace will describe the SESA. Figure 2.6a illustrates the difference between these last 2 surfaces.

In 3 dimensions, rolling sphere programs obtain the SASA by placing the probe in contact with 3 atoms at the same time, without intersecting any, as shown in Figure 2.6c. Then, a tetrahedron is defined by the center of the 3 atoms and of the probe. The intersections between the probe and the tetrahedron's edges define the vertices of the spherical section of the probe that forms a patch of SESA. This is illustrated in Figure 2.6c. Then the probe is rolled over 2 or 1 atoms until it finds another point in space where it can be in contact with a new unique set of 3 atoms. Along the roll, new patches of SESA are defined, and the center of the probe traces the SASA as can be seen in Figure 2.6c. The end result will be the 2 surfaces which will naturally depend on the probe radius, especially the SASA. The bigger the probe is the more space will remain between it and the surface of the protein. For the same reason, if the probe radius becomes infinitesimal —that is, it becomes a 3D point, rather than a sphere—, it will discard every possible groove since it will travel the surface of every atom. In this

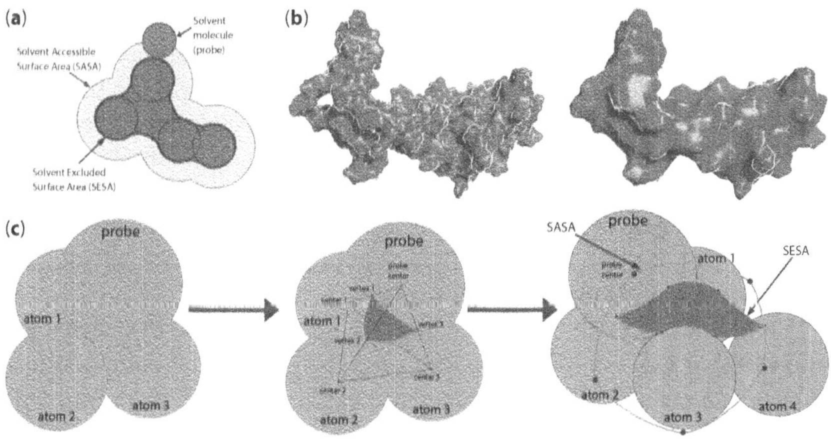

Figure 2.6 (a) SASA (red line) and SESA (blue bold line) in 2 dimensions with circles as atoms and a circular red probe. (b) The effect of the change of probe radius from 1.4Å (left) to 4Å (right) on the C terminal section of the HER2 ectodomain (P04626). (c) Steps in a rolling probe program. 3 contiguous atoms (brown spheres) of a protein in contact with the probe (purple sphere) which define the red spherical patch of the SESA. Then, the probe rolls and defines more patches of the SESA and the SASA (green outline, not filled for clarity). We thank Dr. Michel Sanner for kindly allowing us to adapt figures (a) and (c) from his seminal work [92].

limit, the 3 surfaces: VdWS, SAS and SES, are identical. Figure 2.6b shows how a change of probe radius affects the resulting SASA.

For this reason, different probe sizes are often alternated. First, a 1.4 Å probe that simulates water defines a SASA for the protein and then another larger probe (sometimes called shell probe), will differentiate the volume close to the protein from the rest of the solvent by defining a new larger Accessible Surface Area. The voids enclosed between the 2 Accessible Surface Areas are the protein voids. A usual second step is to discretize this void space with the help of a grid in order to calculate volume, surface area, depth and other cavity parameters. As mentioned before, most tools employ some form of grid at one point or another.

Although these programs do not tend to be the most efficient and have a limited field of application, grooves (shallow pockets) are usually well characterized by these methods and so rolling probe based methods are great options for analyzing this type of voids as they approximate the true cavity shape with good precision.

Also, the same probe can be used as a model of a ligand of interest to obtain an approximation of the possible interactions between the protein and its ligands.

Finally, the *tessellation* methods. They subdivide the 3D space into geometric figures (polygons), without overlap or empty spaces. More specifically, the triangulation of a set of points is the subdivision of the space between them with triangles and although these methods work in 3 dimensions and thus divide the space in tetrahedra, we will use the terms tessellation and triangulation interchangeably, as the literature often does.

In the case of a protein this method implies, as in methods above, a model of the protein composed of a set of spheres centered on their atoms and of equal radius to their respective Van der Waals radio. The tessellation of the centers of these spheres will be a set of polyhedra that will allow to infer structural information of the protein.

While Sanners method for obtaining the SASA was based on a triangulation [92], it was Edelsbrunner who used the methods of computational geometry intensively to detect and analyze cavities [93–96]. Beginning with Edelsbrunner's CAST; many programs such as Fpocket, CAVER, MOLE, ANA, etc. were developed based on a few computational geometry concepts with a nice common property: since they are mathematically related it is possible to calculate one of them by post-processing another. More importantly, one of them, the Voronoi Diagram, allowed the development of programs tailored for the discovery and characterization of tunnels and channels, which are highly important in terms of biological relevance but were not analyzable before, since these voids have a special property: they imply a path.

The Convex Hull (CH) of a set of points is the smallest convex polygon—that is, defined by the fewest number of points—, which contains all points of the set. Figure 2.7a illustrates an analogy between points in two-dimensional space and nails on a table, surrounded by a rubber band. The CH can be obtained for a set of points in any number of dimensions and in the case of proteins, is a first and rudimentary approximation to their topology. CAVER [99] uses the CH of a protein to define a boundary between the protein and the solvent in order to determine if a found tunnel is solvent exposed. ANA [100] is another program that makes use of the CH. In the same way grid based methods (POVME or Epock [98, 101]) use cylinders or spheres to select the region where the cavity lies, ANA uses a CH to let the user pinpoint the cavity to be calculated; this method has the added advantage of a higher flexibility, since a CH can take the shape of any convex polyhedron.

The Voronoi Diagram (VD) of a set of points is a subdivision of space such that each partition (Voronoi face) contains 1 point and all the space whose closest point is that same contained point. Figure 2.7b shows a simple example in two dimensions. The main feature of interest is that the edges lie at the same distance of 2 points and the vertices are located at the point of equal distance between 3 points.

By modelling a protein as a set of points (representing its atoms) in 3D space, the VD of the protein will be determined by the edges and facets of

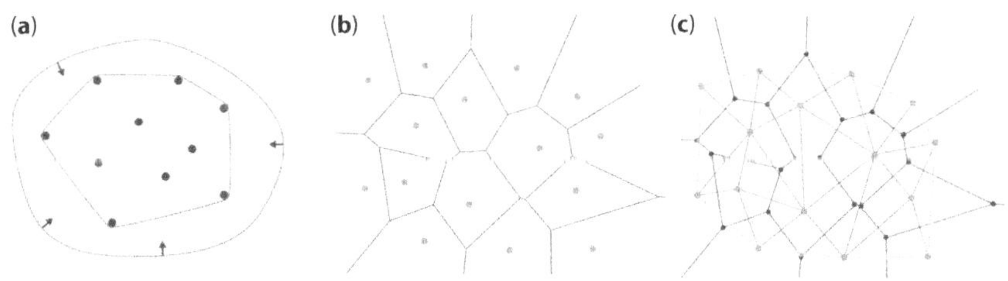

Figure 2.7 (a) The nails and elastic band analogy for the CH. The series of nails (points) that are in contact with the blue elastic band (CH) and the order in which they must be connected are sufficient to define the CH. This is equivalent to defining the CH segments. (b) VD in blue and the set of points in green. Notice the number of edges of the polygons are not fixed but depend on the point set topology. Points on the frontier of the point set are not contained in a polygon, but instead are just separated by edges. (c) A set of points (green dots), its DT in blue and its VD in pink. The vertices of the VD are in black and they correspond to the circumcenters of the pink triangles. The outer edges of the DT (highlighted) define the CH of the set of points.

the polyhedra. Facets will lie at an equivalent distance between 2 atoms, edges will be in between 3 atoms and vertices will be at the same distance of 4 atoms. Thus, a continuous trace of a subset of edges is the natural precursor of a potential tunnel axis and the distance between the atoms that lie on the sides is the radius of this tunnel, if the minimum radius along this tunnel is larger than a potential ligand, then an actual tunnel is found and this minimum radius is called the "bottleneck radius," the main parameter characterizing a tunnel or channel. This is the basic idea behind tunnel detection software such as CAVER [99] and MOLE [102].

We will succinctly define the Delaunay Triangulation since it connects all the previously mentioned constructs, the Alpha Shapes, the Convex Hull and the Voronoi Diagram.

The Delaunay Triangulation (DT) of a set of points in 2 dimensions is a triangulation such that no point is inside the circumcircle of any triangle, the circumcircle being the circle defined by the 3 vertices (points) of the triangle. This definition is already a hint of the usefulness of this triangulation when searching for voids in proteins, if the points are atoms, then we have found putative empty spheres inside our protein, although these are not entirely empty, since the volume of the atoms Van der Waals radii have to be accounted for.

But the most important fact about DTs is their relationship to other tessellation methods. The set of alpha shapes, that is, the approximation of the shape of the set of points can be obtained from the DT. The CH can also be obtained from the DT, it is the subset of edges that lie on the outside of the triangulation, as Figure 2.7c shows. The VD can also be obtained, since its vertices are the circumcenters of the DT's triangles, that is, the centers of the triangles' circumcircles.

Many tessellation programs use this triangulation as the first step, obtaining tetrahedrons with 4 atoms as vertices, since they operate in 3D.

While some tunnel-specific tools are not based on Voronoi Diagrams (e.g.: CHUNNEL [103] and PoreWalker [104]), modern ones tend to be based on these concepts. Some examples include CHEXVIS [105], MolAxis [106], CAVER [99] and MOLE [102].

Tunnel and channel detection and characterization turned out to be a subfield in its own, since these kinds of voids have the added concept of "path," which does not apply to other voids, such as clefts or pockets. As mentioned, these programs tend to be based on the Voronoi diagram of the atoms, since the edges of the resulting polyhedra trace the center of potential tunnels and make it easy to calculate important tunnel variables as the bottleneck radius (the radius of the tunnel at its most narrow section). Also due to the need of determining potential paths a ligand would take along the tunnel, they also tend to incorporate shortest path algorithms, such as Dijkstra's.

The fact that all these programs can be clustered, does not mean they are identical in any way. They all use different strategies and each of them approach the problem in a different way and utilize their base methods (grid, rolling probe, triangulation), in radically different ways. Some programs, like HOLLOW [107], mostly care about visualization. More modern ones, like Epock [98], make emphasis on control and efficiency, something which was not present at the beginning of the field (HOLE's paper [108] was the first to emphasize its performance).

It is the diversity and complexity of protein voids that drove this plethora of cavity calculation software; each researcher finding that the available tools were insufficient to conduct their research and consequently turned themselves into software developers.

We now devote ourselves to Machine Learning approaches, starting off with one of the most basic ML methods and one which, as we said in Chapter 2, was designed to be a classification method from the beginning, Support Vector Machines (SVMs).

2.3.3 Machine Learning Approaches

2.3.3.1 SVM-Based Approaches

ATPint [109] (Table 2.2) is the first surveyed method, it was published in 2009 and was specifically designed to predict ATP binding residues. The feature vector comprised 7 groups of features: hydrophobicity, beta strand propensity, polarity, solvation potential (to represent the probability of the

Table 2.2 Survey of ML methods for LBS prediction.

Method	Software
SVM	ATPint [109], ATPsite [112], MetaDBSite [115], NsitePred [113], vitapred [116], COACH [117], eFindSite [122], TargetS [123], OSML [126], ATPbind [138], n/n [125]
RF	LigandRFs [127], PRANK [130]
CNN	DeepSite [133], DeepCSeqSite [135], DELIA [135, 136], Kalasanty [139]
Ensemble classifier	TargetATPSite [114]

amino acid type to be exposed), interface propensity (propensity of the amino acid type to be part of the interface of a complex with another molecule), net charge and average accessible surface area.

ATPint was trained on primary sequence and its data was augmented by performing a Multiple Sequence Alignment (MSA) of the input sequence using PSI-BLAST [110]. Given an input sequence, PSI-BLAST returns a Position Specific Scoring Matrix (PSSM), also called Profile. Profiles are matrices of 21 rows (1 + 20 for each amino acid type) and n columns (1 for each alignment column), that condense the information of a MSA. They contain the probability of occurrence of each type of amino acid at each position along with insertion/deletion. Knowing that function is more conserved than sequence, this technique allows to expand the available information for the ML model. Indeed, ATPint reached a MCC score of 0.33 when processing the input sequence and a MCC score of 0.51, when dealing with the PSSM. A noticeable improvement that all the following sequence-based methods take advantage of. The first step in most, if not all, sequence based LBS is to obtain a PSSM. It is important to emphasize that the method only learned how to weight each feature, but how each feature was calculated was fixed by the researchers. For each feature, the 20 amino acids were assigned a score, calculated from first principles, based on previous literature. Current techniques tend to favor learning over this approach and for good reason. For example, the feature of residue interface propensity was calculated with a formula that came from a Thornton paper [111] from 1996 that dealt with protein-protein interactions, not with proteins and small ligands. These scores are now being used to predict the interaction of a protein with a small ligand as a nucleotide, an unexpected application of previous work, resulting in parameters that the ML model could not adapt to the data. We also notice that ATPint's features have a high degree of overlap, since they are all related to hydrophobicity.

ATPsite [112] was developed with the same goal as ATPint, but had some key differences, for example, being trained using protein-ATP complexes from the PDB and adding new features like the residue's dihedral angles. These were calculated by predicting its secondary structure, an extra previous step that served to augment the input data. Another new feature are the residue conservation scores, which are present in the PSSM but were not used by ATPint. This is key information, since ATP binding residues are expected to be conserved due to their relevance. With all of this, ATPsite achieves a MCC score of 0.43, which is lower to ATPint's reported MCC score of 0.51. But, ATPsite authors report a MCC score of 0.078 for ATPint. We are unaware of further attempts at reproducing these results. Though there have been further attempts at predicting ATP binding sites [113, 114], we will continue onto other topics.

MetaDBSite [115] is a DNA binding site predictor that, like the previous predictors, works at the residue level, but instead of following a first principles methodology to build its input feature vector, MetaDBSite uses a more straightforward approach; it is a meta predictor that uses a SVM to aggregate the result of six previous predictive tools, giving an output of higher quality. The authors of MetaDBSite report a MCC score of 0.33. When previous methods are available, it is often better to take advantage of them, than to derive a new model, with new fixed features derived from first principles.

VitaPred [116] is a good example of how domain knowledge can guide ML engineering. The authors classified vitamins in 4 groups: vitamin A, vitamin B, vitamin B6 and other vitamins. Then studied which residues tend to interact with each vitamin class and after noticing there were significant differences among each class, decided to build 4 separate SVMs to predict their binding sites. They report MCC scores of 0.48 for vitamin A, 0.61 for vitamin B, 0.81 for vitamin B6, and 0.53 for other vitamins.

COACH [117] is one of the most successful ML methods for LBS prediction. It combines 5 different methods. The first 2 were developed by the authors to work with COACH: TM-SITE, which is based in template structures and S-SITE which is sequence based and as previous sequence-based methods, builds a PSSM. The remaining methods are FINDSITE [118], which is also based on template structures; ConCavity [119], which combines structural models with evolutionary sequence conservation estimates and COFACTOR [120], a method that was also developed by the authors to use a query structure to find similar structures with known LBS. This way, COACH incorporates 3 methods that are based on structural information, 1 sequence-based method and 1 method that comprises both approaches. The authors report a MCC score of 0.54 for COACH.

In 2018 the authors updated COACH and published a new web server, COACH-D [121]. This new tool can also take in a ligand and perform docking on the predicted LBS. It is also noted that one of the methods used by COACH (FINDSITE), released a new version [122] which incorporates a SVM in its final step when classifying residues as ligand binding residues or non-ligand binding residues.

TargetS [123] developers followed an inverse approach. Instead of using one SVM as a last step in the prediction workflow, they integrated several SVM base classifiers into an ensemble classifier. This approach fits nicely with the random undersampling method that is often necessary to compensate for the highly imbalanced datasets that plague bioinformatics. The authors fed the base classifiers with balanced sets of positive samples (proteins with known binding sites), and a random selection of negative samples. Thus, the positive samples were used and reused to train the base classifiers while the set of negative samples among different base classifiers was quite heterogeneous.

The authors also developed a variation of the AdaBoost [124] boosting scheme for their ensemble classifier. AdaBoost scheme beggins training and evaluation with a subset of a single base classifier and then iterates, expanding the set by 1 base classifier at a time until all base classifiers are incorporated into the set. At each step, the subset of base classifiers are evaluated with the same data that was used for training, those samples that were evaluated poorly will bear a higher weight in the next iteration. This was the aspect of AdaBoost that the authors decided was more difficult. These evaluations were too lenient which resulted in over optimist self-evaluation on the training data and poor performance on the evaluation data set. Thus, they separated the sequences from their training data set in pure training data and evaluation data, while keeping low homology between the sequences of the 2 sets, to reduce generalization error. The authors report MCC scores of 0.53 (ATP) to 0.74 (GDP) for the prediction of nucleotide binding sites, depending on the nucleotide.

After describing the most relevant SVM programs, we turn our attention to programs based on another popular classification method: Random Forests (RFs) [71]. Other SVM methods [125, 126] were surveyed and they are all displayed on Table 2.2.

2.3.3.2 Random Forest–Based Approaches

LigandRfs [127] replicates the successful strategy of TargetS. An ensemble of base classifiers is fed randomly undersampled training data. Each of them receives the full positive subset of the data (sequences with binding sites) and a random sample of the non-binding site subset. The goal is the same as before, to reduce False Negatives due to an imbalance in the training data set. The authors reported MCC scores of 0.40 for the CASP9 [128] data set and of 0.44 for the CASP8 [129] data set.

PRANK [130, 131] is one of the few methods that does not work at the residue level, but instead predicts LBS based on voids reported by previously reviewed cavity programs (FPocket [132] and ConCavity [119]). From each reported void, it extracts points that are close to the surface and then constructs a feature vector for each point, characterizing its surroundings with variables such as hydrophobicity or ligand-binding propensities of neighboring amino acids; variables at the atomic level, like physico-chemical properties, are also taken into account. Then, PRANK calculates “ligandability” of each point using RF classifiers and, finally, clusters points based on closeness and relatively high ligandability score; these clusters will be putative LBS and will each be ranked by their "ligandability score" (ligand binding propensity score). The top-1 or top-3 ranked pockets will be classified as LBSs.

2.3.3.3 Deep Learning-Based Approaches

DeepSite [133] is currently the most cited deep learning algorithm in the LBS prediction field. The authors make use of a grid to subdivide the whole protein in 1Å cubic voxels and use the tools from computer vision to analyze this 3D representation as if it were a 2D image. Each voxel works as a pixel and its channels, instead of being colors, are the properties of the atoms that occupy the voxel: hydrophobicity, aromaticity, whether it can be hydrogen donor or acceptor, etc. In the same way computer vision uses a sliding window, DeepSite works with a sliding box that groups voxels, is the input for the layers and becomes smaller as it advances through them until predictions for each voxel are achieved. Voxels then are clustered into putative binding pockets. The authors report different metrics than MCC and compare instead the reported cavities with other methods (FPocket, ConCavity), when analyzing the structures from the scPDB database [134] and, predictably, find their method to perform better than previous methods.

DeepCSeqSite's [135] input is a sequence, instead of a structure and though its architecture is completely different to the traditional ML methods we just surveyed, there are many resemblances on the way of modelling: several features are collected for each residue (PSSM, dihedral angles, secondary structure, etcetera), and then feed into the CNN which outputs a binary classification of each residue, classifying them as ligand binding or not. The authors evaluate their method on different data sets and report MCCs ranging from 0.43 to 0.47, while COACH MCC scores range from 0.34 to 0.42 on the same data sets, according to the authors. A significant difference, considering DeepCSeqSite is sequence only.

DELIA [136] is also a sequence based method, but it augments its data by building the 2D distance matrix (contact map), from the sequence and using both sequence and contact map as the input to the Neural Networks. The authors then established strategies like performing a MSA of the input sequence to build the PSSM (profile) and undersampling their training data to deal with a highly imbalanced data set.

The authors compare their method against established tools like COACH and ATPBind, both being SVM methods that, unlike DELIA, take advantage of structural information. Ions, heme and nucleotides were used in the benchmarks. For example, when predicting binding of nucleotides, DELIA scores a MCC of 0.68, while COACH's MCC is 0.62 and ATPbind is 0.68. It should also be noted that the nucleotide LBS prediction was benchmarked with the same data set ATPbind authors built and used to benchmark their own tool. DELIA matched ATPbind MCC score for nucleotides while being a more general method and working with sequence only information.

We conclude this section with a table of the traditional ML and more recent deep learning methods for LBS prediction. A comparison with the previous classical methods reveals less emphasis on the geometric characteristics of voids and a focus on the protein sequence itself. The lack of MD support in ML methods should not be surprising. These methods are large scale methods in nature, and if the number of structures pales in comparison to that of sequences, the number of available good quality MD trajectories is negligible, as initiatives to make these available do not seem to take off just yet. So, authors instead focus their methods on the most abundant form of biological information: sequences. Although, this may change in the near future with the release and success of AlphaFold2 [137].

This still leaves the discovery of cryptic LBS to the classical methods. Cryptic binding pockets are absent in unliganded protein structures but open due to protein dynamics. So geometric approaches will still be needed in the future.

2.4 Lead Discovery

2.4.1 The Relevance of Predict Binding Affinity

Predicting and studying the interactions between ligands and proteins is a key step in the drug development process. The recognition of a target protein and a small molecule, peptide, or protein capable of modulating the activity involves complex thermodynamics, mediated by both intermolecular interactions and by entropic effects (e.g., desolvation). From a drug-design perspective, a key aspect is the evaluation of thousands of drug candidates in terms of binding affinity, to achieve an efficient overall drug discovery process. Here, the challenge is to quickly eliminate the number of potential candidates [140].

Nowadays, in order to evaluate which potential molecules can bind protein targets, the use of computational tools (like structure based virtual screening) allows analyzing thousands of potential drugs, instead of the old expensive and time-consuming experimental screenings. Between them, docking, QSAR and Molecular Dynamics simulations are among the most common to discover new drugs based on targets like protein structures.

Nevertheless, these techniques from a classical approach are ineffective to use in large sets of potential ligands, since they require a unique set-up for each chemical system [141].

In addition, binding prediction not only focuses on the energy enveloped in the binding itself but also in the correct ligand conformation (or "pose") and it is used in virtual high throughput screening to discriminate between potential ligands [142]. As we pointed up, the ligand-binding phenomena is determined by both chemical interactions and entropic effects. The enthalpic factors involve atom-atom interactions like coulombic forces, hydrogen bonds, and Van der Waals interactions. The entropic factor involves the conformational diversity and the rearrangements of the receptor and drug solvation shell. These entropic aspects are often difficult to determine directly since they include physicochemical properties like hydrophobicity and accessibility of the solvent area among others.

2.4.2 The Concept of Docking

Molecular Docking is a bunch of techniques for the prediction of the best binding between a drug and its associated receptor. Depending on the level of bond treatment of the molecular docking approach, an ensemble of conformations, orientations, or poses are generated. As we need the three-dimensional structure of the receptor, docking is considered a structure-based drug-design methodology. The first docking implementation was published by Kuntz [143]. Using spheres, they explore many binding geometries to optimize the steric overlap, within a fully rigid model. Using this approach, they generated conformations with optimal steric fits for heme-myoglobin and prealbumin ligands.

Docking techniques are useful to predict the best matching between ligands (small organic molecules, peptides, protein, cofactors, etc.) and a defined target. These techniques can be classified as (i) rigid docking, (ii) semi-flexing docking, or (iii) flexible docking. For the first approach both protein and ligand are considered as rigid structures (as in the classical lock-key model). This approach is more suitable to analyze small organic molecule-protein or protein-protein interactions. On the other hand, in the semi-flexing docking approach, protein is a rigid entity and the ligand is flexible (peptide-protein interaction). All ligand conformers are evaluated against the protein and those with better scoring are selected. Finally, flexible docking where both, ligand and protein, are flexible counterparts [19]. There are free docking tools with different approaches (some consider molecules as rigid and others flexible) that bring preliminary information to understand protein-ligand interaction. Some docking methods are available on the Internet, such as: SwissDock [144]; DockThor [145]; ZDOCK [146]; pepATTRACT [147], FlexPepDock [148]; pep-SiteFinder [149]; ModPep [150]; HPEPDOCK [151], among others.

2.4.3 The Scoring Function

In docking, we need to generate an ensemble of conformations, orientations or poses, and then evaluate quantitatively the quality of the binding. This quantitative evaluation is carried out by the **scoring function (SF)**, the mathematical core, and the key step of docking methodologies [152]. Scoring functions estimate the Protein-Ligand free energy of binding in the molecular interaction. They are used in virtual screening, de novo ligand design, lead optimization, pharmacophore modeling, and many other tools related to drug discovery. Improving the accuracy of SFs for structure-based binding affinity prediction or virtual screening has proven to be a challenging task for any class of method.

Traditionally, SFs were separated into 3 categories: those based on molecular mechanics forcefields [153], empirical [154] and knowledge-based [155]. The **molecular mechanics model** describes the system in terms of mainly non-bonded interactions and (sometimes) some bonded interactions, especially for torsional conformations. This approach, as is focused on the enthalpic component, undervalue the entropic contributions to the protein-ligand interaction [156]. Popular and well-proven forcefields for proteins and small organic molecules are CHARMM [157] or AMBER [158], used extensively for molecular dynamics simulations. Docking implementations like *DOCK* [143], *Gold* [159], or *LigandFit* [160] differ in aspects like the ligand placement strategy, but all of them use forcefield-based SF. The **empirical methods** are based on forcefield types, but adding other physicochemical features like solvent accessibility, hydrophobicity, desolvation, entropy, etc; with the terms properly weighted with some regression analysis. Some empirical implementations are *Autodock Vina* [161], *GlideScore* [162], *ChemScore* [163], and *X-Score* [164]. In **knowledge-based approaches**, the 3D coordinates of a large set of protein–ligand complexes are regarded as a knowledge base, and then the relative occurrence frequencies of some features, such as atom–atom pairwise contacts, are calculated. Popular implementations of knowledge-based SFs include PMF [165], DrugScore [166], and ASP [167].

To develop new scoring functions, the databases with experimental information about protein-ligand complexes are very useful. *PDBbind* is a popular resource of this kind. This collection is manually curated, based on the biomolecular complexes taken from the PDB data bank, so is a reliable source of experimental data. Another useful source of data are the datasets with *decoys*. A "decoy" is an **artificially generated compound** with physicochemical properties similar to the ligand. *The Directory of Useful Decoys (DUD)*, the *Database of Useful Decoys-Enhanced (DUD-E)* and the *Maximum Unbiased Validation (MUV)* are representative examples of databases with decoy information. For each molecular target, a set of dozens of decoys are generated.

For the validation or the assessment of a scoring function strength, the *comparative assessment of scoring functions (CASF)* benchmark is a useful tool [168]. CASF is designed as a "scoring benchmark," and aims to evaluate four metrics: *scoring power*, *ranking power*, *docking power*, and *screening power*. The *scoring power* is the correlation between the predicted affinity and the experimental one, the *ranking power* is the capability of properly rank the different evaluated ligands with the receptor, the *docking power* represents the ability of the SF to reach the ligand pose among the different decoys and the *screening power* evaluate the capability to identify the correct binders of a target among a set of random molecules. Here, we

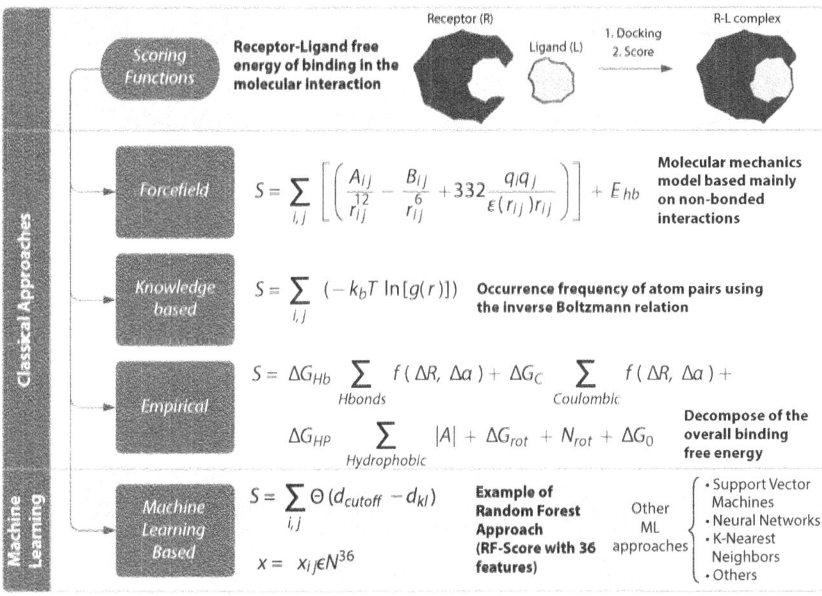

Figure 2.8 Generalization of the main categories between scoring functions. A forcefield potential example taken from GoldScore [159], a generic knowledge based using an inverse Boltzmann relation, an empirical example of SF taken from LUDI [170] and a machine learning SF by using a RF implementation in RF-Score [171].

will focus mainly on *scoring power*, despite the fact that ML methods were applied to all of these docking aspects.

However, these classical approaches to develop SFs have some limitations. The traditional SFs are constructed following linear relationships between the features of proteins and ligands and the characteristics of the protein-ligand complex. But, taking into account the complex nature of the physics involved in the drug-target interactions, SFs normally fit better with non-linear methods. In that sense, the machine learning methods as RF, SVM, and ANN, among others, are very useful for fitting the SF parameters. These methods will statistically analyze the correlation between chemical structures and interaction status of known ligand-receptor pairs to derive statistical models for predicting the status of other unknown compounds. Nevertheless, there are some concerns about these ML scoring functions about the usage of oversimplified descriptors or the excessively biased approaches depending on the training dataset used (Figure 2.8) [169].

2.4.4 Developing of Novels Scoring Functions by Machine Learning

2.4.4.1 Random Forests

As we pointed out, Random Forest (RF) is one of the most popular techniques to develop scoring functions. RF-Score, B2BScore, and SFCscore^{RF} are examples of this. RF-Score has three versions: RF-Score-v1, a knowledge-based SF that utilizes nine different heavy atoms (CNOSP and the halogens) to count occurrences within a given distance range. This model was trained with the PDBbind v2007b database, reaching a high accuracy (R = 0.776, RMSE = 1.58 log K unit) [171]. In the improved version, RF-Score-v2 [172] they achieve the best performance, with Rp = 0.803 by tuning some additional parameters. RF-Score-v3 [173] (With an Rp of 0.803) adds empirical energy terms trained with RF from AutoDock Vina, the aforementioned docking software. On the other hand, B2BScore is an SF that integrates two physicochemical properties for protein-ligand affinity calculation: the *beta-contacts*, which includes the interactions between atoms; and the *B-factors*, a measure of the atom flexibility [174]. Another interesting case is *SFCscore*^{RF} [175], a ML optimization from the classical *SFCscore* [176], where the linear fitting was replaced by an improved SF that uses RF for regression. The descriptors are taken from the classical *SFCscore*, but the use of RF enhanced the scoring power, increasing the

Rp from 0.644 (classical SFCscore) to 0.779 (*SFCscore*^{RF}). As in the case of *SFCscore*^{RF}, many classical SFs have been used as a basis to develop RF-based scoring functions. For example, the simple replacement of the linear regression function for a RF regression improved the performance of the traditional *Cyscore* scoring function [177].

2.4.4.2 Support Vector Machines

Another popular ML technique used for developing SFs is the Support Vector Machine (SVM). Support vector machine was originally designed for classification (for example, for the cases treated in the LBS section), but it also can be used for regression problems (SVR). For example, Kinning *et al.* [178] used a SVM to determine the optimal weights of the empirical SF to improve the affinity prediction for Enoyl-[Acyl-Carrier-Protein] reductase. Koppisetty *et al.* [179] used SVM for developing a SF to compute binding energies and their enthalpy and entropy components of protein–ligand complexes, including several protein–ligand interactions or ligand-based descriptors generated with AutoDock and the Schrödinger's suite. Similarly, Li *et al.* [180] developed a SF based on SMV called *ID-Score. ID-Score* uses a set of descriptors that cover molecular interactions, desolvation effect, entropic loss effect, shape matching, and surface property matching. *SVR-KB* and *SVR-EP* are scoring functions released on the same publication. Both apply SVM-based SFs in regression mode (SVR). The first are knowledge-based pairwise potentials, while SVR-EP is based on physicochemical properties. The same group developed SVR-Gen and other SMV applications on protein-ligand binding.

An interesting article of Ashtaway *et al.* [181] develops and compares many ML methods to construct SFs, in order to evaluate them and seek the approach that better fits the data. To develop the different SF, they used multiple linear regression (MLR), RF, and SVM, in addition to other different ML techniques such as multivariate adaptive regression splines (MARS), kNN, and boosted regression trees (BRT). The results found more accuracy in the RF and BRT approaches, with a Pearson correlation coefficient of 0.806 between predicted and measured binding affinities compared to 0.644 achieved by a traditional SF. The same authors evaluate the same techniques to improve SF for pose prediction. Here, the MARS approach had a success rate of nearly 80%, in comparison a 70% obtained with the empirical-conventional SF model GOLD, and evaluated on the same test set [182].

2.4.4.3 Neural Networks

The application of ANN was also useful for the creation of novel Scoring Functions. For example, *NNScore* [183] is a SF deployed by the use of ANN. The original method had as output a binary classification of ligand potency, by rescoring the docked poses of candidate ligands; while the improved *NNScore 2.0* [184] includes an estimation of the pKd. *CScore* [185] uses systematic element-pair distance-based features and the Cerebellar Model Articulation Controller (CMAC), a kind of network model based on the mammalian cerebellum to predict binding affinity, with R = 0.7668 and RMSE = 1.4540. Similarly, *BgN-score* and *BsN-score* are SFs that conjugate a set of physicochemical and geometrical features with ANN using bagging and boosting ensemble techniques to predict binding affinity (Pearson correlation of 0.804 and 0.816) [186].

From a deep learning approach, *AtomNet* [187] was designed to predict the bioactivity of small molecules for targets with no previously known modulators, achieving an AUC greater than 0.9 on 57.8% of the targets in the DUDE benchmark. Similarly, *DeepVS* [188, 189] is an improvement of Docking-based Virtual Screening (DBVS). The docking results are used as input for a Deep Neural Network which extracts the relevant features from the basic data, achieving an interesting AUC ROC of 0.81. Ragoza also uses CNN to predict not only binding but also pose [188]. As DeepVS, Ragoza uses a 3D representation of a protein–ligand interaction, and the scoring function automatically learns the key features of protein–ligand interactions that correlate with binding.

Finally, *Deepdrug3D* [190] is not exactly a docking suite, but it is worth a brief mention since it is a fitting end to our review of existing approaches. *Deepdrug3D* takes a protein-ligand complex, builds a classical 3D grid around the ligand, discards the voxels that are occupied by protein atoms and uses the remaining voxels as input to a CNN. This tool was developed for rational drug design, and the approach is also valuable for LBS classification and the potential prediction of a putative ligand for the known void. The authors argue that their approach leads to better results than purely geometric metrics such as void volume or shape treated previously in the LBS section.

2.4.4.4 Gradient Boosting Decision Tree

The aforementioned *RF-Score-v3* was also improved with the aim of the ML tool *Gradient Boosting Decision Tree*, being called *XGB-Score* [191], with a significant improvement of the RF-based SF. The same ML tool was used to implement three novel SFs for scoring, docking, and screening called *BT-Score*, *BT-Dock* and *BT-Screen*, respectively [192]. The testing results on CASF-2013 indicated that BT-Score, BT-Dock and BT-Screen could yield the higher scoring power (Rp = .825 vs. .627), docking power (S_2 Docking Accuracy of 96.87% vs. 82.05%) and screening power (Screening enrichment $EF_{1\%}$ of 33.90 vs. 19.54) than other conventional SFs. The Gradient Boosting Decision Trees also were applied by Wang *et al.* [193] to develop a feature functional theory-binding predictor (FFT-BP). Wang *et al.* developed a feature functional theory-binding predictor (FFT-BP) for protein–ligand binding affinity prediction based on six types of microscopic features, including reaction field features, electrostatic binding features, atomic coulombic interactions, atomic van der Waals interactions, atomic solvent-excluded surface area and molecular volume.

2.5 Lead Optimization

2.5.1 QSAR and Proteochemometrics

Alexander Crum Brown, a Scottish organic chemist was one of the first to remark the connection between chemical constitution and physiological action. Besides the concept of "chemical constitution-physiological action" relation itself, he proposed a mathematical function to model the relationship [194]. In the words of Brown and Fraser:

> "To use a mathematical analogy, if we represent the constitution by C and the physiological action by Φ, (Φ is some unknown function of C, say f(C); to discover this we produce a known change on the constitution by which it becomes C + ΔC, and examine the corresponding change of physiological action which has become (Φ + ΔΦ)." [195]

Nowadays, the same concept models the *Quantitative structure–activity relationship (QSAR)* technique. QSAR is a quantitative approach that establishes a correlation between some chemical properties of a molecule and the biological activity [196]. QSAR derives from the molecular information *descriptors*, mathematical values that describe the structure and physicochemical properties of a molecule. Depending on the system and the aim of the calculation, descriptors can be more or less complex, classified into different "dimensional" categories. For instance, the representation of only basic chemical information like the elemental composition of the compound is defined as zerodimentional or 0D-QSAR, while a list of specific pools of atoms like organic functional groups or atomtypes corresponds to

1D-QSAR. The topological information of the molecule adds another layer of information, called 2D-QSAR; and the spatial configuration defines a 3D-QSAR. Four or even more dimensions may include interaction energies or additional spatial information, like binding cavities, similar to the LBS approaches treated in the former section (4D-QSAR or higher) [197]. The descriptors can include also important physicochemical properties in drug design, like the octanol/water partition coefficient or *log(P)*, a measure of the lipophilicity and hence the capability of the drug to migrate from an aqueous phase to the lipophilic bilayer core of cell membrane, for example [198]. This physicochemical property affects, for example, the absorption of an oral drug in the gastrointestinal system. In this way, the QSAR approaches are extensively used in the pharma industry not only to study drug-receptor interactions, but also for toxicology and ADME (Absorption, Distribution, Metabolism and Elimination) properties [199].

From the mathematically point of view, a generic QSAR model can be defined as:

$$P = f(x1, x2, \ldots, xp)$$

where P is the molecular activity and x_1, x_2, x_n are the descriptors, with a function f that is the QSAR relationship itself.

The oldest and most common algorithm applied in QSAR is the mentioned *Multiple Linear Regression* (MLR) which is nothing more than a classical linear regression with multiple variables. As expected, this approach presents some problems and limitations, like a tendency to overfitting [200]. Another regression technique is the Partial Least Squares (PLS), used with a large number of descriptors, like the *4D-QSAR* as *GRID* and *CoMFA* [197]. PLS reduce dimensionality as other related technique, the *Principal Component Regression* (PCR), that converts numerous correlated features to a few uncorrelated variables called principal components. As we pointed out previously, these techniques reveal linear relations between variables, so they are not able to capture nonlinear relationships. In this context, ML approaches are useful to identify new correlations.

2.5.2 Machine Learning Algorithms in Deriving Descriptors

As we see with the Scoring Functions, RF and SVM techniques are very popular and versatile implementations within the ML toolbox. In the same way, RF and SVM were extensively used to develop novel descriptors for QSAR, where the aim is to identify key chemical features of the drug.

The utility of RF for predicting biological activity was first evaluated by Svetnik *et al.* [201] in six different chemoinformatics datasets. These datasets present both classification problems (for example, permeability across Blood-Brain Barrier, among others) or regression problems (like the dopamine receptor binding affinity). Similarly, RF classification was also used to find the best chemical fingerprints for Epidermal Growth Factor Receptor (EGFR) inhibitors, a well-characterized cancer drug target [202]. Likewise, RF was used to construct toxicity profiles for drug vehicles [203] and to identify potential drug targets in human proteins based on sequence information [204]. Cano *et al.* used a RF approach to automatically select molecular descriptors of training data for ligands of kinases, nuclear hormone receptors, and other enzymes [205].

As we noted, classification can be carried out also by using SVM techniques. For example, to predict anti-HIV-1 peptides [206]; inhibitors of activator protein (AP)-1 and nuclear factor (NF)-kB [207]; or to select descriptors for selective inhibitors of VEGFR-2, in combination with genetic algorithms [208].

Another common ML algorithm is the k-Nearest Neighbors (KNN). In QSAR they were mainly used to cluster sets of molecules based on chemical similarity. For example, KNN was used to group receptors in terms of their ligands [209], for drug target profiling [210] or for target prediction based on fingerprint similarity and explicit bioactivity [211]. Neural Networks are also useful for predicting activity from structure, and in an inverse manner to predict structure from activity. Particularly for binding affinity, ANN were used to design antagonists for 5-hydroxtryptamine subtype 6 receptor (5-HT_6R), a target for Alzheimer's Disease [212] and sigma-1 receptor antagonists for the treatment of neuropathic pain [213]. The use of ANN in combination with RF was used to predict half-maximal effective concentration (EC_{50}) of reverse transcriptase inhibitors, using as descriptors target drug interactions [214]. Other interesting applications of ANN in drug discovery were the prediction of biophysical properties of monoclonal antibodies [215], or to evaluate systemic toxicity of different analogs of valproic acid [216].

The ANN is useful also to do *inverse-QSAR*. As the name suggests, the aim of inverse-QSAR is to infer chemical structures from given chemical activities or properties (the term QSPR is often used to refer to "structure-property relationship"). Ito *et al.* use this approach to generate monocyclic compounds based on physic or chemical desired properties such as heat of atomization, heat of combustion, or octanol/water partition coefficient [217]. *Multitask neural networks* can be used to improve the performance of the model, by using related information as an inductive bias.

This approach was used to train QSAR models for multiple target learning on a family of biological targets [218] or predict activities of compounds from multiple assays simultaneously [219].

The prediction of binding affinity using CNN is another interesting example of the use of neural networks. *DeepDTA* [220] uses simply unidimensional sequence information of both targets and receptors to predict novel drug-target interactions; or *DeepConv-DTI* [221], which captures local residues patterns of target proteins that participate in the drug-protein interaction. Another CNN application was the ranking of potential drug molecules in terms of potency for lead optimization [222].

Other ML tools described in the present book chapter and applied to model QSAR are the *Gaussian Process* for ADME (to modeling properties like blood-brain barrier, hERG inhibition, and aqueous solubility) [223]; the XGBoost to infer refractive index and viscosity of ionic liquids [224]; or PCR for evaluating the inhibitory activity of dipeptides [225], among many others.

Recently, the algorithms reviewed here, such as SVM, RF, KNN, ANN, and XGBoost (among others), were evaluated for 14 datasets comprising nine physicochemical properties and five toxicity endpoints to study the performance of each method. The SVM and XGBoost approaches were better in terms of prediction accuracy and computational efficiency for small datasets, while XGBoost was better for the large ones [200].

2.6 Peptides in Pharmaceuticals

2.6.1 Peptide Natural and Synthetic Sources

Peptides, polypeptides and proteins are the main components of life and can present different pharmaceutical activities, for example antimicrobial activity (Figure 2.9). They can be isolated from their natural source or chemically synthesized. Since the use of peptides purified from animal tissue such as Insulin or Adrenocorticotrophic Hormone to the chemically synthesized peptide hormone like oxytocin, peptides had been part of the medicine strategies for decades [33]. Peptides can present anti-inflammatory properties like melittin, discovered in bee venom [226] and is therefore approved by the FDA for relieving pain and swelling associated with rheumatoid arthritis, tendinitis, bursitis and multiple sclerosis [227].

On the other hand, antimicrobial peptides (AMPs) have been found in animals (mammals and amphibians), plants, bacteria, insects and marine organisms [228–235]. Also, they are present in several insect and reptile

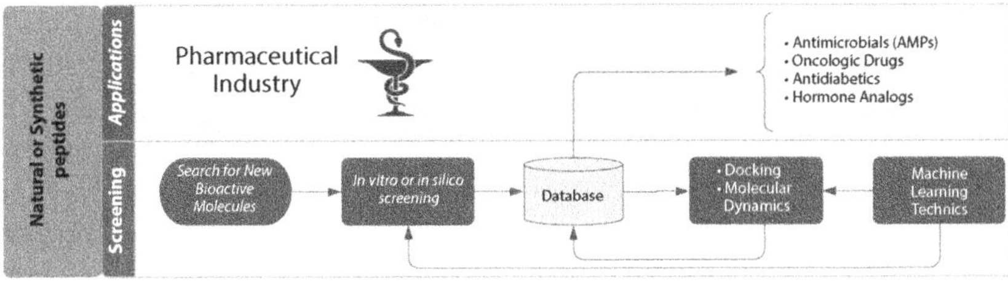

Figure 2.9 Machine learning techniques applied to peptide-based drug development.

venoms. Animal derived AMPs were initially discovered in invertebrates and later in vertebrates. Mammals, including humans, have an arsenal of AMPs, each displaying a distinct, specific expression pattern [228, 236, 237]. Milk proteins are considered the most important source of bioactive peptides in mammals and their production and properties have been reviewed in many articles [238–240]. Nevertheless, the main source of AMPs are amphibians, and especially frogs. Till today, new peptides from frogs are identified as AMPs [36, 241]. Recently, insect AMPs have also been used for anti-biofilm-based strategies [242] (Table 2.3).

The emergence of antibiotic-resistant microbes has stimulated research worldwide seeking new biologically active molecules. In this respect, synthetic AMPs have been suggested to overcome this problem.

In order to study the antimicrobial activity and the molecular mechanism of natural or synthetic AMPs, molecular dynamics simulations have been extensively used [243, 244], besides the traditional experimental

Table 2.3 Survey of some ML methods for SF.

Method	SF
RFw	RF-Score-v1 [171], RF-Score-v2 [172], RF-Score-v3 [173], B2BScore [174], SFCscore^{RF} [175], Cyscore [177],
SVM	SVR-KB [180], SVR-EP [180], ID-Score [180], n/n [179], n/n (application of many techniques besides SVM) [181, 182]
NN	NNScore [183], NNScore 2.0 [184], CScore [185], BgN-score [186], BsN-score [186], AtomNet [187], DeepVS [189], Deepdrug3D [190], n/n [188]
Gradient Boost Decision Tree	XGB-Score [191], BT-Score [192], BT-Dock [192], BT-Screen [192]

approaches [245]. Once the structure of a given bioactive peptide is known, it is possible to synthesize it. Three main approaches are available at present: (1) chemical synthesis; (2) recombinant DNA technology; and (3) enzymatic synthesis [246]. The length and quantity of the desired peptide are the two criteria that mainly determine the most suitable method for peptide synthesis. Chemical synthesis is the most popular method for short peptides in a laboratory, while recombinant DNA technology is the preferred choice for large peptides [247, 248]. The bioactive peptide is used as a template to develop more suitable structures to be used as drugs. Several strategies, both biological or chemical, can be implemented for the library synthesis [249–251]. One chemical approach is solid phase peptide synthesis developed by Merrifield in 1963 [252] and specially, the "divide-coupling-recombined" (also known as "split and mix" or "portion-mixing" technique) [253–255] to synthesize a one-bead-one-compound (OBOC) library is the better approach. This methodology, using Fmoc/tBu strategy, allows the synthesis of tens of thousands to millions peptides over resin beads (solid phase). First, the resin is divided into so many vessels as different amino acids are wanted to be in the first position, then those amino acids are coupled to the resin, finally the vessels are combined and separated again so many times, as long peptide sequences are [253, 256, 257]. Once the library is finished, and with a previous step of conditioning, it can be submitted to an incubate step, putting together the library with the target protein. The protein has to be complex with a label, for example, a fluorescent tag to perform a screening [258]. Those beads with fluorescence are isolated manually or by flow cytometry equipment and their peptide sequences determined using soft mass spectrometry techniques like electrospray ionization (ESI) and matrix-assisted laser desorption ionization (MALDI) mass spectrometry (MS) [259]. The sequence can be identified by peptide fragmentation using tandem mass spectrometry (MS/MS) [258, 260]. Also, to improve OBOC library screening, in the last years various strategies have been developed to avoid the selection of false positive beads and to obtain selective ligands [261–265]. In this way, combinatorial libraries have been widely used to find ligands with pharmacological and analytical uses, and to purify or detect proteins in complex mixtures [250, 266].

2.6.2 Applications and Market for Peptides-Based Drugs

Peptide-drugs possess high specificity, affinity, ability to stay in target areas longer due to their size, and ability to be easily degraded. In the last three years, several peptide-based drugs have been approved [267]: 1) bremelanotide, a cyclic heptapeptide developed from a peptide hormone (melanotan II) has been applied to treat female Hypoactive Sexual Desire Disorder [268]; semaglutide an anti-diabetic drug is a 94 % analogue of human glucagon-like peptide-1 [269]; afamelanotide a synthetic analogue of α-melanocyte stimulating hormone, is used to prevent sun damage in persons with erythropoietic protoporphyria disease [270]; octreotide an octapeptide that mimics natural somatostatin is used, for example, in acromegaly disorder and voclosporin is an analogue of the ciclosporin, and it is used in lupus nephritis [271].

Many natural peptides have been used as potential drugs thanks to their antimicrobial properties. Some of these properties are: 1) a broad spectrum of activity, 2) multi-hit, non-specific and rapid mode of action, 3) potential immunomodulatory properties, and 4) synergistic interactions with conventional antibiotics [272]. All these properties make peptides the principal candidates for the pharmaceutical industry. Some of them have unique structures. For example, macrocyclic θ-defensins are the only known ribosomally synthesized cyclic peptides in mammals and are distinguished by their unique immunomodulating properties [273, 274]. Cyclic peptides constitute a class of compounds used in the treatment of certain diseases. Examples of cyclic peptides with pharmacological activity are: a) insulin, for diabetic disease treatment; b) cyclosporine, a natural product used as an immunosuppressant medication; and c) gramicidin, which has strong antibiotic activity [275]. Many other peptides have been successfully approved as efficient drugs, and currently, nisin, polymyxins, daptomycin, and melittin are in clinical use as alternatives to antibiotics because of their antimicrobial potency [272, 276]. In 2010 alone, there were between 500 and 600 peptides in preclinical phases [277]. Today, more than 60 peptide drugs have reached the market and several hundreds of novel therapeutic peptides are in preclinical and clinical development [278]. Oncology, with 5 drugs, metabolism with 3 peptides, and endocrinology with 2 are currently the most frequent medical indications for peptide drugs [5]. Europe and North America are the leading regions in the global AMP market. The European AMP market was valued USD 0.39 billion in 2016, and the European Union announced that will invest USD 1.7 billion to develop AMP drugs to tackle drug-resistant bacteria [279]. The results from pre-clinical studies using AMPs revealed that they could be used for the prevention and treatment of various clinical conditions. Based on promising preclinical results, numerous AMPs have been investigated in human clinical trials to demonstrate efficacy and safety [272]. The activity of AMPs can be divided into different categories that can be summarized as antibacterial, antiviral, antifungal, antiparasitic, and anti-tumor peptides [236].

More than 3,000 AMPs have been discovered, 7 of these peptides (gramicidin, daptomycin, colistin, vancomycin, oritavancin, dalbavancin, and telavancin) have been approved by the U.S. FDA and utilized for topical medications [280]. These peptides, together with bacitracin, polymyxin B, and teicoplanin, are today commercially available [53, 281]. After the discovery of nisin, naturally produced by *Lactococcus lactis*, several other AMPs such as gramicidin, tyrocidine, alamethicin, purothionin, and defensins were isolated from bacteria, fungi, plants, invertebrates and vertebrates [282, 283].

Another approach is targeting protein–protein interactions (PPIs) as a new strategy for the development of new drugs. In the past few decades, the modulation of PPIs has been recognized as one of the most challenging drug discovery tasks. In recent years, some PPIs modulators have entered clinical studies, some of which have been approved for marketing [18].

2.6.3 Challenges to Become a Peptide Into a Drug

Peptide-drugs have high specificity, high affinity (both characteristic are advantageous over drug based on small organic molecules), low molecular weight (making them better than proteins and antibodies), they are safe and well tolerated, less immunogenic and they may retain physicochemical properties from their template proteins, when they have been designed from them [18, 31, 272]. For all these reasons, they are the principal candidates for the pharmaceutical industry. Once a peptide has been selected for further development as drug, it needs to be produced in large quantities with consistent quality. A variety of technologies such as chemical synthesis, recombinant DNA technologies, cell-free expression systems (*in vitro* translation) and transgenic plants or animals have been adopted for this purpose. The majority of peptide pharmaceuticals are produced in high volumes using solution phase chemistry which is preferably employed for small to medium-sized peptides.

There are many challenges in effective drug production using peptides, which physicochemical properties can generate poor oral bioavailability [284, 285]. Peptides have great potential as therapeutics. However, the major problem encountered with the use of peptide drugs is related to its absorption after oral intake and its bioavailability. Oral peptide bioavailability is limited by degradation in the gastrointestinal tract as well as their inability to cross the epithelial barrier. To solve this problem, one structural strategy is cyclization. PEGylation is other option for some peptides not amenable to cyclization [31, 286]. Other methods to increase oral peptide bioavailability are the coadministration with enzyme inhibitors, or the use of absorption enhancers. Examples of absorption enhancers are chitosan, medium-chain fatty acids, lectins, and some toxins [286]. Coadministration of cell-penetrating peptides with therapeutic peptides has also been attempted in order to increase absorption [287]. Many drug carrier systems are currently being developed in an attempt to increase the oral bioavailability of peptide drugs, for example, hydrophilic mucoadhesive polymers [288], nanoemulsions [289], hydrogels [290], liposome systems [291], and nanoparticles [292]. In transdermal administration, small and highly hydrophobic peptides have been successfully delivered. Large and potentially hydrophilic peptides require some type of physical and/or chemical enhancement. Conventional enhancements in transdermal delivery generally aim to bypass the main physical barrier [293, 294].

Due to their hydrophilicity, peptides exhibit limited ability to cross physiological barriers. Aside from the classic subcutaneous, intramuscular and intravenous administration, alternative routes have been developed as nasal or pulmonary new technological approaches for enhanced peptide-based drug delivery. They also present a short half-life and lower potency than antibodies [31, 33, 286, 295]. A number of excipients protect the peptide against peptidases and facilitate its paracellular uptake through the intestinal wall into the systemic circulation [285].

Some strategies to increase peptide stability are to modify enzymatic cleavage sites such as acetylating the N-terminal or amidating the C-terminal, replacing L-amino acids by D-amino acids, unnatural ones or other organic structures (like lipids), cyclizing them, etc. [272, 283, 296–298]. Muttenthaler *et al.* summarize in their review more and very interesting strategies to enhance peptides stability [283]. Several strategies to make peptides better drugs exist, for example selecting from a known peptide the sequences with better antimicrobial and less hemolytic activity; to develop peptides that can target specifically a given microorganism; improve the delivery system; combinate peptides with other drugs; change the contra-ion or introduce chemical modifications to improve their performance as drugs; among others [31, 272]. Due to the increasing number of antibiotic resistant bacteria, there has been a renewed interest in peptides and proteins as a potential alternative to conventional antibiotics [399].

2.6.4 Improving Peptide Drug Development Using Machine Learning Techniques

However, challenges during the process in which a peptide turns into a drug appears. Drug discovery is a cost and time-intensive process that is often assisted by computational methods, such as virtual screening, to speed up and guide the design of new compounds. Recently, thanks to the rise of novel technologies, machine learning methods have been successfully applied in the context of computer-aided drug discovery [300].

Computational techniques have been a useful alternative to solve these problems. Different computational methods have improved the screening to find the best candidates for new drugs. Virtual screening and molecular docking had been used to reduce time and cost during drug design. For example, Pant *et al.* used all of the above and PDB (Table 2.3), FDA approved or under clinical trial drugs, ZINC and CHEMBL databases to evaluate peptides and small molecule inhibitors against SARS-CoV-2 [301]. But they also bring some inaccuracy and inefficiency making the search for new techniques needed [11, 302]. Another approach is to discover a new generation of peptides from non-natural sources focused on computational design by screening libraries. Significant advances in peptide computational design have been developed in the last years [273]. Some free online servers have been created to, for example, predict and characterize synthetic AMPs [303, 304]. By using those servers, it is possible to prospect for synthetic AMPs from any protein sequence. Then, employing some criteria from natural AMPs/proteins, those servers can predict sequences with antimicrobial potential [305]. The interest in machine learning techniques (MLT) application for drug design have been growing in the last decades. It was first used for the development of small molecule drugs, but it is increasingly being applied in the development of peptide-based drugs, although more slowly given the difficulties of using molecules with more complex chemical structures as a model [39]. That requires the use of hybrid techniques for peptide-based drugs. Nowadays, an increasing number of studies in medical chemistry employs these techniques. The models obtained from MLT can be used in virtual screening studies as well as filters to develop and discover new chemicals. An important challenge in the drug design field is the prediction of pharmacokinetic and toxicity properties. This challenge can be easily resolved with MLT models [306, 307]. Machine learning models normally used to find peptides with certain activity are random forest (RF), support vector machine (SVM), deep-learning, artificial neural network (ANN), among others. Capecchi and Raymond propose that MLT can be used mainly to predict properties of peptides or to design peptides *de novo*. For the first task supervised MLT is used and peptide sequence, spatial distribution, and structure, among others, can be used as input information. In response, the ML will provide information on whether it complies with the evaluated parameter. To be efficient, the data entered must be curated and the use of two datasets, one positive and the other negative for training the system is recommended. The goal of the second task is to train the system to return peptide sequences with a given characteristic as output [308, 309].

It has been proposed to use SVM to evaluate the solubility of a peptide based on the solubility of a motif exhibiting the peptide sequence or its hydrophobicity/hydrophilicity and its secondary structure [310, 311].

Narayanan *et al.* in their review explained that MLT can replace molecular dynamics in peptide-based drug design and can be applied on peptides rationally designed, directed evolution or de novo designed to find peptides to be used as drugs. They gave some examples on antimicrobial peptides and cell-penetrating peptides to be used in drug delivery and had been designed using MLT [39]. Giguère *et al.* proposed an algorithm-based ML and string kernel methods to evaluate peptide bioactivity to be used as drugs and validated their results against *in vitro* finding new AMPs [312]. Also, IBM company (https://research.ibm.com/blog/ai-finds-new-peptides) has interest in the use of ML to find better AMP drugs. They joined Das group to design a deep learning to generate new antimicrobial therapeutic peptides with good broad-spectrum potency and low toxicity. In just over 45 days, they managed to obtain 2 peptides with great potency against $gram^{+}$ and $gram^{-}$ bacteria with low toxicity [313]. Also, Khosravia *et al.* used ML models to predict AMPs but they used SVM and contrasted their finding using *in vitro* experiments with good results [314]. Plisson *et al.* developed a ML QSAR/QSPR approach to evaluate hemolytic activity of AMP. Most AMPs are also hemolytic, reducing the possibility of administering them only topically. Their ML model allowed them to quickly and efficiently determine if an AMP is also hemolytic *in silico*, saving time and in turn allowing them to design new peptides taking these findings into account [315]. Van oort *et al.* used a generative adversarial network (GAN) as ML model and were able to generate new AMP sequences different from the peptide dataset but maintain key features of AMPs [316]. In GAN ML two neural networks compete one against the other, one producing new examples, while the other determining whether or not they belong to that classification. Casey *et al.* developed new anti-diabetic short peptides (less than 16 amino acids) with the possibility to replace hormone or longer peptides with good safety performance using graph-based techniques [317]. Puentes *et al.* explained that the better tool to discover new AMP is probably deep learning because they do not only learn from manually entered models but also from features they discover. Furthermore, if additional properties are known, they allow them to be entered to improve performance. Other machine learning tools depend so much on manually entered information that they hardly propose a structure that differs from those already known that act as antimicrobial peptides [299]. Yan *et al.* designed Deep-AmPEP30 by using deep convolutional neural network models to evaluate peptide candidates as AMPs [318]. Thomas *et al.* used SVMs, random forest (RF), and discriminant analysis (DA) based on its dataset CAMP (Table 2.3) to predict AMPs [319]. Müller *et al.* used Recurrent Neural Network Model to first predict and then design cationic peptides forming amphipathic helices with AMP activity because of its ability to cross bacterial membranes [320]. For more examples, Basith *et al.* in their review describe very broadly and systematically the different ways in which ML can be used to determine the therapeutic possibilities of a peptide. They also describe how to avoid reaching bad results: the dataset used to train the ML model has to be adequate and curated, with high quality and quantity; it has to be balanced. Overfitting or underfitting the training data can lead to the development of a biased model [321].

In some diseases the endogenous interaction between proteins must be blocked by a drug to exert a pharmacological action. Peptides are both rigid and flexible structures, whereas small organic molecules are only rigid. They are also smaller than proteins like antibodies and can be designed to cross membranes. Peptides can interfere with such association with high affinity and specificity. All this proposes them as ideal candidates. Peptides with the possibility to interfere with protein-protein interaction can be used in cancer therapy: antimicrobial peptides (because they can produce pores in cell-membranes), cell-permeable peptides (CPPs) (can be used to cargo other drug or peptide inside the cells) and tumor-targeting peptides (TTPs) (its target is a receptor in the tumor-cell) [322]. Both flexible-docking tools and ML contribute to understanding and designing peptides to reach this goal [323]. Taherzadeh *et al.* used the RF ML model called SPRINT-Str to predict protein-peptide interaction and binding sites with similar prediction performance than experimentally approaches [324]. Obarska-Kosinska *et al.* designed PepComposer based on Monte Carlo model but, sadly, currently its web servers are down (http://biocomputing.it/pepcomposer/webserver and https://cassandra.med.uniroma1.it/pepcomposer/webserver/pepcomposer.php) [323, 325].

Furthermore, ML has been used to predict CPPs. CPPs are peptides with the possibility of crossing the plasma membrane, a characteristic that makes them interesting when designing peptide drugs. As mentioned above, some of the drawbacks of using peptides as drugs are their inability to be administered orally and their low ability to cross membranes, which would not be a drawback in these cases. Holton *et al.* used neural networks [326] and Wei *et al.* used RF ML models to predict CPPs [327]. Also, Sanders *et al.* used

SVM with a balanced dataset with positive and negative examples to find new CPPs. One hundred percent of the CPP predicted by its model showed good performance when it was experimentally evaluated [328]. Manavalan *et al.* used both SVM and RF to predict TTPS [329].

On the other hand, the use of publicly available bioinformatics tools on the Internet is helping to quickly identify amino acid sequences for different disease treatments, including COVID-19 [330–333], making the study of sequences easier for new diagnosis assays or as potential vaccines. Different developments to produce SARS-CoV-2 vaccines are based on computing and bioinformatics platforms [334]. Computational approaches have been used for the production of vaccines by the identification of B and T cell epitopes [335, 336], the prediction of continuous epitopes [337], discontinuous epitopes [338], and also the design of *in silico* peptide vaccines [339]. In this way, ML and AI are essential tools for the screening, prediction and forecast of new drugs and vaccines [340]. New computational models in ML are continuously developing to overcome the limitations traditional techniques could have in vaccine development. Immunoinformatic approaches are more beneficial, and thus modern technologies such as ML and AI are more in demand to develop the potential new vaccine candidates [341–345].

Ashkenazy *et al.* used *Motifier* to study epitopes (peptides)-monoclonal antibodies (mAbs) recognition, a computational tool able to study peptide libraries to find the better match for a given mAb based on RF [342]. Liu *et al.* used combinatorial MLT to evaluate and optimize anti-SARS CoV-2 peptide-based vaccines: OptiVax and EvalVax, previously designed by MIT - Massachusetts Institute of Technology [343]. OptiVax uses MLT to score peptide ability to elicit an immune response and they are then selected to maximize population coverage. Instead, EvalVax analyzed genetic variation across the population [346]. Yang *et al.* develop a new multi-epitope *in silico* vaccine designer: DeepVacPred based on a DNN architecture. The input data are peptide sequences and the system can predict if it is a good subunit candidate for a multi-epitope vaccine development [345]. Also, Yazdani *et al.* designed a multi-epitope vaccine against SARS-CoV-2 based on MLT. They used SVM and multilayer perceptron to screen potential epitope candidates [347].

2.7 Conclusions

Throughout this chapter, the need to search for more efficient alternatives when designing and developing less expensive and more efficient drugs has been evidenced. Different classical tools used for drug design have been listed and how they can be combined with ML tools to accelerate their performance. The urgency for the discovery of new and more effective drugs has motivated the entire world to found new strategies and methodologies. Faster and avoiding or reducing time-consuming wet lab experiments currently are giving results, as previously mentioned. Also, computational tools like docking and molecular dynamics provide information to MLT, and new result achievement can feed classical tools too.

The use of MLT has increased in the last decades and this indicates a tendency in the chemistry field. As the world increasingly moves into an age of large medical datasets, from clinical studies to massive cell line-omics databases, there is clearly an opportunity for application of ML to biology. For this reason, the ML models, methods, predictions and applications described in this chapter demonstrated their important contribution to medicine. However, it is important to mention that ML is imperfect. Experimental and computational methods working together could change the rules in drug discovery.

We have focused on the implementation of MLT for the study of drug-target interaction, but ML tools are being implemented in other aspects of the design and manufacture of classic or biosimilar drugs. MLT had been used to improve biosimilars fermentation process and formulation. Also, with aim to improve and accelerate clinical diagnosis. Clearly, this is only the first step in a long run that only the future will disclose.

References

1. Réda, C., Kaufmann, E., Delahaye-Duriez, A., Machine learning applications in drug development. *Comput. Struct. Biotechnol. J.*, 18, 241, 2020.
2. Van Norman, G.A., Drugs, Devices, and the FDA: Part 1: An overview of approval processes for drugs. *JACC Basic Transl. Sci.*, 1, 170, 2016.
3. Voss, L., Guttek, K., Reddig, A., Reinhold, A., Voss, M., Schraven, B., Reinhold, D., Screening of FDA-approved drug library identifies adefovir dipivoxil as highly potent inhibitor of T cell proliferation. *Front. Immunol.*, 11, 616570, 2020.
4. Ng, Y.L., Salim, C.K., Chu, J.J.H., Drug repurposing for COVID-19: Approaches, challenges and promising candidates. *Pharmacol. Ther.*, 228, 107930, 2021.
5. de la Torre, B.G. and Albericio, F., Peptide therapeutics 2.0. *Molecules*, 25, 2293, 2020.

6. Wouters, O.J., McKee, M., Luyten, J., Estimated research and development investment needed to bring a new medicine to market, 2009-2018. *JAMA*, 323, 844, 2020.
7. Won, J.-H. and Lee, H., Can the COVID-19 pandemic disrupt the current drug development practices? *Int. J. Mol. Sci.*, 22, 5457, 2021.
8. Karki, N., Verma, N., Trozzi, F., Tao, P., Kraka, E., Zoltowski, B., Predicting potential SARS-COV-2 drugs-in depth drug database screening using deep neural network framework SSnet, classical virtual screening and docking. *Int. J. Mol. Sci.*, 22, 1573, 2021.
9. Rifaioglu, A.S., Cetin Atalay, R., Cansen Kahraman, D., Doğan, T., Martin, M., Atalay, V., MDeePred: Novel multi-channel protein featurization for deep learning-based binding affinity prediction in drug discovery. *Bioinformatics*, 37, 693, 2021.
10. Winkler, D.A., Use of artificial intelligence and machine learning for discovery of drugs for neglected tropical diseases. *Front. Chem.*, 9, 614073, 2021.
11. Gupta, R., Srivastava, D., Sahu, M., Tiwari, S., Ambasta, R.K., Kumar, P., Artificial intelligence to deep learning: Machine intelligence approach for drug discovery. *Mol. Divers.*, 25, 1315, 2021.
12. Vamathevan, J., Clark, D., Czodrowski, P., Dunham, I., Ferran, E., Lee, G., Li, B., Madabhushi, A., Shah, P., Spitzer, M., Zhao, S., Applications of machine learning in drug discovery and development. *Nat. Rev. Drug Discovery*, 18, 463, 2019.
13. Mak, K.-K. and Pichika, M.R., Artificial intelligence in drug development: Present status and future prospects. *Drug Discovery Today*, 24, 773, 2019.
14. Jones, D., Kim, H., Zhang, X., Zemla, A., Stevenson, G., Bennett, W.F.D., Kirshner, D., Wong, S.E., Lightstone, F.C., Allen, J.E., Improved protein-ligand binding affinity prediction with structure-based deep fusion inference. *J. Chem. Inf. Model.*, 61, 1583, 2021.
15. Hu, F., Jiang, J., Wang, D., Zhu, M., Yin, P., Multi-PLI: Interpretable multi-task deep learning model for unifying protein-ligand interaction datasets. *J. Cheminform.*, 13, 30, 2021.
16. Verma, N., Qu, X., Trozzi, F., Elsaied, M., Karki, N., Tao, Y., Zoltowski, B., Larson, E.C., Kraka, E., SSnet: A deep learning approach for protein-ligand interaction prediction. *Int. J. Mol. Sci.*, 22, 1392, 2021.
17. Fang, Y.-M., Lin, D.-Q., Yao, S.-J., Review on biomimetic affinity chromatography with short peptide ligands and its application to protein purification. *J. Chromatogr. A*, 1571, 1, 2018.
18. Lu, H., Zhou, Q., He, J., Jiang, Z., Peng, C., Tong, R., Shi, J., Recent advances in the development of protein-protein interactions modulators: Mechanisms and clinical trials. *Signal Transduct Target Ther.*, 5, 213, 2020.
19. Salmaso, V. and Moro, S., Bridging molecular docking to molecular dynamics in exploring ligand-protein recognition process: An overview. *Front. Pharmacol.*, 9, 923, 2018.

20. Siebenmorgen, T. and Zacharias, M., Computational prediction of protein-protein binding affinities. *WIREs Comput. Mol. Sci.*, 10, e1448, 2020.
21. Tomasella, C., Floris, M., Guccione, S., Pappalardo, M., Basile, L., Peptidomimetics *in silico. Mol. Inform.*, 40, 2000087, 2021.
22. Zhao, J., Cao, Y., Zhang, L., Exploring the computational methods for protein-ligand binding site prediction. *Comput. Struct. Biotechnol. J.*, 18, 417, 2020.
23. Whitfield, T.W., Ragland, D.A., Zeldovich, K.B., Schiffer, C.A., Characterizing protein-ligand binding using atomistic simulation and machine learning: Application to drug resistance in HIV-1 protease. *J. Chem. Theory Comput.*, 16, 1284, 2020.
24. Yang, J., Shen, C., Huang, N., Predicting or pretending: artificial intelligence for protein-ligand interactions lack of sufficiently large and unbiased datasets. *Front. Pharmacol.*, 11, 69, 2020.
25. Raschka, S. and Kaufman, B., Machine learning and AI-based approaches for bioactive ligand discovery and GPCR-ligand recognition. *Methods*, 180, 89, 2020.
26. Center for drug evaluation, research, transcript: definition of a drug, 2017. https://www.fda.gov/drugs/information-health-care-professionals-drugs/transcript-definition-drug-april-2017.
27. Macielag, M.J., Chemical properties of antimicrobials and their uniqueness, in: *Antibiotic discovery and development*, T.J. Dougherty and M.J. Pucci (Eds.), pp. 793–820, Springer US, Boston, MA, 2012.
28. Veber, D.F., Johnson, S.R., Cheng, H.-Y., Smith, B.R., Ward, K.W., Kopple, K.D., Molecular properties that influence the oral bioavailability of drug candidates. *J. Med. Chem.*, 45, 2615, 2002.
29. Samanen, J., Chapter 5 - Similarities and differences in the discovery and use of biopharmaceuticals and small-molecule chemotherapeutics, in: *Introduction to biological and small molecule drug research and development*, R. Ganellin, S. Roberts, R. Jefferis (Eds.), pp. 161–203, Elsevier, Oxford, 2013.
30. Craik, D.J., Fairlie, D.P., Liras, S., Price, D., The future of peptide-based drugs. *Chem. Biol. Drug Des.*, 81, 136, 2013.
31. Sachdeva, S., Peptides as "drugs": The journey so far. *Int. J. Pept. Res. Ther.*, 23, 49, 2017.
32. De, A., *Application of peptide-based prodrug chemistry in drug development*, pp. 1–60, Springer, New York, 2012.
33. Lau, J.L. and Dunn, M.K., Therapeutic peptides: Historical perspectives, current development trends, and future directions. *Bioorg. Med. Chem.*, 26, 2700, 2018.
34. Makarova, O., Rodríguez-Rojas, A., Eravci, M., Weise, C., Dobson, A., Johnston, P., Rolff, J., Antimicrobial defence and persistent infection in insects revisited. *Philos. Trans. R. Soc Lond. B Biol. Sci.*, 371, 20150296, 2016.
35. Xu, X. and Lai, R., The chemistry and biological activities of peptides from amphibian skin secretions. *Chem. Rev.*, 115, 1760, 2015.

36. Romero, S.M., Cardillo, A.B., Martínez Ceron, M.C., Camperi, S.A., Giudicessi, S.L., Temporins: an approach of potential pharmaceutic candidates. *Surg. Infect.*, 21, 309, 2020.
37. Craik, D.J. and Kan, M.-W., How can we improve peptide drug discovery? Learning from the past. *Expert Opin. Drug Discovery*, 4, 1, 2021.
38. Fosgerau, K. and Hoffmann, T., Peptide therapeutics: Current status and future directions. *Drug Discovery Today*, 20, 122, 2015.
39. Narayanan, H., Dingfelder, F., Butté, A., Lorenzen, N., Sokolov, M., Arosio, P., Machine learning for biologics: Opportunities for protein engineering, developability, and formulation. *Trends Pharmacol. Sci.*, 42, 151, 2021.
40. Joosten, R.P., Te Beek, T.A.H., Krieger, E., Hekkelman, M.L., Hooft, R.W.W., Schneider, R., Sander, C., Vriend, G., A series of PDB related databases for everyday needs. *Nucleic Acids Res.*, 39, D411, 2011.
41. Wishart, D.S., Feunang, Y.D., Guo, A.C., Lo, E.J., Marcu, A., Grant, J.R., Sajed, T., Johnson, D., Li, C., Sayeeda, Z., Assempour, N., Iynkkaran, I., Liu, Y., Maciejewski, A., Gale, N., Wilson, A., Chin, L., Cummings, R., Le, D., Pon, A., Knox, C., Wilson, M., DrugBank 5.0: a major update to the DrugBank database for 2018. *Nucleic Acids Res.*, 46, D1074, 2018.
42. Chang, A., Jeske, L., Ulbrich, S., Hofmann, J., Koblitz, J., Schomburg, I., Neumann-Schaal, M., Jahn, D., Schomburg, D., BRENDA, the ELIXIR core data resource in 2021: new developments and updates. *Nucleic Acids Res.*, 49, D498, 2021.
43. Mendez, D., Gaulton, A., Bento, A.P., Chambers, J., De Veij, M., Félix, E., Magariños, M.P., Mosquera, J.F., Mutowo, P., Nowotka, M., Gordillo-Marañón, M., Hunter, F., Junco, L., Mugumbate, G., Rodriguez-Lopez, M., Atkinson, F., Bosc, N., Radoux, C.J., Segura-Cabrera, A., Hersey, A., Leach, A.R., ChEMBL: Towards direct deposition of bioassay data. *Nucleic Acids Res.*, 47, D930, 2019.
44. Chen, X., Lin, Y., Gilson, M.K., The binding database: Overview and user's guide. *Biopolymers*, 61, 127, 2001.
45. Wang, R., Fang, X., Lu, Y., Yang, C.-Y., Wang, S., The PDBbind database: Methodologies and updates. *J. Med. Chem.*, 48, 4111, 2005.
46. Wen, Z., He, J., Tao, H., Huang, S.-Y., PepBDB: A comprehensive structural database of biological peptide-protein interactions. *Bioinformatics*, 35, 175, 2019.
47. Martins, P.M., Santos, L.H., Mariano, D., Queiroz, F.C., Bastos, L.L., Gomes, I., de, S., Fischer, P.H.C., Rocha, R.E.O., Silveira, S.A., de Lima, L.H.F., de Magalhães, M.T.Q., Oliveira, M.G.A., de Melo-Minardi, R.C., Propedia: A database for protein-peptide identification based on a hybrid clustering algorithm. *BMC Bioinf.*, 22, 1, 2021.
48. Laskowski, R.A., Jabłońska, J., Pravda, L., Vařeková, R.S., Thornton, J.M., PDBsum: Structural summaries of PDB entries. *Protein Sci.*, 27, 129, 2018.
49. Teyra, J., Kelil, A., Jain, S., Helmy, M., Jajodia, R., Hooda, Y., Gu, J., D'Cruz, A.A., Nicholson, S.E., Min, J., Sudol, M., Kim, P.M., Bader, G.D., Sidhu, S.S.,

Large-scale survey and database of high affinity ligands for peptide recognition modules. *Mol. Syst. Biol.*, 16, e9310, 2020.
50. Kardani, K. and Bolhassani, A., Cppsite 2.0: an available database of experimentally validated cell-penetrating peptides predicting their secondary and tertiary structures. *J. Mol. Biol.*, 433, 166703, 2021.
51. Waghu, F.H., Barai, R.S., Gurung, P., Idicula-Thomas, S., CAMPR3: A database on sequences, structures and signatures of antimicrobial peptides. *Nucleic Acids Res.*, 44, D1094, 2016.
52. Usmani, S.S., Bedi, G., Samuel, J.S., Singh, S., Kalra, S., Kumar, P., Ahuja, A.A., Sharma, M., Gautam, A., Raghava, G.P.S., THPdb: Database of FDA-approved peptide and protein therapeutics. *PloS One*, 12, e0181748, 2017.
53. D'Aloisio, V., Dognini, P., Hutcheon, G.A., Coxon, C.R., PepTherDia: Database and structural composition analysis of approved peptide therapeutics and diagnostics. *Drug Discovery Today*, 26, 1409, 2021.
54. Hammami, R., Zouhir, A., Le Lay, C., Ben Hamida, J., Fliss, I., BACTIBASE second release: A database and tool platform for bacteriocin characterization. *BMC Microbiol.*, 10, 22, 2010.
55. Zhao, X., Wu, H., Lu, H., Li, G., Huang, Q., LAMP: A database linking antimicrobial peptides. *PloS One*, 8, e66557, 2013.
56. Pirtskhalava, M., Gabrielian, A., Cruz, P., Griggs, H.L., Squires, R.B., Hurt, D.E., Grigolava, M., Chubinidze, M., Gogoladze, G., Vishnepolsky, B., Alekseyev, V., Rosenthal, A., Tartakovsky, M., DBAASP v.2: An enhanced database of structure and antimicrobial/cytotoxic activity of natural and synthetic peptides. *Nucleic Acids Res.*, 44, D1104, 2016.
57. Zhao, Z., Peng, Z., Yang, J., Improving sequence-based prediction of protein-peptide binding residues by introducing intrinsic disorder and a consensus method. *J. Chem. Inf. Model.*, 58, 1459, 2018.
58. Zaidman, D. and Wolfson, H.J., PinaColada: Peptide-inhibitor ant colony ad-hoc design algorithm. *Bioinformatics*, 32, 2289, 2016.
59. Chaudhary, A., Bhalla, S., Patiyal, S., Raghava, G.P.S., Sahni, G., FermFooDb: A database of bioactive peptides derived from fermented foods. *Heliyon*, 7, e06668, 2021.
60. Kumar, R., Chaudhary, K., Sharma, M., Nagpal, G., Chauhan, J.S., Singh, S., Gautam, A., Raghava, G.P.S., AHTPDB: A comprehensive platform for analysis and presentation of antihypertensive peptides. *Nucleic Acids Res.*, 43, D956, 2015.
61. Panyayai, T., Ngamphiw, C., Tongsima, S., Mhuantong, W., Limsripraphan, W., Choowongkomon, K., Sawatdichaikul, O., FeptideDB: A web application for new bioactive peptides from food protein. *Heliyon*, 5, e02076, 2019.
62. Nielsen, S.D., Beverly, R.L., Qu, Y., Dallas, D.C., Milk bioactive peptide database: A comprehensive database of milk protein-derived bioactive peptides and novel visualization. *Food Chem.*, 232, 673, 2017.
63. Wang, J., Yin, T., Xiao, X., He, D., Xue, Z., Jiang, X., Wang, Y., StraPep: A structure database of bioactive peptides. *Database*, 2018 bay038, 2018.

64. Das, D., Jaiswal, M., Khan, F.N., Ahamad, S., Kumar, S., PlantPepDB: A manually curated plant peptide database. *Sci. Rep.*, 10, 2194, 2020.
65. Kunz, M., Liang, C., Nilla, S., Cecil, A., Dandekar, T., The drug-minded protein interaction database (DrumPID) for efficient target analysis and drug development. *Database*, 2016, baw041, 2016.
66. Wang, C., Hu, G., Wang, K., Brylinski, M., Xie, L., Kurgan, L., PDID: Database of molecular-level putative protein-drug interactions in the structural human proteome. *Bioinformatics*, 32, 579, 2016.
67. Chollet, F., *Deep learning with python*, pp. 1–384, Manning Publications, Shelter Island, NY, 2017.
68. Cortes, C. and Vapnik, V., Support-vector networks. *Mach. Learn.*, 20, 273, 1995.
69. Vapnik, V.N., An overview of statistical learning theory. *IEEE Trans. Neural Netw.*, 10, 988, 1999.
70. Brereton, R.G. and Lloyd, G.R., Support vector machines for classification and regression. *Analyst.*, 135, 230, 2010.
71. Breiman, L., Random forests. *Mach. Learn.*, 45, 5, 2001.
72. Friedman, J.H., Greedy function approximation: A gradient boosting machine. *Ann. Stat.*, 29, 1189, 2001.
73. Friedman, J.H., Stochastic Gradient Boosting. *Comput. Stat. Data Anal.*, 38, 367, 1999.
74. Mason, L., Baxter, J., Bartlett, P., Frean, M., Boosting algorithms as gradient descent, in: *Proceedings of the 12th international conference on neural information processing systems*, MIT Press, Cambridge, MA, USA, pp. 512–518, 1999.
75. Fix, E. and Hodges, J.L., Discriminatory analysis, nonparametric discrimination: consistency properties, in: *USAF school of aviation medicine*, vol. 4, Randolph Field, Texas, Tech. Report, 1951.
76. Cover, T. and Hart, P., Nearest neighbor pattern classification. *IEEE Trans. Inf. Theory*, 13, 21, 1967.
77. Altman, N.S., An introduction to kernel and nearest-neighbor nonparametric regression. *Am. Stat.*, 46, 175, 1992.
78. Rumelhart, D.E., Hinton, G.E., Williams, R.J., Learning representations by back-propagating errors. *Nature*, 323, 533, 1986.
79. Rasmussen, C.E. and Williams, C.K.I., *Gaussian processes for machine learning*, pp. 2–266, MIT Press, Cambridge, MA, 2006.
80. Seeger, M., Gaussian processes for machine learning. *Int. J. Neural Syst.*, 14, 69, 2004.
81. Pearson, K., Notes on regression and inheritance in the case of two parents. *Proc. R. Soc. Lond.*, 58, 240, 1895.
82. Draper, N.R. and Smith, H., *Applied regression analysis*, pp. 1–736, John Wiley & Sons, Hoboken, New Jersey, USA, 1998.

83. Roche, D.B., Tetchner, S.J., McGuffin, L.J., The binding site distance test score: A robust method for the assessment of predicted protein binding sites. *Bioinformatics*, 26, 2920, 2010.
84. Levinthal, C., Wodak, S.J., Kahn, P., Dadivanian, A.K., Hemoglobin interaction in sickle cell fibers. I: Theoretical approaches to the molecular contacts. *Proc. Natl. Acad. Sci.U. S. A.*, 72, 1330, 1975.
85. Fischer, E., Einfluss der Configuration auf die Wirkung der Enzyme. *Ber. Dtsch. Chem. Ges.*, 27, 2985, 1894.
86. Goodford, P.J., A computational procedure for determining energetically favorable binding sites on biologically important macromolecules. *J. Med. Chem.*, 28, 849, 1985.
87. Ho, C.M. and Marshall, G.R., Cavity search: An algorithm for the isolation and display of cavity-like binding regions. *J. Comput. Aided Mol. Des.*, 4, 337, 1990.
88. Lee, B. and Richards, F.M., The interpretation of protein structures: Estimation of static accessibility. *J. Mol. Biol.*, 55, 379, 1971.
89. Shrake, A. and Rupley, J.A., Environment and exposure to solvent of protein atoms. Lysozyme and insulin. *J. Mol. Biol.*, 79, 351, 1973.
90. Connolly, M.L., Analytical molecular surface calculation. *J. Appl. Crystallogr.*, 16, 548, 1983.
91. Connolly, M.L., Molecular surface Triangulation. *J. Appl. Crystallogr.*, 18, 499, 1985.
92. Sanner, M.F., Olson, A.J., Spehner, J.C., Reduced surface: An efficient way to compute molecular surfaces. *Biopolymers*, 38, 305, 1996.
93. Edelsbrunner, H., Kirkpatrick, D., Seidel, R., On the shape of a set of points in the plane. *IEEE Trans. Inf. Theory*, 29, 551, 1983.
94. Edelsbrunner, H. and Mücke, E.P., Three-dimensional alpha shapes. *ACM Trans. Graph.*, 13, 43, 1994.
95. Edelsbrunner, H., Shah, N.R., Avis, D., Incremental topological flipping works for regular triangulations, in: *Proceedings of the eighth annual symposium on Computational geometry - SCG*, vol. *92*, ACM Press, New York, NY, pp. 223–241, 1992.
96. Liang, J., Edelsbrunner, H., Woodward, C., Anatomy of protein pockets and cavities: measurement of binding site geometry and implications for ligand design. *Protein Sci.*, 7, 1884, 1998.
97. Radhakrishnan, S., Kolippakkam, D., Mathura, V.S., Introduction to algorithms, in: *Bioinformatics: A concept-based introduction*, V. Mathura and P. Kangueane (Eds.), pp. 27–37, Springer US, Boston, MA, 2008.
98. Laurent, B., Chavent, M., Cragnolini, T., Dahl, A.C.E., Pasquali, S., Derreumaux, P., Sansom, M.S.P., Baaden, M., Epock: Rapid analysis of protein pocket dynamics. *Bioinformatics*, 31, 1478, 2015.
99. Petrek, M., Otyepka, M., Banás, P., Kosinová, P., Koca, J., Damborský, J., CAVER: A new tool to explore routes from protein clefts, pockets and cavities. *BMC Bioinf.*, 7, 316, 2006.

100. Barletta, G.P. and Fernandez-Alberti, S., Protein fluctuations and cavity changes relationship. *J. Chem. Theory Comput.*, 14, 998, 2018.
101. Wagner, J.R., Sørensen, J., Hensley, N., Wong, C., Zhu, C., Perison, T., Amaro, R.E., POVME 3.0: Software for mapping binding pocket flexibility. *J. Chem. Theory Comput.*, 13, 4584, 2017.
102. Petrek, M., Kosinová, P., Koca, J., Otyepka, M., MOLE: A Voronoi diagram-based explorer of molecular channels, pores, and tunnels. *Structure*, 15, 1357, 2007.
103. Coleman, R.G. and Sharp, K.A., Finding and characterizing tunnels in macromolecules with application to ion channels and pores. *Biophys. J.*, 96, 632, 2009.
104. Pellegrini-Calace, M., Maiwald, T., Thornton, J.M., PoreWalker: A novel tool for the identification and characterization of channels in transmembrane proteins from their three-dimensional structure. *PloS Comput. Biol.*, 5, e1000440, 2009.
105. Masood, T.B., Sandhya, S., Chandra, N., Natarajan, V., CHEXVIS: A tool for molecular channel extraction and visualization. *BMC Bioinf.*, 16, 119, 2015.
106. Yaffe, E., Fishelovitch, D., Wolfson, H.J., Halperin, D., Nussinov, R., MolAxis: Efficient and accurate identification of channels in macromolecules. *Proteins*, 73, 72, 2008.
107. Ho, B.K. and Gruswitz, F., HOLLOW: Generating accurate representations of channel and interior surfaces in molecular structures. *BMC Struct. Biol.*, 8, 49, 2008.
108. Smart, O.S., Neduvelil, J.G., Wang, X., Wallace, B.A., Sansom, M.S., HOLE: A program for the analysis of the pore dimensions of ion channel structural models. *J. Mol. Graph.*, 14, 354, 376, 1996.
109. Chauhan, J.S., Mishra, N.K., Raghava, G.P.S., Identification of ATP binding residues of a protein from its primary sequence. *BMC Bioinf.*, 10, 434, 2009.
110. Altschul, S.F., Madden, T.L., Schäffer, A.A., Zhang, J., Zhang, Z., Miller, W., Lipman, D.J., Gapped, BLAST, and PSI-BLAST: a new generation of protein database search programs. *Nucleic Acids Res.*, 25, 3389, 1997.
111. Jones, S. and Thornton, J.M., Principles of protein-protein interactions. *Proc. Natl. Acad. Sci. U. S. A.*, 93, 13, 1996.
112. Chen, K., Mizianty, M.J., Kurgan, L., ATPsite: Sequence-based prediction of ATP-binding residues. *Proteome Sci.*, 9, Suppl 1, 2011.
113. Chen, K., Mizianty, M.J., Kurgan, L., Prediction and analysis of nucleotide-binding residues using sequence and sequence-derived structural descriptors. *Bioinformatics*, 28, 331, 2012.
114. Yu, D.-J., Hu, J., Huang, Y., Shen, H.-B., Qi, Y., Tang, Z.-M., Yang, J.-Y., TargetATPsite: A template-free method for ATP-binding sites prediction with residue evolution image sparse representation and classifier ensemble. *J. Comput. Chem.*, 34, 974, 2013.

115. Si, J., Zhang, Z., Lin, B., Schroeder, M., Huang, B., MetaDBSite: A meta approach to improve protein DNA-binding sites prediction. *BMC Syst. Biol.*, 5, Suppl 1, 2011.
116. Panwar, B., Gupta, S., Raghava, G.P.S., Prediction of vitamin interacting residues in a vitamin binding protein using evolutionary information. *BMC Bioinf.*, 14, 44, 2013.
117. Yang, J., Roy, A., Zhang, Y., Protein-ligand binding site recognition using complementary binding-specific substructure comparison and sequence profile alignment. *Bioinformatics*, 29, 2588, 2013.
118. Brylinski, M. and Skolnick, J., A threading-based method (FINDSITE) for ligand-binding site prediction and functional annotation. *Proc. Natl. Acad. Sci. U. S. A.*, 105, 129, 2008.
119. Capra, J.A., Laskowski, R.A., Thornton, J.M., Singh, M., Funkhouser, T.A., Predicting protein ligand binding sites by combining evolutionary sequence conservation and 3D structure. *PloS Comput. Biol.*, 5, e1000585, 2009.
120. Roy, A., Yang, J., Zhang, Y., COFACTOR: an accurate comparative algorithm for structure-based protein function annotation. *Nucleic Acids Res.*, 40, W471, 2012.
121. Wu, Q., Peng, Z., Zhang, Y., Yang, J., COACH-D: Improved protein-ligand binding sites prediction with refined ligand-binding poses through molecular docking. *Nucleic Acids Res.*, 46, W438, 2018.
122. Brylinski, M. and Feinstein, W.P., eFindSite: improved prediction of ligand binding sites in protein models using meta-threading, machine learning and auxiliary ligands. *J. Comput. Aided Mol. Des.*, 27, 551, 2013.
123. Yu, D.-J., Hu, J., Yang, J., Shen, H.-B., Tang, J., Yang, J.-Y., Designing template-free predictor for targeting protein-ligand binding sites with classifier ensemble and spatial clustering. *IEEE/ACM Trans. Comput. Biol. Bioinform.*, 10, 994, 2013.
124. Freund, Y. and Schapire, R.E., A decision-theoretic generalization of on-line learning and an application to boosting. *J. Comput. System Sci.*, 55, 119, 1997.
125. Wong, G.Y., Leung, F.H.F., Ling, S.S.H., Identification of protein-ligand binding site using multi-clustering and support vector machine, in: *IECON 2016 - 42nd Annual Conference of the IEEE Industrial Electronics Society*, IEEE, Florence, It, pp. 939–944, 2016.
126. Yu, D.-J., Hu, J., Li, Q.-M., Tang, Z.-M., Yang, J.-Y., Shen, H.-B., Constructing query-driven dynamic machine learning model with application to protein-ligand binding sites prediction. *IEEE Trans. Nanobioscience*, 14, 45, 2015.
127. Chen, P., Huang, J.Z., Gao, X., LigandRFs: Random forest ensemble to identify ligand-binding residues from sequence information alone. *BMC Bioinf.*, 15, Suppl 15, 2014.
128. Schmidt, T., Haas, J., Gallo Cassarino, T., Schwede, T., Assessment of ligand-binding residue predictions in CASP9. *Proteins*, 79, 126, 2011.

129. López, G., Ezkurdia, I., Tress, M.L., Assessment of ligand binding residue predictions in CASP8. *Proteins*, 77, 138, 2009.
130. Krivák, R. and Hoksza, D., Improving protein-ligand binding site prediction accuracy by classification of inner pocket points using local features. *J. Cheminform.*, 7, 12, 2015.
131. Krivák, R. and Hoksza, D., P2Rank: Machine learning based tool for rapid and accurate prediction of ligand binding sites from protein structure. *J. Cheminform.*, 10, 39, 2018.
132. Le Guilloux, V., Schmidtke, P., Tuffery, P., Fpocket: An open source platform for ligand pocket detection. *BMC Bioinf.*, 10, 168, 2009.
133. Jiménez, J., Doerr, S., Martínez-Rosell, G., Rose, A.S., De Fabritiis, G., DeepSite: Protein-binding site predictor using 3D-convolutional neural networks. *Bioinformatics*, 33, 3036, 2017.
134. Desaphy, J., Bret, G., Rognan, D., Kellenberger, E., sc-PDB: A 3D-database of ligandable binding sites–10 years on. *Nucleic Acids Res.*, 43, D399, 2015.
135. Cui, Y., Dong, Q., Hong, D., Wang, X., Predicting protein-ligand binding residues with deep convolutional neural networks. *BMC Bioinf.*, 20, 93, 2019.
136. Xia, C.-Q., Pan, X., Shen, H.-B., Protein-ligand binding residue prediction enhancement through hybrid deep heterogeneous learning of sequence and structure data. *Bioinformatics*, 36, 3018, 2020.
137. Jumper, J., Evans, R., Pritzel, A., Green, T., Figurnov, M., Ronneberger, O., Tunyasuvunakool, K., Bates, R., Žídek, A., Potapenko, A., Bridgland, A., Meyer, C., Kohl, S.A.A., Ballard, A.J., Cowie, A., Romera-Paredes, B., Nikolov, S., Jain, R., Adler, J., Back, T., Petersen, S., Reiman, D., Clancy, E., Zielinski, M., Steinegger, M., Pacholska, M., Berghammer, T., Bodenstein, S., Silver, D., Vinyals, O., Senior, A.W., Kavukcuoglu, K., Kohli, P., Hassabis, D., Highly accurate protein structure prediction with AlphaFold. *Nature*, 596, 583, 2021.
138. Hu, J., Li, Y., Zhang, Y., Yu, D.-J., ATPbind: Accurate protein-ATP binding site prediction by combining sequence-profiling and structure-based comparisons. *J. Chem. Inf. Model.*, 58, 501, 2018.
139. Stepniewska-Dziubinska, M.M., Zielenkiewicz, P., Siedlecki, P., Improving detection of protein-ligand binding sites with 3D segmentation. *Sci. Rep.*, 10, 5035, 2020.
140. Lorber, D.M., Computational drug design. *Chem. Biol.*, 6, R227, 1999.
141. D'Souza, S., Prema, K.V., Balaji, S., Machine learning models for drug–target interactions: Current knowledge and future directions. *Drug Discovery Today*, 25, 748, 2020.
142. Ellingson, S.R., Davis, B., Allen, J., Machine learning and ligand binding predictions: A review of data, methods, and obstacles. *Biochim. Biophys. Acta - Gen. Subjects.*, 1864, 129545, 2020.
143. Kuntz, I.D., Blaney, J.M., Oatley, S.J., Langridge, R., Ferrin, T.E., A geometric approach to macromolecule-ligand interactions. *J. Mol. Biol.*, 161, 269, 1982.

144. Grosdidier, A., Zoete, V., Michielin, O., SwissDock, a protein-small molecule docking web service based on EADock DSS. *Nucleic Acids Res.*, 39, W270, 2011.
145. Guedes, I.A., Barreto, A.M.S., Marinho, D., Krempser, E., Kuenemann, M.A., Sperandio, O., Dardenne, L.E., Miteva, M.A., New machine learning and physics-based scoring functions for drug discovery. *Sci. Rep.*, 11, 3198, 2021.
146. Pierce, B.G., Wiehe, K., Hwang, H., Kim, B.-H., Vreven, T., Weng, Z., ZDOCK server: interactive docking prediction of protein-protein complexes and symmetric multimers. *Bioinformatics*, 30, 1771, 2014.
147. Schindler, C.E.M., de Vries, S.J., Zacharias, M., Fully blind peptide-protein docking with pepATTRACT. *Structure*, 23, 1507, 2015.
148. London, N., Raveh, B., Cohen, E., Fathi, G., Schueler-Furman, O., Rosetta FlexPepDock web server–high resolution modeling of peptide-protein interactions. *Nucleic Acids Res.*, 39, W249, 2011.
149. Camproux, A.C., Gautier, R., Tufféry, P., A hidden markov model derived structural alphabet for proteins. *J. Mol. Biol.*, 339, 591, 2004.
150. Han, K.-L., Zhang, X., Yang, M.-J., *Protein conformational dynamics*, pp. 1–488, Springer Science & Business Media, New York, US, 2014.
151. Remmert, M., Biegert, A., Hauser, A., Söding, J., HHblits: Lightning-fast iterative protein sequence searching by HMM-HMM alignment. *Nat. Methods*, 9, 173, 2011.
152. Moro, S., Sturlese, M., Ciancetta, A., Floris, M., Benfenati, E., pp. 23–35, Springer Linf, New York, US, 2016.
153. Huang, N., Kalyanaraman, C., Bernacki, K., Jacobson, M.P., Molecular mechanics methods for predicting protein-ligand binding. *Phys. Chem. Chem. Phys.*, 8, 5166, 2006.
154. Krammer, A., Kirchhoff, P.D., Jiang, X., Venkatachalam, C.M., Waldman, M., LigScore: A novel scoring function for predicting binding affinities. *J. Mol. Graph. Model.*, 23, 395, 2005.
155. Gohlke, H., Hendlich, M., Klebe, G., Knowledge-based scoring function to predict protein-ligand interactions. *J. Mol. Biol.*, 295, 337, 2000.
156. Shen, C., Ding, J., Wang, Z., Cao, D., Ding, X., Hou, T., From machine learning to deep learning: Advances in scoring functions for protein–ligand docking. *Wiley Interdiscip. Rev. Comput. Mol. Sci.*, 10, 1, 2020.
157. Huang J, M.A.D. C.OMMAJ.R.X.X.X, CHARMM36 all-atom additive protein force field: Validation based on comparison to NMR data. *J. Comput. Chem.*, 34, 2135, 2013.
158. Sprenger, K.G., Jaeger, V.W., Pfaendtner, J., The general AMBER force field (GAFF) can accurately predict thermodynamic and transport properties of many ionic liquids. *J. Phys. Chem. B.*, 119, 5882, 2015.
159. Jones, G., Willett, P., Glen, R.C., Leach, A.R., Taylor, R., Development and validation of a genetic algorithm for flexible docking. *J. Mol. Biol.*, 267, 727, 1997.

160. Venkatachalam, C.M., Jiang, X., Oldfield, T., Waldman, M., LigandFit: A novel method for the shape-directed rapid docking of ligands to protein active sites. *J. Mol. Graph. Model.*, 21, 289, 2003.
161. Trott, O. and Olson, A.J., AutoDock Vina: Improving the speed and accuracy of docking with a new scoring function, efficient optimization, and multi-threading. *J. Comput. Chem.*, 31, 455, 2010.
162. Friesner, R.A., Banks, J.L., Murphy, R.B., Halgren, T.A., Klicic, J.J., Mainz, D.T., Repasky, M.P., Knoll, E.H., Shelley, M., Perry, J.K., Shaw, D.E., Francis, P., Shenkin, P.S., Glide: A new approach for rapid, accurate docking and scoring. 1. Method and assessment of docking accuracy. *J. Med. Chem.*, 47, 1739, 2004.
163. Eldridge, M.D., Murray, C.W., Auton, T.R., Paolini, G.V., Mee, R.P., Empirical scoring functions: I. The development of a fast empirical scoring function to estimate the binding affinity of ligands in receptor complexes. *J. Comput. Aided Mol. Des.*, 11, 425, 1997.
164. Wang, R., Lai, L., Wang, S., Further development and validation of empirical scoring functions for structure-based binding affinity prediction. *J. Comput. Aided Mol. Des.*, 16, 11, 2002.
165. Muegge, I., Martin, Y.C., General, A., and fast scoring function for protein–ligand interactions: A simplified potential approach. *J. Med. Chem.*, 42, 791, 1999.
166. Velec, H.F.G., Gohlke, H., Klebe, G., DrugScore(CSD)-knowledge-based scoring function derived from small molecule crystal data with superior recognition rate of near-native ligand poses and better affinity prediction. *J. Med. Chem.*, 48, 6296, 2005.
167. Mooij, W.T.M. and Verdonk, M.L., General and targeted statistical potentials for protein-ligand interactions. *Proteins*, 61, 272, 2005.
168. Su, M., Yang, Q., Du, Y., Feng, G., Liu, Z., Li, Y., Wang, R., Comparative assessment of scoring functions: The CASF-2016 update. *J. Chem. Inf. Model.*, 59, 895, 2019.
169. Soni, A., Bhat, R., Jayaram, B., Improving the binding affinity estimations of protein-ligand complexes using machine-learning facilitated force field method. *J. Comput. Aided Mol. Des.*, 34, 817, 2020.
170. Böhm, H.J., LUDI: rule-based automatic design of new substituents for enzyme inhibitor leads. *J. Comput. Aided Mol. Des.*, 6, 593, 1992.
171. Ballester, P.J. and Mitchell, J.B.O., A machine learning approach to predicting protein–ligand binding affinity with applications to molecular docking. *Bioinformatics*, 26, 1169, 2010.
172. Ballester, P.J., Schreyer, A., Blundell, T.L., Does a more precise chemical description of protein–ligand complexes lead to more accurate prediction of binding affinity? *J. Chem. Inf. Model.*, 54, 944, 2014.
173. Li, H., Leung, K.-S., Wong, M.-H., Ballester, P.J., Improving AutoDock Vina using random forest: The growing accuracy of binding affinity prediction by the effective exploitation of larger data sets. *Mol. Inform.*, 34, 115, 2015.

174. Liu, Q., Keong Kwoh, C., Li, J., Binding affinity prediction for protein–ligand complexes based on β contacts and B factor. *J. Chem. Inf. Model.*, 53, 3076, 2013.
175. Zilian, D. and Sotriffer, C., A., SFCscoreRF: A random forest-based scoring function for improved affinity prediction of protein–ligand complexes. *J. Chem. Inf. Model.*, 53, 1923, 2013.
176. Sotriffer, C.A., Sanschagrin, P., Matter, H., Klebe, G., SFCscore: Scoring functions for affinity prediction of protein-ligand complexes. *Proteins*, 73, 395, 2008.
177. Li, H., Leung, K.-S., Wong, M.-H., Ballester, P.J., Substituting random forest for multiple linear regression improves binding affinity prediction of scoring functions: Cyscore as a case study. *BMC Bioinf.*, 15, 291, 2014.
178. Kinnings, S.L., Liu, N., Tonge, P.J., Jackson, R.M., Xie, L., Bourne, P.E., A machine learning-based method to improve docking scoring functions and its application to drug repurposing. *J. Chem. Inf. Model.*, 51, 408, 2011.
179. Koppisetty, C.A.K., Frank, M., Kemp, G.J.L., Nyholm, P.-G., Computation of binding energies including their enthalpy and entropy components for protein–ligand complexes using support vector machines. *J. Chem. Inf. Model.*, 53, 2559, 2013.
180. Li, G.-B., Yang, L.-L., Wang, W.-J., Li, L.-L., Yang, S.-Y., ID-Score: A new empirical scoring function based on a comprehensive set of descriptors related to protein–ligand interactions. *J. Chem. Inf. Model.*, 53, 592, 2013.
181. Ashtawy, H.M. and Mahapatra, N.R., A comparative assessment of predictive accuracies of conventional and machine learning scoring functions for protein-ligand binding affinity prediction. *IEEE/ACM Trans. Comput. Biol. Bioinform.*, 12, 335, 2015.
182. Ashtawy, H.M. and Mahapatra, N.R., Machine-learning scoring functions for identifying native poses of ligands docked to known and novel proteins. *BMC Bioinf.*, 16, S3, 2015.
183. Durrant, J.D. and McCammon, J.A., NNScore: A neural-network-based scoring function for the characterization of protein-ligand complexes. *J. Chem. Inf. Model.*, 50, 1865, 2010.
184. Durrant, D. and Andrew McCammon, J., NNScore 2.0: A neural-network receptor–ligand scoring function. *J. Chem. Inf. Model.*, 51, 2897, 2011.
185. Ouyang, X., Handoko, S.D., Kwoh, C.K., CScore: A simple yet effective scoring function for protein ligand binding affinity prediction using modified cmac learning architecture. *J. Bioinform. Comput. Biol.*, 9, 1, 2011.
186. Ashtawy, H.M. and Mahapatra, N.R., BgN-Score and BsN-Score: Bagging and boosting based ensemble neural networks scoring functions for accurate binding affinity prediction of protein-ligand complexes. *BMC Bioinf.*, 16, 1, 2015.
187. Wallach, I., Dzamba, M., Heifets, A., AtomNet: a deep convolutional neural network for bioactivity prediction in structure-based drug discovery, arXiv:1510.02855. 2015.

188. Ragoza, M., Hochuli, J., Idrobo, E., Sunseri, J., Ryan Koes, D., Protein–ligand scoring with convolutional neural networks. *J. Chem. Inf. Model.*, 57, 942, 2017.
189. Pereira, J.C., Caffarena, E.R., Dos Santos, C.N., Boosting docking-based virtual screening with deep learning. *J. Chem. Inf. Model.*, 56, 2495, 2016.
190. Pu, L., Govindaraj, R.G., Lemoine, J.M., Wu, H.-C., Brylinski, M., DeepDrug3D: Classification of ligand-binding pockets in proteins with a convolutional neural network. *PloS Comput. Biol.*, 15, e1006718, 2019.
191. Li, H., Peng, J., Sidorov, P., Leung, Y., Leung, K.-S., Wong, M.-H., Lu, G., Ballester, P.J., Classical scoring functions for docking are unable to exploit large volumes of structural and interaction data. *Bioinformatics*, 35, 3989, 2019.
192. Ashtawy, H.M. and Mahapatra, N.R., Task-specific scoring functions for predicting ligand binding poses and affinity and for screening enrichment. *J. Chem. Inf. Model.*, 58, 119, 2018.
193. Wang, B., Zhao, Z., Nguyen, D.D., Wei, G.-W., Feature functional theory–binding predictor (FFT–BP) for the blind prediction of binding free energies. *Theor. Chem. Acc.*, 136, 55, 2017.
194. Smith, E.F., Dunstan, W.R., Keen, B.A., Clarke, F.W., Obituary notices: Charles Baskerville, 1870–1922; Alexander Crum Brown, 1838–1922; Charles Mann Luxmoore, 1857–1922; Edward Williams Morley, 1838–1923; William Thomson, 1851–1923. *J. Chem. Soc, Trans.*, 123, 3421, 1923.
195. Brown, A.C. and Fraser, T.R., On the connection between chemical constitution and physiological action; with special reference to the physiological action of the salts of the ammonium bases derived from Strychnia, Brucia, Thebaia, Codeia, Morphia, and Nicotia. *J. Anat. Physiol.*, 2, 224, 1868.
196. Balatti, G.E. and Flórez-Zapata, N.V., Bioinformática para la creación y fortalecimiento de empresas de base tecnológica: Conceptos y aplicaciones, in: *Biotecnología y emprendimientos: herramientas, perspectivas y desafíos*, P.A. Pellegrini (Ed.), pp. 42–62, Universidad Nacional de Quilmes, Bernal, 2019.
197. Todeschini, R., Consonni, V., Ballabio, D., Grisoni, F., Brown, S., Tauler, R., Walczak, B., Chemometrics for QSAR modeling, in: *Comprehensive Chemometrics*, pp. 129–172, Elsevier Inc., Amsterdam, 2020.
198. Danishuddin, and Khan, A.U., Descriptors and their selection methods in QSAR analysis: Paradigm for drug design. *Drug Discovery Today*, 21, 1291, 2016.
199. Sprous, D.G., Palmer, R.K., Swanson, J.T., Lawless, M., QSAR in the pharmaceutical research setting: QSAR models for broad, large problems. *Curr. Top. Med. Chem.*, 10, 619, 2010.
200. Wu, Z., Zhu, M., Kang, Y., Leung, E.L.-H., Lei, T., Shen, C., Jiang, D., Wang, Z., Cao, D., Hou, T., Do we need different machine learning algorithms for QSAR modeling? A comprehensive assessment of 16 machine learning algorithms on 14 QSAR data sets. *Brief. Bioinform.*, 22, bbaa321, 2021.

201. Svetnik, V., Liaw, A., Tong, C., Christopher Culberson, J., P. Sheridan, R., P. Feuston, B., Random forest: A classification and regression tool for compound classification and QSAR modeling. *J. Chem. Inf. Comput. Sci.*, 43, 1947, 2003.
202. Singh, H., Singh, S., Singla, D., Agarwal, S.M., Raghava, G.P.S., QSAR based model for discriminating EGFR inhibitors and non-inhibitors using random forest. *Biol. Direct.*, 10, 10, 2015.
203. Mistry, P., Neagu, D., Trundle, P.R., Vessey, J.D., Using random forest and decision tree models for a new vehicle prediction approach in computational toxicology. *Soft Computing.*, 20, 2967, 2016.
204. Kumari, P., Nath, A., Chaube, R., Identification of human drug targets using machine-learning algorithms. *Comput. Biol. Med.*, 56, 175, 2015.
205. Cano, G., Garcia-Rodriguez, J., Garcia-Garcia, A., Perez-Sanchez, H., Benediktsson, J.A., Thapa, A., Barr, A., Automatic selection of molecular descriptors using random forest: Application to drug discovery. *Expert Syst. Appl.*, 72, 151, 2017.
206. Poorinmohammad, N., Mohabatkar, H., Behbahani, M., Biria, D., Computational prediction of anti HIV-1 peptides and *in vitro* evaluation of anti HIV-1 activity of HIV-1 P24-derived peptides. *J. Pept. Sci.*, 21, 10, 2015.
207. Liu, H.X., Zhang, R.S., Yao, X.J., Liu, M.C., Hu, Z.D., Fan, B.T., QSAR Study of Ethyl 2-[(3-Methyl-2,5-dioxo(3-pyrrolinyl))amino]-4-(trifluoromethyl) pyrimidine-5-carboxylate: An Inhibitor of AP-1 and NF-κB Mediated Gene Expression Based on Support Vector Machines. *J. Chem. Inf. Comput. Sci.*, 43, 1288, 2003.
208. Nekoei, M., Mohammadhosseini, M., Pourbasheer, E., QSAR study of VEGFR-2 inhibitors by using genetic algorithm-multiple linear regressions (GA-MLR) and genetic algorithm-support vector machine (GA-SVM): A comparative approach. *Med. Chem. Res.*, 24, 3037, 2015.
209. Keiser, M.J., Roth, B.L., Armbruster, B.N., Ernsberger, P., Irwin, J.J., Shoichet, B.K., Relating protein pharmacology by ligand chemistry. *Nat. Biotechnol.*, 25, 197, 2007.
210. Lo, Y.-C., Senese, S., Li, C.-M., Hu, Q., Huang, Y., Damoiseaux, R., Torres, J.Z., Large-scale chemical similarity networks for target profiling of compounds identified in cell-based chemical screens. *PloS Comput. Biol.*, 11, e1004153, 2015.
211. Huang, T., Mi, H., Lin, C.-Y., Zhao, L., Zhong, L.L.D., Liu, F.-B., Zhang, G., Lu, A.-P., Bian, Z.-X., MOST: Most-similar ligand based approach to target prediction. *BMC Bioinf.*, 18, 1, 2017.
212. da Silva, A.P., Chiari, L.P.A., Guimaraes, A.R., Honorio, K.M., da Silva, A.B.F., Drug design of new 5-HT6R antagonists aided by artificial neural networks. *J. Mol. Graph. Model.*, 104, 107844, 2021.
213. Chiari, L.P.A., da Silva, A.P., de Oliveira, A.A., Lipinski, C.F., Honório, K.M., da Silva, A.B.F., Drug design of new sigma-1 antagonists against neuropathic

pain: A QSAR study using partial least squares and artificial neural networks. *J. Mol. Struct.*, 1223, 129156, 2021.
214. Mozafari, Z., Arab Chamjangali, M., Beglari, M., Doosti, R., The efficiency of ligand-receptor interaction information alone as new descriptors in QSAR modeling via random forest artificial neural network. *Chem. Biol. Drug Des.*, 96, 812, 2020.
215. Gentiluomo, L., Roessner, D., Augustijn, D., Svilenov, H., Kulakova, A., Mahapatra, S., Winter, G., Streicher, W., Rinnan, Å., Peters, G.H.J., Harris, P., Frieß, W., Application of interpretable artificial neural networks to early monoclonal antibodies development. *Eur. J. Pharm. Biopharm.*, 141, 81, 2019.
216. Hisaki, T., Kaneko, M.A.N., Hirota, M., Matsuoka, M., Kouzuki, H., Integration of read-across and artificial neural network-based QSAR models for predicting systemic toxicity: A case study for valproic acid. *J. Toxicol. Sci.*, 45, 95, 2020.
217. Ito, R., Azam, N.A., Wang, C., Shurbevski, A., Nagamochi, H., Akutsu, T., Arabnia, H.R., Deligiannidis, L., Shouno, H., Tinetti, F.G., Tran, Q.N., A novel method for the inverse QSAR/QSPR to monocyclic chemical compounds based on artificial neural networks and integer programming, in: *Advances in computer vision and computational biology*, pp. 641–655, Springer, Cham, New York, 2021.
218. Erhan, D., L'Heureux, P.J., Yue, S.Y., Bengio, Y., Collaborative filtering on a family of biological targets. *J. Chem. Inf. Model.*, 46, 626, 2006.
219. Dahl, G.E., Jaitly, N., Salakhutdinov, R., Multi-task neural networks for QSAR predictions, arXiv:1406.1231. 2014.
220. Öztürk, H., Ozkirimli, E., Özgür, A., DeepDTA: deep drug-target binding affinity prediction, arXiv:1801.10193. 2018.
221. Lee, I., Keum, J., Nam, H., DeepConv-DTI: Prediction of drug-target interactions via deep learning with convolution on protein sequences. *PloS Comput. Biol.*, 15, e1007129, 2019.
222. Jiménez-Luna, J., Pérez-Benito, L., Martínez-Rosell, G., Sciabola, S., Torella, R., Tresadern, G., De Fabritiis, G., DeltaDelta neural networks for lead optimization of small molecule potency. *Chem. Sci.*, 10, 10911, 2019.
223. Obrezanova, O., Csányi, G., Gola, J.M.R., Segall, M.D., Gaussian processes: A method for automatic QSAR modeling of ADME properties. *J. Chem. Inf. Model.*, 47, 1847, 2007.
224. Ding, Y., Chen, M., Guo, C., Zhang, P., Wang, J., Molecular fingerprint-based machine learning assisted QSAR model development for prediction of ionic liquid properties. *J. Mol. Liq.*, 326, 115212, 2021.
225. Hemmateenejad, B., Miri, R., Elyasi, M., A segmented principal component analysis—Regression approach to QSAR study of peptides. *J. Theor. Biol.*, 305, 37, 2012.

226. Lee, G. and Bae, H., Anti-inflammatory applications of melittin, a major component of bee venom: Detailed mechanism of action and adverse effects. *Molecules*, 21, 616, 2016.
227. Alves, E.M., Heneine, L.G.D., Pesquero, J.L., Merlo, L.D.E.A., Pharmaceutical composition containin an apitoxin fraction and use thereof, WO2011041865A1, assigned to Universidade Federal De Minas Gerais - Ufmg. *Fundação Ezequiel Dias - Funed, Fundação Amparo À Pesquisa Do Estado Minas Gerais – Fapemig*, 2011.
228. Datta, S. and Roy, A., Antimicrobial peptides as potential therapeutic agents: A review. *Int. J. Pept. Res. Ther.*, 27, 555, 2021.
229. Buonocore, F., Fausto, A.M., Della Pelle, G., Roncevic, T., Gerdol, M., Picchietti, S., Attacins: A promising class of insect antimicrobial peptides. *Antibiotics*, 10, 212, 2021.
230. Sperstad, S.V., Haug, T., Blencke, H.-M., Styrvold, O.B., Li, C., Stensvåg, K., Antimicrobial peptides from marine invertebrates: Challenges and perspectives in marine antimicrobial peptide discovery. *Biotechnol. Adv.*, 29, 519, 2011.
231. Semreen, M.H., El-Gamal, M.I., Abdin, S., Alkhazraji, H., Kamal, L., Hammad, S., El-Awady, F., Waleed, D., Kourbaj, L., Recent updates of marine antimicrobial peptides. *Saudi Pharm. J.*, 26, 396, 2018.
232. Paiva, A.D. and Breukink, E., Antimicrobial peptides produced by microorganisms, in: *Antimicrobial Peptides and Innate Immunity. Progress in Inflammation Research*, P. Hiemstra and S. Zaat (Eds.), pp. 53–95, Springer, Basel, 2013.
233. Riley, M.A. and Wertz, J.E., Bacteriocin diversity: Ecological and evolutionary perspectives. *Biochimie.*, 84, 357, 2002.
234. Goyal, R.K. and Mattoo, A.K., *Plant Antimicrobial Peptides, in: Host Defense Peptides and Their Potential as Therapeutic Agents*, R.M. Epand (Ed.), pp. 111–136, Springer, Cham, 2016.
235. Montesinos, E., Antimicrobial peptides and plant disease control. *FEMS Microbiol. Lett.*, 270, 1, 2007.
236. Huan, Y., Kong, Q., Mou, H., Yi, H., Antimicrobial peptides: Classification, design, application and research progress in multiple fields. *Front. Microbiol.*, 11, 2559, 2020.
237. Brogden, K.A., Ackermann, M., McCray, P.B., Tack, B.F., Antimicrobial peptides in animals and their role in host defences. *Int. J. Antimicrob. Agents.*, 22, 465, 2003.
238. Clare, D.A. and Swaisgood, H.E., Bioactive milk peptides: A prospectus. *J. Dairy Sci.*, 83, 1187, 2000.
239. Korhonen, H., Milk-derived bioactive peptides: From science to applications. *J. Funct. Foods.*, 1, 177, 2009.
240. Bhat, Z.F., Kumar, S., Bhat, H.F., Bioactive peptides of animal origin: A review. *J. Food Sci. Technol.*, 52, 5377, 2015.

241. Cancelarich, N.L., Wilke, N., Fanani, M.L., Moreira, D.C., Pérez, L.O., Alves Barbosa, E., Plácido, A., Socodato, R., Portugal, C.C., Relvas, J.B., de la Torre, B.G., Albericio, F., Basso, N.G., Leite, J.R., Marani, M.M., Somuncurins: Bioactive peptides from the skin of the endangered endemic patagonian frog Pleurodema somuncurense. *J. Nat. Prod.*, 83, 972, 2020.
242. Sahoo, A., Swain, S.S., Behera, A., Sahoo, G., Mahapatra, P.K., Panda, S.K., Antimicrobial peptides derived from insects offer a novel therapeutic option to combat biofilm: A review. *Front. Microbiol.*, 12, 661195, 2021.
243. Balatti, G.E., Ambroggio, E.E., Fidelio, G.D., Martini, M.F., Pickholz, M., Differential interaction of antimicrobial peptides with lipid structures studied by coarse-grained molecular dynamics simulations. *Molecules*, 22, 1775, 2017.
244. Balatti, G.E., Domene, C., Martini, M.F., Pickholz, M., Differential stability of Aurein 1.2 pores in model membranes of two probiotic strains. *J. Chem. Inf. Model.*, 60, 5142, 2020.
245. Szymanowski, F., Balatti, G.E., Ambroggio, E., Hugo, A.A., Martini, M.F., Fidelio, G.D., Gómez-Zavaglia, A., Pickholz, M., Pérez, P.F., Differential activity of lytic α-helical peptides on lactobacilli and lactobacilli-derived liposomes. *Biochim. Biophys. Acta Biomembr.*, 1861, 1069, 2019.
246. Korhonen, H. and Pihlanto, A., Food-derived bioactive peptides - opportunities for designing future Foods. *Curr. Pharm. Des.*, 9, 1297, 2005.
247. Narai-Kanayama, A., Shikata, Y., Hosono, M., Aso, K., High level production of bioactive di- and tri-tyrosine peptides by protease-catalyzed reactions. *J. Biotechnol.*, 150, 343, 2010.
248. Dziuba, B. and Dziuba, M., Milk proteins-derived bioactive peptides in dairy products: Molecular, biological and methodological aspects. *Acta Sci. Pol. Technol. Aliment.*, 13, 5, 2014.
249. Quartararo, A.J., Gates, Z.P., Somsen, B.A., Hartrampf, N., Ye, X., Shimada, A., Kajihara, Y., Ottmann, C., Pentelute, B.L., Ultra-large chemical libraries for the discovery of high-affinity peptide binders. *Nat. Commun.*, 11, 3183, 2020.
250. Bozovičar, K. and Bratkovič, T., Evolving a peptide: Library platforms and diversification strategies. *Int. J. Mol. Sci.*, 21, 215, 2019.
251. Chandrudu, S., Simerska, P., Toth, I., Chemical methods for peptide and protein production. *Molecules*, 18, 4373, 2013.
252. Merrifield, R.B., Solid phase peptide synthesis. I. The synthesis of a tetrapeptide. *J. Am. Chem. Soc*, 85, 2149, 1963.
253. Lam, K.S., Salmon, S.E., Hersh, E.M., Hruby, V.J., Kazmierski, W.M., Knapp, R.J., A new type of synthetic peptide library for identifying ligand-binding activity. *Nature*, 354, 82, 1991.
254. Houghten, R.A., Pinilla, C., Blondelle, S.E., Appel, J.R., Dooley, C.T., Cuervo, J.H., Generation and use of synthetic peptide combinatorial libraries for basic research and drug discovery. *Nature*, 354, 84, 1991.

255. Furka, A., Sebestyen, F., Asgedom, M., Dibo, G., General method for rapid synthesis of multicomponent peptide mixtures. *Int. J. Pept. Protein Res.*, 37, 487, 1991.
256. Lam, K.S., Lehman, A.L., Song, A., Doan, N., Enstrom, A.M., Maxwell, J., Liu, R., Synthesis and screening of "one-bead one-compound" combinatorial peptide libraries. *Methods Enzymol.*, 369, 298, 2003.
257. Lam, K.S. and Lebl, M., Streptavidin and avidin recognize peptide ligands with different motifs. *Immunomethods*, 1, 11, 1992.
258. Camperi, S.A., Giudicessi, S.L., Martínez-Ceron, M.C., Gurevich-Messina, J.M., Saavedra, S.L., Acosta, G., Cascone, O., Erra-Balsells, R., Albericio, F., Combinatorial library screening coupled to mass spectrometry to identify valuable cyclic peptides. *Curr. Protoc. Chem. Biol.*, 8, 109, 2016.
259. Marani, M.M., Martínez Ceron, M.C., Giudicessi, S.L., De Oliveira, E., Côté, S., Erra-Balsells, R., Albericio, F., Cascone, O., Camperi, S.A., Screening of one-bead-one-peptide combinatorial library using red fluorescent dyes. Presence of positive and false positive beads. *J. Comb. Chem.*, 11, 146, 2009.
260. Martínez-Ceron, M.C., Giudicessi, S.L., Saavedra, S.L., Gurevich-Messina, J.M., Erra-Balsells, R., Albericio, F., Cascone, O., Camperi, S.A., Latest advances in OBOC peptide libraries. Improvements in screening strategies and enlarging the family from linear to cyclic libraries. *Curr. Pharm. Biotechnol.*, 17, 449, 2016.
261. Martínez-Ceron, M.C., Giudicessi, S.L., Kruszyn, J.N., Marani, M.M., Albericio, F., Cascone, O., Camperi, S.A., Two-stage screening of combinatorial peptide libraries. Application to bovine serum albumin ligand selection. *Rev. CENIC Cienc. Biológicas*, 46, 77, 2015.
262. Cha, J., Lim, J., Zheng, Y., Tan, S., Ang, Y.L., Oon, J., Ang, M.W., Ling, J., Bode, M., Lee, S.S., Process automation toward ultra-high-throughput screening of combinatorial one-bead-one-compound (OBOC) peptide libraries. *J. Lab. Autom.*, 17, 186, 2012.
263. Doran, T.M., Gao, Y., Mendes, K., Dean, S., Simanski, S., Kodadek, T., Utility of redundant combinatorial libraries in distinguishing high and low quality screening hits. *ACS Comb. Sci.*, 16, 259, 2014.
264. Hintersteiner, M. and Auer, M., A two-channel detection method for autofluorescence correction and efficient on-bead screening of one-bead one-compound combinatorial libraries using the COPAS fluorescence activated bead sorting system. *Methods Appl. Fluoresc.*, 1, 17001, 2013.
265. Martínez Ceron, M.C., Ávila, L., Giudicessi, S.L., Minoia, J.M., Fingermann, M., Camperi, S.A., Albericio, F., Cascone, O., Fully automated screening of a combinatorial library to avoid false positives: Application to tetanus toxoid ligand identification. *ACS Omega*, 6, 18756, 2021.
266. Gray, B.P. and Brown, K.C., Combinatorial peptide libraries: Mining for cell-binding peptides. *Chem. Rev.*, 114, 1020, 2014.
267. Peptide Therapeutics Market. https://www.globenewswire.com/news-release/2021/07/08/2259717/0/en/Peptide-Therapeutics-Market.html.

268. Kingsberg, S.A., Clayton, A.H., Portman, D., Williams, L.A., Krop, J., Jordan, R., Lucas, J., Simon, J.A., Bremelanotide for the treatment of hypoactive sexual desire disorder: Two randomized phase 3 trials. *Obstet. Gynecol.*, 134, 899, 2019.
269. Lau, J., Bloch, P., Schäffer, L., Pettersson, I., Spetzler, J., Kofoed, J., Madsen, K., Knudsen, L.B., McGuire, J., Steensgaard, D.B., Strauss, H.M., Gram, D.X., Knudsen, S.M., Nielsen, F.S., Thygesen, P., Reedtz-Runge, S., Kruse, T., Discovery of the once-weekly glucagon-like peptide-1 (GLP-1) analogue Semaglutide. *J. Med. Chem.*, 58, 7370, 2015.
270. New Drug Therapy Approvals 2019, FDA. https://www.fda.gov/drugs/new-drugs-fda-cders-new-molecular-entities-and-new-therapeutic-biological-products/new-drug-therapy-approvals-2019.
271. Rovin, B.H., Teng, Y.K.O., Ginzler, E.M., Arriens, C., Caster, D.J., Romero-Diaz, J., Gibson, K., Kaplan, J., Lisk, L., Navarra, S., Parikh, S.V., Randhawa, S., Solomons, N., Huizinga, R.B., Efficacy and safety of voclosporin versus placebo for lupus nephritis (AURORA 1): a double-blind, randomised, multicentre, placebo-controlled, phase 3 trial. *Lancet*, 397, 2070, 2021.
272. Dijksteel, G.S., Ulrich, M.M.W., Middelkoop, E., Boekema, B.K.H.L., Review: Lessons learned from clinical trials using antimicrobial peptides (AMPs). *Front. Microbiol.*, 12, 616979, 2021.
273. Conibear, A.C., Rosengren, K.J., Harvey, P.J., Craik, D.J., Structural characterization of the cyclic cystine ladder motif of θ-defensins. *Biochemistry*, 51, 9718, 2012.
274. Schaal, J.B., Maretzky, T., Tran, D.Q., Tran, P.A., Tongaonkar, P., Blobel, C.P., Ouellette, A.J., Selsted, M.E., Macrocyclic θ-defensins suppress tumor necrosis factor-α (TNF-α) shedding by inhibition of TNF-α–converting enzyme. *J. Biol. Chem.*, 293, 2725, 2018.
275. Matsoukas, J., Apostolopoulos, V., Zulli, A., Moore, G., Kelaidonis, K., Moschovou, K., Mavromoustakos, T., From Angiotensin II to cyclic peptides and angiotensin receptor blockers (ARBs): Perspectives of ARBs in COVID-19 therapy. *Molecules*, 26, 618, 2021.
276. Wang, G., Structures of human host defense Cathelicidin LL-37 and its smallest antimicrobial peptide KR-12 in lipid micelles. *J. Biol. Chem.*, 283, 32637, 2008.
277. Lax, R., The future of peptide development in the pharmaceutical industry. https://www.polypeptide.com/wp-content/uploads/2019/10/1401702726538c49464a6f5.pdf.
278. Boparai, J.K. and Sharma, P.K., Mini review on antimicrobial peptides, sources, mechanism and recent applications. *Protein Pept. Lett.*, 27, 4, 2019.
279. Goldstein Market Intelligence, Anti-microbial peptides market: Potential chronic diseases drug and alternatives for antibiotics. https://www.goldsteinresearch.com/pressrelease/anti-microbial-peptides-market-potential-chronic-diseases-drug-and-alternatives-for-antibiotics.

280. Chen, C.H. and Lu, T.K., Development and challenges of antimicrobial peptides for therapeutic applications. *Antibiotics*, 9, 24, 2020.
281. Browne, K., Chakraborty, S., Chen, R., Willcox, M.D., Black, D.S., Walsh, W.R., Kumar, N., A new era of antibiotics: The clinical potential of antimicrobial peptides. *Int. J. Mol. Sci.*, 21, 7047, 2020.
282. Bahar, A.A. and Ren, D., Antimicrobial peptides. *Pharmaceuticals*, 6, 1543, 2013.
283. Muttenthaler, M., King, G.F., Adams, D.J., Alewood, P.F., Trends in peptide drug discovery. *Nat. Rev. Drug Discovery*, 20, 309, 2021.
284. Uhlig, T., Kyprianou, T., Martinelli, F.G., Oppici, C.A., Heiligers, D., Hills, D., Calvo, X.R., Verhaert, P., The emergence of peptides in the pharmaceutical business: From exploration to exploitation. *EuPA Open Proteomics.*, 4, 58, 2014.
285. DRUG DELIVERY - oral delivery of peptides by peptelligence technology. https://drug-dev.com/oral-delivery-of-peptides-by-peptelligence-technology/, last accessed 2021/08/31.
286. Bruno, B.J., Miller, G.D., Lim, C.S., Basics and recent advances in peptide and protein drug delivery. *Ther. Deliv.*, 4, 1443, 2013.
287. Morishita, M., Kamei, N., Ehara, J., Isowa, K., Takayama, K., A novel approach using functional peptides for efficient intestinal absorption of insulin. *J. Control. Releas*, 118, 177, 2007.
288. Asane, G.S., Nirmal, S.A., Rasal, K.B., Naik, A.A., Mahadik, M.S., Rao, Y.M., Polymers for mucoadhesive drug delivery system: A current status. *Drug Dev. Ind. Pharm.*, 34, 1246, 2008.
289. Shah, P., Bhalodia, D., Shelat, P., Nanoemulsion: A pharmaceutical review. *Sys. Rev. Pharm.*, 1, 24, 2010.
290. Peppas, N.A., Wood, K.M., Blanchette, J.O., Hydrogels for oral delivery of therapeutic proteins. *Expert Opin. Biol. Ther.*, 4, 881, 2004.
291. Chen, Y., Ping, Q., Guo, J., Lv, W., Gao, J., The absorption behavior of cyclosporin A lecithin vesicles in rat intestinal tissue. *Int. J. Pharm.*, 261, 21, 2003.
292. Jung, T., Kamm, W., Breitenbach, A., Kaiserling, E., Xiao, J.X., Kissel, T., Biodegradable nanoparticles for oral delivery of peptides: Is there a role for polymers to affect mucosal uptake? *Eur. J. Pharm. Biopharm.*, 50, 147, 2000.
293. Arora, A., Prausnitz, M.R., Mitragotri, S., Micro-scale devices for transdermal drug delivery. *Int. J. Pharm.*, 364, 227, 2008.
294. Bloom, B.S., Brauer, J.A., Geronemus, R.G., Ablative fractional resurfacing in topical drug delivery: An update and outlook. *Dermatol. Surg.*, 39, 839, 2013.
295. Otvos, L. C.OMMAJ.R.X.X.X and Wade, J.D., Current challenges in peptide-based drug discovery. *Front. Chem.*, 2, 62, 2014.
296. Giudicessi, S.L., Salum, M.L., Saavedra, S.L., Martínez-Ceron, M.C., Cascone, O., Erra-Balsells, R., Camperi, S.A., Simple method to assess stability of immobilized peptide ligands against proteases. *J. Pept. Sci.*, 23, 685, 2017.

297. Ree, R., Varland, S., Arnesen, T., Spotlight on protein N-terminal acetylation. *Exp. Mol. Med.*, 50, 90, 2018.
298. Buckton, L.K., Rahimi, M.N., McAlpine, S.R., Cyclic peptides as drugs for intracellular targets: The next frontier in peptide therapeutic development. *Chem. Eur. J.*, 27, 1487, 2021.
299. Puentes, P.R., Henao, M.C., Torres, C.E., Gómez, S.C., Gómez, L.A., Burgos, J.C., Arbeláez, P., Osma, J.F., Muñoz-Camargo, C., Reyes, L.H., Cruz, J.C., Design, screening, and testing of non-rational peptide libraries with antimicrobial activity: *In silico* and experimental approaches. *Antibiotics*, 9, 1, 2020.
300. Kimber, T.B., Chen, Y., Volkamer, A., Deep learning in virtual screening: recent applications and developments. *Int. J. Mol. Sci.*, 22, 4435, 2021.
301. Pant, S., Singh, M., Ravichandiran, V., Murty, U.S.N., Srivastava, H.K., Peptide-like and small-molecule inhibitors against Covid-19. *J. Biomol. Struct. Dyn.*, 39, 2904, 2021.
302. Hassanzadeh, P., Atyabi, F., Dinarvand, R., The significance of artificial intelligence in drug delivery system design. *Adv. Drug Deliv. Rev.*, 151, 169, 2019.
303. Gautam, A., Chaudhary, K., Kumar, R., Raghava, G.P.S., Computer-aided virtual screening and designing of cell-penetrating peptides, in: *Cell-Penetrating Peptides: Methods and Protocols*, pp. 59–69, Humana Press, New York, NY, 2015.
304. Sharma, A., Gupta, P., Kumar, R., Bhardwaj, A., dPABBs: A Novel *in silico* approach for predicting and designing anti-biofilm peptides. *Sci. Rep.*, 6, 21839, 2016.
305. Souza, P.F.N., Marques, L.S.M., Oliveira, J.T.A., Lima, P.G., Dias, L.P., Neto, N.A.S., Lopes, F.E.S., Sousa, J.S., Silva, A.F.B., Caneiro, R.F., Lopes, J.L.S., Ramos, M.V., Freitas, C.D.T., Synthetic antimicrobial peptides: From choice of the best sequences to action mechanisms. *Biochimie.*, 175, 132, 2020.
306. Gertrudes, J.C., Maltarollo, V.G., Silva, R.A., Oliveira, P.R., Honorio, K.M., da Silva, A.B.F., Machine learning techniques and drug design. *Curr. Med. Chem.*, 19, 4289, 2012.
307. Zhong, F., Xing, J., Li, X., Liu, X., Fu, Z., Xiong, Z., Lu, D., Wu, X., Zhao, J., Tan, X., Li, F., Luo, X., Li, Z., Chen, K., Zheng, M., Jiang, H., Artificial intelligence in drug design. *Sci. China Life Sci.*, 61, 1191, 2018.
308. Wu, Q., Ke, H., Li, D., Wang, Q., Fang, J., Zhou, J., Recent progress in machine learning-based prediction of peptide activity for drug discovery. *Curr. Top. Med. Chem.*, 19, 4, 2019.
309. Capecchi, A. and Reymond, J.-L., Peptides in chemical space. *Med. Drug Discovery.*, 9, 100081, 2021.
310. Agostini, F., Cirillo, D., Livi, C.M., Delli Ponti, R., Tartaglia, G.G., cc SOL omics: A webserver for solubility prediction of endogenous and heterologous expression in Escherichia coli. *Bioinformatics,30*, 2975, 2014.

311. Smialowski, P., Doose, G., Torkler, P., Kaufmann, S., Frishman, D., PROSO II – a new method for protein solubility prediction. *FEBS J.*, 279, 2192, 2012.
312. Giguère, S., Laviolette, F., Marchand, M., Tremblay, D., Moineau, S., Liang, X., Biron, É., Corbeil, J., Machine learning assisted design of highly active peptides for drug discovery. *PloS Comput. Biol.*, 11, e1004074, 2015.
313. Das, P., Sercu, T., Wadhawan, K., Padhi, I., Gehrmann, S., Cipcigan, F., Chenthamarakshan, V., Strobelt, H., dos Santos, C., Chen, P.-Y., Yang, Y.Y., Tan, J.P.K., Hedrick, J., Crain, J., Mojsilovic, A., Accelerated antimicrobial discovery via deep generative models and molecular dynamics simulations. *Nat. Biomed. Eng.*, 5, 613, 2021.
314. Khosravian, M., Faramarzi, F.K., Beigi, M.M., Behbahani, M., Mohabatkar, H., Predicting antibacterial peptides by the concept of Chou's pseudo-amino acid composition and machine learning methods. *Protein Pept. Lett.*, 20, 180, 2013.
315. Plisson, F., Ramírez-Sánchez, O., Martínez-Hernández, C., Machine learning-guided discovery and design of non-hemolytic peptides. *Sci. Rep.*, 10, 16581, 2020.
316. Van Oort, C.M., Ferrell, J.B., Remington, J.M., Wshah, S., Li, J., AMPGAN v2: Machine learning-guided design of antimicrobial peptides. *J. Chem. Inf. Model.*, 61, 2198, 2021.
317. Casey, R., Adelfio, A., Connolly, M., Wall, A., Holyer, I., Khaldi, N., Discovery through Machine Learning and preclinical validation of novel anti-diabetic peptides. *Biomedicines*, 9, 276, 2021.
318. Yan, J., Bhadra, P., Li, A., Sethiya, P., Qin, L., Tai, H.K., Wong, K.H., Siu, S.W.I., Deep-AmPEP30: Improve short antimicrobial peptides prediction with deep learning. *Mol. Ther. Nucleic Acids*, 20, 882, 2020.
319. Thomas, S., Karnik, S., Barai, R.S., Jayaraman, V.K., Idicula-Thomas, S., CAMP: A useful resource for research on antimicrobial peptides. *Nucleic Acids Res.*, 38, D774, 2010.
320. Müller, A.T., Hiss, J.A., Schneider, G., Recurrent neural network model for constructive peptide design. *J. Chem. Inf. Model.*, 58, 472, 2018.
321. Basith, S., Manavalan, B., Hwan Shin, T., Lee, G., Machine intelligence in peptide therapeutics: A next-generation tool for rapid disease screening. *Med. Res. Rev.*, 40, 1276, 2020.
322. Marqus, S., Pirogova, E., Piva, T.J., Evaluation of the use of therapeutic peptides for cancer treatment. *J. Biomed. Sci.*, 24, 21, 2017.
323. Lee, A.C.-L., Harris, J.L., Khanna, K.K., Hong, J.-H., A comprehensive review on current advances in peptide drug development and design. *Int. J. Mol. Sci.*, 20, 2383, 2019.
324. Taherzadeh, G., Zhou, Y., Liew, A.W.-C., Yang, Y., Structure-based prediction of protein–peptide binding regions using random forest. *Bioinformatics*, 34, 477, 2018.

325. Obarska-Kosinska, A., Iacoangeli, A., Lepore, R., Tramontano, A., PepComposer: Computational design of peptides binding to a given protein surface. *Nucleic Acids Res.*, 44, W522, 2016.
326. Holton, T.A., Pollastri, G., Shields, D.C., Mooney, C., CPPpred: Prediction of cell penetrating peptides. *Bioinformatics*, 29, 3094, 2013.
327. Wei, L., Xing, P., Su, R., Shi, G., Ma, Z.S., Zou, Q., CPPred-RF: A sequence-based predictor for identifying cell-penetrating peptides and their uptake efficiency. *J. Proteome Res.*, 16, 2044, 2017.
328. Sanders, W.S., Johnston, C.I., Bridges, S.M., Burgess, S.C., Willeford, K.O., Prediction of cell penetrating peptides by support vector machines. *PloS Comput. Biol.*, 7, e1002101, 2011.
329. Manavalan, B., Basith, S., Shin, T.H., Choi, S., Kim, M.O., Lee, G., MLACP: Machine-learning-based prediction of anticancer peptides. *Oncotarget*, 8, 77121, 2017.
330. Wang, J., Fast identification of possible drug treatment of Coronavirus Disease-19 (COVID-19) through computational drug repurposing study. *J. Chem. Inf. Model.*, 60, 3277, 2020.
331. Patiyal, S., Kaur, D., Kaur, H., Sharma, N., Dhall, A., Sahai, S., Agrawal, P., Maryam, L., Arora, C., Raghava, G., A web-based platform on COVID-19 to maintain predicted diagnostic, drug and vaccine candidates. *Monoclon. Antib. Immunodiagn. Immunother.*, 39, 204, 2020.
332. Kong, R., Yang, G., Xue, R., Liu, M., Wang, F., Hu, J., Guo, X., Chang, S., COVID-19 Docking Server: An interactive server for docking small molecules, peptides and antibodies against potential targets of COVID-19. *Bioinformatics*, 36, 5109, 2020.
333. Robson, B., Computers and viral diseases. Preliminary bioinformatics studies on the design of a synthetic vaccine and a preventative peptidomimetic antagonist against the SARS-CoV-2 (2019-nCoV, COVID-19) coronavirus. *Comput. Biol. Med.*, 119, 103670, 2020.
334. Slathia, P., Sharma, P., Singh Slathia, P., Prediction of T and B cell epitopes in the proteome of SARS-CoV-2 for potential use in diagnostics and vaccine design. *ChemRxiv.*, 2020.
335. Vashi, Y., Jagrit, V., Kumar, S., Understanding the B and T cells epitopes of spike protein of severe respiratory syndrome coronavirus-2: A computational way to predict the immunogens. *Infection, Genetics and Evolution*, 84, 104382, 2020.
336. Joshi, A., Joshi, B.C., Mannan, M.A.-U., Kaushik, V., Epitope based vaccine prediction for SARS-COV-2 by deploying immuno-informatics approach. *Inform Med. Unlocked*, 19, 100338, 2020.
337. Jespersen, M.C., Peters, B., Nielsen, M., Marcatili, P., BepiPred-2.0: Improving sequence-based B-cell epitope prediction using conformational epitopes. *Nucleic Acids Res.*, 45, W24, 2017.

338. Ponomarenko, J., Bui, H.H., Li, W., Fusseder, N., Bourne, P.E., Sette, A., Peters, B., ElliPro: A new structure-based tool for the prediction of antibody epitopes. *BMC Bioinf.*, 9, 514, 2008.
339. Biswas, S., Chatterjee, S., Dey, T., Dey, S., Manna, S., Nandy, A., Basak, S., *In silico* approach for peptide vaccine design for COVID 19, in: *Proceedings of MOL2NET 2020, International Conference on Multidisciplinary Sciences*, 6th, MDPI, Basel, Switzerland, p. 6787, 2020.
340. Lalmuanawma, S., Hussain, J., Chhakchhuak, L., Applications of machine learning and artificial intelligence for Covid-19 (SARS-CoV-2) pandemic: A review. *Chaos Solitons Fractals*, 139, 110059, 2020.
341. Ong, E., Wong, M.U., Huffman, A., He, Y., COVID-19 coronavirus vaccine design using reverse vaccinology and machine learning. *Front. Immunol.*, 11, 1581, 2020.
342. Ashkenazy, H., Avram, O., Ryvkin, A., Roitburd-Berman, A., Weiss-Ottolenghi, Y., Hada-Neeman, S., Gershoni, J.M., Pupko, T., Motifier: An IgOme profiler based on peptide motifs using machine learning. *J. Mol. Biol.*, 433, 167071, 2021.
343. Liu, G., Carter, B., Bricken, T., Jain, S., Viard, M., Carrington, M., Gifford, D.K., Computationally optimized SARS-CoV-2 MHC Class I and II vaccine formulations predicted to target human haplotype distributions. *Cell Syst.*, 11, 131, 2020.
344. Kamalov, F., Cherukuri, A. K. and Thabtah, F., Machine learning applications to Covid-19: A state-of-the-art survey. *ASET*, 1, 1, 2022.
345. Yang, Z., Bogdan, P., Nazarian, S., An *in silico* deep learning approach to multi-epitope vaccine design: A SARS-CoV-2 case study. *Sci. Rep.*, 11, 3238, 2021.
346. Liu, G., Dimitrakakis, A., Carter, B., Gifford, D., Maximum n-times coverage for vaccine design, arXiv:2101.10902. 1, 2021.
347. Yazdani, Z., Rafiei, A., Yazdani, M., Valadan, R., Design an efficient multi-epitope peptide vaccine candidate against SARS-CoV-2: An *in silico* analysis. *Infect. Drug Resist.*, 13, 3007, 2020.

3

Machine Learning Applications in Rational Drug Discovery

Hemanshi Chugh and Sonal Singh*

Delhi Technological University, Shahbad Daulatpur, Main Bawana Road, Delhi, India

Abstract

Artificial intelligence (AI) has transformed industries around the world and has been promising in revolutionizing health care for approximately 30 years now. The scientific advancement of AI in the latest years state this as a fact of how AI could radically transform patient care and diagnosis. Machine learning in medicinal drug system can result in accurate diagnostic algorithms and individual patient remedy. The capability to collect huge data units and predictive models helps physicians in hopefully diagnosing the diseases, expecting the side effects and thereby dealing with the patients in a more confident way. Deploying AI in health care requires integration into the existing medical surroundings and a platform to accumulate, store, and process the data, and to deliver the outputs to users in a well-timed way. AI programs provide substantial capacity to enhance patient care, from figuring out new drug targets to supporting scientific drug selection making and way of life modifications for sickness prevention. AI makes viable applications, which can learn, adapt, and expect drug outcomes. In medicine, that is starting to have an impact at three stages: for clinicians, predominantly thru fast, accurate photo interpretation; for health structures, by using enhancing workflow and the potential for lowering medical errors; and for patients, through permitting them to method their own data to practice fitness. Machine learning techniques that underpin artificial intelligence provide promise in improving health care structures and services.

***Keywords*:** Machine learning, artificial intelligence, adverse drug reactions (ADR), polypharmacology, drug repurposing

**Corresponding author*: sonalsingh@dtu.ac.in

Inamuddin, Tariq Altalhi, Jorddy N. Cruz and Moamen Salah El-Deen Refat (eds.) Drug Design Using Machine Learning, (97–116) © 2022 Scrivener Publishing LLC

3.1 Introduction

Mr. Arthur Lee Samuel, a leading pioneer in the field of computer gaming and artificial intelligence, popularized the term machine learning (ML) in the year 1959. AI is a wide-ranging branch of computer science which concerns in building smart machines capable of performing tasks that apparently require human intelligence. These machines are also known as "intelligent agents" while Samuel popularized machine learning (ML) as the study of computer algorithms which improve automatically through experience and by the use of the data provided to them (i.e., making decisions without being programmed explicitly) [1]. The terms artificial intelligence (AI) and machine learning (ML) are frequently used synonymously, albeit incorrectly. Machine learning is a specific application or discipline of AI—but not the only one. The main proposition of ML algorithms is to build a model based on the sample data, learn from these data, identify its trends and patterns, and then make decisions within an admissible range of precision with minimal human intervention [2].

Humans can recognize patterns and regularities in data, which is known as pattern recognition. Machines are better at recognition as they can use more amount of data. Machines can learn in more than 100 dimensions and thereby make predictions much more accurately than humans. Machine learning is a branch that uses algorithms to learn from the information and make possible predictions. Artificial intelligence is the intelligence demonstrated by machines involving consciousness and emotionality. AI supports in building smart machines, which can execute tasks that require human intelligence [3].

Artificial intelligence basically uses incorporated understanding and acquires further knowledge from the answers it generates to cope with both unique and additionally complicated issues [2]. The progress in AI may be thought of as a mixed blessing. On one hand, it creates a doubt that it is going to jeopardize the employment; and on the other hand, each improvement in AI when accessed deeply is well known because it helps in contributing to the upgradation of society vastly. The significant advancements in the processing capacity combined with improvements in AI techniques may be put to use effectively to transform the drug improvement technique [3]. Artificial intelligence in health care, also known as deep medicine, is the usage of machine learning algorithms or AI to imitate human cognition in analysis, presentation and comprehension of complex scientific, and health care records. The exquisite concept of embracing AI in the health care system can be seen as a transfer from hype to hope.

Applying AI to medical analysis offers numerous benefits to the developing of the health care industry [4].

3.2 The Drug Development and Approval Process

The evolution of advanced medicines is a cumbersome and exquisite process. With the aim of ensuring the patients' safety and effectiveness of the drug, the proposed drugs need to go through a competitive and long series of steps. The entire drug advancement outline [5] is illustrated in Figure 3.1. Drug development can be broadly divided in four significant tiers, commonly known as phases (Table 3.1). The first phase, phase 0 accommodates primary studies/drug analysis and diagnosis assessments, which strive to assess the ability and body activity of the drug prospect. The further three phases are clinical trials: such that in phase I, the observation of dose-toxicity and short-term aftereffects are assessed; in phase II, the kinetic relationships ascertainment of drug performance is made and contrast of the molecule to the standard-of-care is studied in phase III. An alternative phase IV is usually done postdrug marketing to keep the track of the persistent aftereffects of the drugs and drug amalgamation with other remedial treatments. The minimum quantity of time to cover the setup of the phases from 0 up to III, i.e., the preclinical and clinical assessments may be accomplished in a minimum span of 5 years [6] but may also last as long as 15 years (Table 3.1) [7]. It is estimated that from 5,000 to 10,000 compounds only one new drug reaches the market [4, 8, 9].

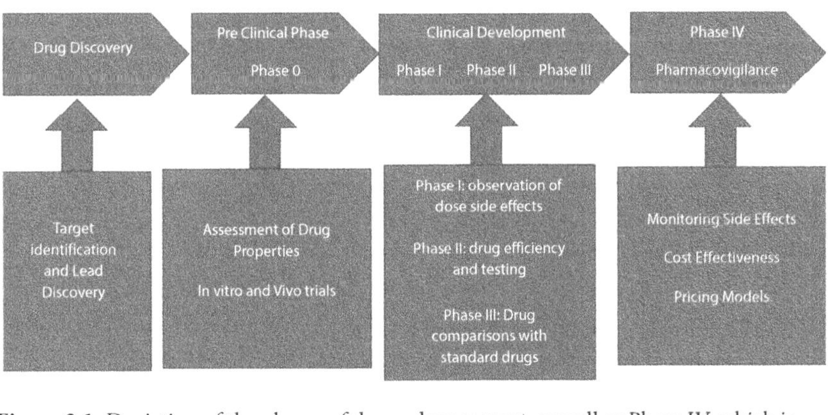

Figure 3.1 Depiction of the phases of drug advancement, as well as Phase IV, which is done postdrug advertising (redrawn from [5]).

Table 3.1 Drug discovery and development phases.

	Drug discovery	**Preclinical phase (phase 0)**	**Clinical development (phase 1–3)**	**Pharmaco-vigilance (phase 4)**
Test population	Laboratory studies	*Vitro* and *vivo* trials	Patient volunteers	Postmarketing testing by FDA
Timeline	3–5 years	1–3 years	6–7 years	1–2 years
Success rate	5000-10000 compounds sampled	250 compounds evaluated	5 compounds enter trials	1 approved drug

Table 3.1 shows a summary of drug approval process, with phase 0 focussing on drug analysis and diagnosis, phase I concentrating on drug safety, phase II on efficacy, and phase III on confirming the outcomes from a larger population. Positive results from clinical trials lead to a new drug application submitted for further review (phase IV) and approval by the FDA and other regulatory agencies [8, 10].

Drug safety can be observed at all stages of preclinical and clinically advanced primary candidates through postmarketing surveillance. And it can intelligently generate important metrics at each step to provide insight into important decisions, traversing thousands or hundreds of pages which offer important information for better decision making. The overarching goal is to bring more efficient and safer treatments to the patients as quickly as possible after a thorough medical evaluation [11].

This is where AI plays an important role. Safety is confirmed at all levels of drug history. Final testing is performed only after the drug has been declared and is used in clinical practice in most patients, with a variety of drugs and a wider range of symptoms. There is always a risk. However, the more data one can collect, analyze, and transform into real data, the more likely one is to mitigate these risks. The discovery pipeline has the potential to save time, money, and lives by terminating unreliable drug projects in the shortest possible time [10, 12–14].

The goal of drug development is to prevent human and animal pain and suffering whenever possible and find and provide new drugs that we can depend on to improve our health and happiness [11].

3.3 Human-AI Partnership

Proper algorithms may not be the most important factor, but providing higher quality information (Figure 3.2) to facilitate various programs will greatly enhance the field of AI exploration [15]. The lack of high-quality data is a major challenge for machine learning in drug development. Accessing and sharing information is troublesome because of the expense, lawful issues, and hesitance to share information from certain organizations.

The necessity to provide vast amounts of relevant information to AI programs is changing science, and researchers are experimenting more with AI data in consideration [4]. More significant informational collections allow the program to identify more productive research tools and faster development of the drugs (Figure 3.2). The fundamental methodology is to extract data that can be obtained from patient tissue sets, body fluids, and blood tests. This extricated information might incorporate genomics, proteomics, metabolomics, lipidomic, and that is just the beginning—a surprisingly expansive reach to consider in a chase for targets [15].

Artificial intelligence still relies on humans to support and enhance human efforts, generate novel biological knowledge, set research needs and

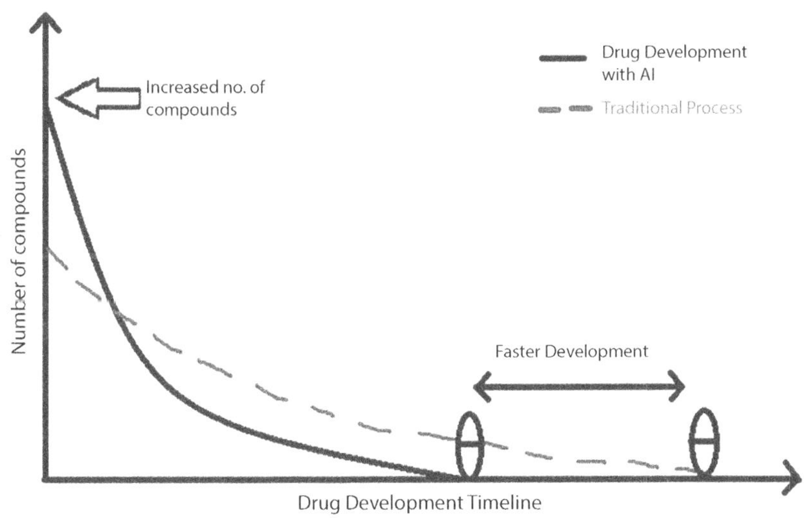

Figure 3.2 Accelerated drug discovery process with machine learning and AI (redrawn from [51]).

considerations, drive and approve results, and generate the necessary data. Many researchers in this field believe that artificial intelligence will further develop drug advancement in a number of means, for example; recognizing favorable drug molecules; increasing the "hit rate" or the number of drug candidates that endure clinical assays and are legally accepted; thereby accelerating the overall development process (Figure 3.2). These findings assist researchers focus on the drug candidates, which are potentially effective and safer in repeated human trials rather than rapidly researching potentially toxic drugs. Artificial intelligence can have an immense effect in knowing which drugs are failing fast before investing in them.

3.4 AI in Understanding the Pathway to Assess the Side Effects

The process may include collecting information, establishing rules or algorithms for utilizing the data and statistics, illustrating estimated or maybe final inferences and self-correction. The more drugs a patient consumes, the possible risk of drug-drug interactions increases extensively. Physicians advising drugs are unable to foresee all the possible side effects that could arise, as there is a lot that is unknown about the possible adverse effects from the amalgamation of different drugs. An AI system can be prepared to predict side effects of different drug combinations in patients. AI system would help the doctors to make informed decisions before prescribing the combinations of drugs to patients with complex or multiple diseases.

In order to bring out a productive and successful AI algorithm, the systems must be provided with enough sets of data. The data required for such a system would be more than 4 million known associations between the drugs and their side effects. The AI system will be designed in a way to infer patterns about drug interactions and side effects, thereby, predicting formerly unidentified consequences from taking two or more drugs together. As predictive models increase in complexity, the number of observations required to train these models increases as well [16].

The algorithmic program usually involves the input of the data to be tested for which the medical doctor is aware of the solution already, letting them verify the algorithms' ability to determine the correct solution. Depending on those testing results, the algorithm could possibly be altered, fed with more data or statistics, or maybe rolled out completely to help make best possible decisions.

3.4.1 Traditional Versus New Strategies in Drug Discovery

Since many years, pharmaceutical research companies have been developing new drugs using a standard drug discovery method [17]. The process generally starts with extensive medical research about a specific disease, which in turn provides the researchers with an ability to understand the target disease and how it may affect the body. The next phase of the drug exploration procedure usually involves the identification and validation of the target (Table 3.2). Generally, drugs fight the disease by targeting a particular molecule or a set of homogeneous molecules within the body. The process begins by recognizing a molecule (often a protein or a gene) that plays a role in that particular disease the researchers are attempting to treat. The target molecule must be able to interact with and be affected by drug molecules. Once a target molecule is identified, scientists conduct a broad range of experiments with living cells and animal models to prove that the target molecule may actually cause the disease and can be affected by drugs. The continuous increase in polypharmacy and the diversity of patients limits the application and reliability of these traditional processes. Thus, the vast amounts of new data available allow artificial intelligence (AI) and machine learning (ML) to be used efficiently to improve the drug safety field. The new strategies in drug development procedure (Table 3.2) work on the principle stating that the development of any disease phenotype

Table 3.2 Traditional versus new strategies in drug development process.

	Target identification and validation	**Lead identification**	**Lead optimization**
Traditional drug development process	Genomic data, basic research, cell-based trials, animal-based trials	HTS (*in vitro* and *vivo*)	Toxicity trials *in vitro* and *vivo*
New strategies in drug development process	Functional and structural genomics, proteomics, bioinformatics	HTS (*in vitro* and *vivo*), *In silico* structure-based design for known compound	Toxicity trials *in vitro* and *vivo*

includes changes in the gene expression in the cells and tissues involved. Research with an intent of identifying a therapeutic target includes continuous assessment of the functional and structural genomics, proteomics, and bioinformatics trials using AI.

3.4.2 Target Identification and Authentication

Target identification acts toward the identification of the role of the proteins or genes of a small molecule also known as a potential molecular target and the function it plays in a disease, which works toward discovering the efficiency of the target of a particular drug [10]. This would require continuous assessment of the structural and functional genetic data, large scale study of proteomes, cell-based, and animal research *in vitro* and *vivo* trials.

In order to examine the entire Drug Information Bank[iii] which includes the drug candidates, expressions of various genes, multiple protein-protein interactions, and medical data reports from an information centre for foreseeing the medicinal and healing potential, AI can be used efficiently [18].

For identification of the possible target site of a drug, individual chemicals can be concealed in a normal chamber with latent vectors, allowing optimization based on gradients in molecular space, and permits predictions using a lattice-based graphical system, depending on the binding strength and several other characteristics.

In an attempt to perceive a comprehensive three-dimensional spatial structure of molecular complexes and proteins, AI procedure also relies on the observations of the two-dimensional structure of cryo-EM microscope data and machine learning representations.

The choice of a particular drug candidate would require a sequence of preferred characteristics such as safe and effective therapeutic management of drugs in an individual patient, study of the body's reaction to drugs and toxicity profile of a drug [18].

3.4.3 Searching the Hit and Lead Molecules with the Help of AI

The initial step for drug improvement is to identify the different chemical compounds having biological reactions. These reactions may come to light through the interaction of compounds with certain enzymes or with whole organisms. "Hit" is described as the first compound that would indicate a reaction against a specified biological target. These hits are frequently discovered in the testing phase of naturally isolated materials viz plants, microorganisms, and fungi, screening of chemical libraries or computer simulations [19]. Secondly, recognizing the lead is the next stage in drug advancement. A lead molecule may be defined as a chemical compound with great hopes that could lead to the improvement of new drugs as cures for certain diseases. To clearly identify the effectiveness of the compound and its anticipated safety profile the hits which are identified previously (Figure 3.3) are concealed in the cell-based evaluations that are diagnostic of the disease state and in the animal models of disease. As soon as a lead is discovered, further modifications are made with the major purpose of identifying compounds with highest medicinal benefits and minimum risk of patients suffering by using the lead compound's chemical structure as an initial point [19, 20]. In the course of lead generation, hit molecules are orderly reformed in order to improve their activity and sensitivity with respect to the particular targets, meanwhile decreasing the undesirable effects and toxicity. Analogs are hereby chemical compounds that are procured from a hit. The process of discovering these analogs is known as hit expansion [21]. The use of artificial intelligence to train small drug molecules limits the use of chemical space. This chemical drug space is spanned by all possible molecules and millions of chemical compounds adhering to a given set of construction principles and boundary conditions providing a platform for identifying different molecules of high quality and enumerating the possible biological molecules [22]. Furthermore, ML technologies and predictive modelling software can also be used to identify the relationship between virtual targets and related targets, in order to improve the safety and efficiency attributes associated with the drug development. Artificial intelligence systems can reduce wear and tear and R&D costs

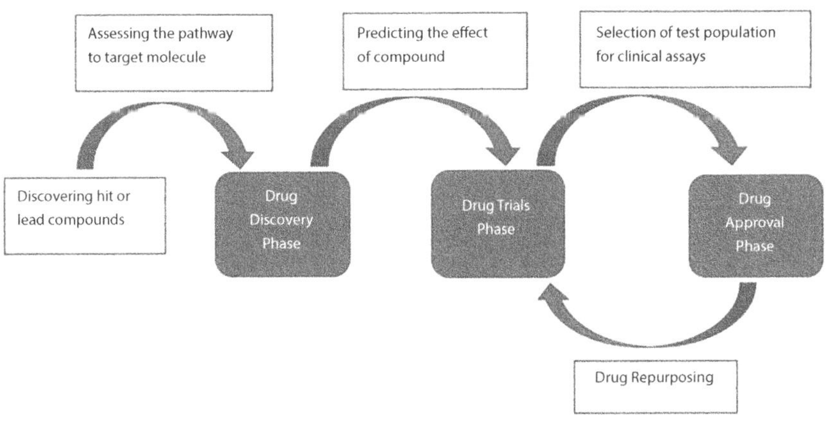

Figure 3.3 Remarkable improvements by using AI in drug development process (redrawn from [31]).

by reducing the number of compounds synthesized that then need to be tested [13, 19].

3.4.4 Discretion of a Population for Medical Trials Using AI

An intelligent method that'd be able to help in clinical trials must be the one that is capable of recognizing the disease in the patient, discovering the genetic targets in them, as well as predicting the on- and off-target effects and after effect of the designed molecule. The most critical process for a specific clinical trial is the patient selection. Thus, cross-examining the correlation between the human biomarkers and *in vitro* reaction phenotypes will provide a better, foreseeable and a computable evaluation of the unpredictability of the medicinal response in a given patient. The AI development aims toward discovering and predicting human-relevant biomarkers of a particular infection, also permitting the recruitment of a particular patient community in the different phases of these clinical assays. This prediction model to select a particular patient population using Artificial Intelligence would thereby lead to a significant increase in the successful clinical trials, thereby enhancing the drug development workflow [23, 24].

3.5 Predicting the Side Effects Using AI

Pharmacovigilance is a medical field that specialises in monitoring, detecting, and hence preventing adverse drug reactions (ADRs). Besides the safety of drugs being tested multiple times during the development process, through clinical experiments and further postmarketing inspection of ADRs in real time patients, the future toxicity and many adverse drug reactions (ADR) may still remain unexplored under certain specific circumstances, for example: long-term use of a drug, when a drug is used in conjunction with other drugs or if it is being used by a section of people which remain excluded from the clinical trials, such as children or pregnant women.

The AI technique will be able to help both the patients and the physicians to make informed decisions related to the selection and setup of a brand-new drug. However, doctors must be very careful as the AI system can only give a rough idea of what might possibly happen (viz not likely to happen). The side effects of a drug are often quoted like "it is likely to happen, but there's a possibility it won't happen" [25]. In other words, the AI system can just warn you regarding a potential risk, so that one can predict and prepare for the exact risk, but it still gives much deeper insight and information which doctors had about the drug initially. Thus, an AI approach in health care could extract information about the different possible drug combinations and thereby predict their possible side effects, which could further be used by physicians or prescribers to assess the potential risks of prescribing a certain combination of drugs to patients. With AI, computational efforts will be efficiently utilized as the lab efforts would be time consuming and ultimately ineffective.

3.6 AI for Polypharmacology and Repurposing

Drug discovery and advancement is a very complicated and an expensive process. As a result of the exponential growth of the vast molecular data and rapid evolution in the technologies, the drug discovery efforts are intensifying [26]. Since many years in drug discovery, the predominant paradigm has been "one target one disease," yet with the drug development, it has become certain that there are various diseases that are too complex to be cured efficiently within this paradigm. A multitarget approach to drug discovery seems to be a favorable method to discover more reliable and safe medicines. The ideology of drug design seems to deviate from "one disease one target" to "one disease several targets" commonly labelled as polypharmacology [27]. Presently, polypharmacology (i.e., 'one-disease–several-targets') rules the "one-disease–single-target" prototype due to the profound understanding at molecular level of pathological processes in various diseases. Polypharmacological phenomena consists of: (a) one drug performing on different targets of a particular pathway of a disease, or (b) one drug impacting more than one target associated with multiple pathways of a disease [26]. Furthermore, polypharmacology in complicated diseases is expected to utilize several drugs acting on unique targets, which would be the part of a network regulating numerous physiological responses. The polypharmacological approach as shown in Figure 3.3 intends to find the unidentified off targets for the currently existing drugs (the process is called drug repurposing). The traditional drug discovery approach includes five phases such as preclinical phase, safety review phase, clinical research, FDA review and postmarketing surveillance (Figure 3.1), which is a time consuming, high risk, and high investment process [28]. On the other hand, drug repurposing requires only four phases which include compound identification, compound collection, development, and postmarket safety surveillance (Table 3.3) [29]. Drug repurposing identifies new pharmacological indications for existing drugs. It is a promising approach due to the possibility of reduced

Table 3.3 Traditional drug development vs drug repurposing process [29].

	Traditional drug development	Drug repurposing
Phases	5	4
Time required	10-17 years	3-12 years
Cost	12 billion $	1.6 billion $

development timelines and overall costs (Table 3.3). Drug repurposing is known to be one of the glorious technologies in the advancement of AI to gain worth recently since abundant information about the drug in trial is already known [30]. Repurposing these earlier studied drugs or late-stage drugs toward new medical fields is in addition a required strategy for many pharmaceutical companies as it is more likely to have a lower risk of unexpected toxicity or side effects in subsequent human trials, and, probably, lesser amount of R&D spent [31]. Thus, drug repurposing offers an opportunity to develop drugs with lower investments [29]. The process basically requires the methodical incorporation of the data that is collected through various fields which include computational modelling, organic and inorganic chemistry, *in vitro/in vivo* pharmacological testing, and other clinical fields. (Figure 3.3). This is especially significant to foresee the probable side effects of the recently developed drugs in the development phase. The several databases (Table 3.4), like Drug Bank[iii] [32, 33], ZINC[iv] [34], ChEMBL[v] [35, 36], PubChem[vi] [37], KEGG[vii] [38], STITCH[viii] [39], BindingDB[ix] [40], Supertarget[x] [41], PDB[xi] [42], LigandExpo[xii] [43], etc are accessible to merge the various information regarding the molecular pathways of drugs, their chemical structures, their binding affinities, their drug targets, the relevance of disease, their chemical properties and the different biological activities [44]. Thus, AI can now be utilized to efficiently examine these databases to plan the polypharmacological agents.

In view of the large amount of data to be processed, the use of computational methods in this field is very essential. Apart from leading to more medicines, AI might even permit the introduction of better medicines. Hence, the advances in AI could be used to modernize the pharma industry resulting in an efficient, automated, cost-effective and extendable solution with more reliable understanding and minimization of harm to patients [13].

Table 3.4 Open-source databases with molecular, or pharmacological information [46].

Name	Description	References	Resource
DrugBank	A comprehensive online database containing extensive biochemical and pharmacological information about drugs, their mechanisms and their targets.	[32, 33]	iii
ZINC	A free database of commercially available compounds for virtual screening	[34]	iv
ChEMBL	A manually curated database of bioactive molecules with drug-like properties	[35, 36]	v
PubChem	An open chemistry database at the National Institutes of Health (NIH)	[37]	vi
KEGG	A database resource for understanding high-level functions and utilities of the biological system, the organism and the ecosystem, from molecular-level information	[38]	vii
STITCH	Search tool for interactions of chemicals	[39]	viii
BindingDB	Public, web-accessible database of measured binding affinities, focusing chiefly on the interactions of protein considered to be drug-targets with small, drug-like molecules	[40]	ix

(*Continued*)

Table 3.4 Open-source databases with molecular, or pharmacological information [46]. (*Continued*)

Name	Description	References	Resource
Supertarget	Database which integrates drug-related information associated with medical indications, adverse drug effects, drug metabolism, pathways and gene ontology terms for target proteins.	[41]	x
PDB	Worldwide archive of structural data of biological macromolecules.	[42]	xi
LigandExpo	The single archive of experimentally determined structures of nucleic acids, proteins and complex assemblies	[43]	xii

In addition, artificial intelligence may also be used to support techniques that use genes to prevent or treat diseases and several other remedial treatments which are not readily accessible in health care currently. The likelihood to combine regenerative medicine (seeks to regrow, repair or replace damaged or diseased cells, organs or tissues) with pharmacology and gene therapies in conjunction with Artificial Intelligence becomes evident [45]. With the rising drug prices and the slow growth in drug development, repurposing the existing drugs to treat diseases other than their originally accepted symptoms is becoming an increasingly attractive proposition. These drugs will soon take over most of the pharmaceutical industry [44].

3.7 The Challenge of Keeping Drugs Safe

Safety trials are initiated during the drug advancement process within *vivo* and *vitro* studies, proceeding through clinical assays, and extending to postmarketing surveillance of adverse drug reactions in the actual population. Future toxicity and safety problems, such as polypharmacy and increased patient diversity, illustrates the limitations of these traditional methodologies. Drug safety becomes a major challenge for bringing novel drugs to the market [46].

Drug safety and its effectiveness is ensured through various clinical trials before a drug has been accepted. When a drug is placed on the market, AE reports keep a track of these drugs to make sure that the drug's safety data is kept updated, a process commonly known as pharmacovigilance. However, due to structural limitations in clinical trials, none of these processes are error proof. For instance, it becomes impossible to test for all the drug effects or to experiment enough on larger populations to identify the rare adverse reactions. Lately, women and senior citizens are considered as special population unit for clinical experiments. These experiments mainly focus on drug designing for an ordinary patient [47] even when there is a rising demand for accurate medication to ensure the "ideal medication at the ideal portion to the right patient" [48]. The safety of the drugs is monitored by the programs once the drugs are approved. Drug toxicity evaluation is done by using different AI techniques to ensure premarket drug safety. These evaluations become essential to avoid toxic drugs from reaching the clinical assessments. Nonetheless, high toxicity is yet a significant contributor to drug failure considering 66% of marketing recalls [49] and 20% of clinical trial failures [50]. Therefore, precise estimation of toxicity becomes essential in order to ensure drug security, which helps in reducing the cost and improvement time it takes to get new drugs on the market. Since there are limits to the safety evaluations in clinical trials, the drug safety must be actively examined throughout the drug life.

3.8 Conclusion

Drug companies invest approximately 10 to 15 years to bring a drug to the market, often at a higher price. In addition to this, multiple clinical trials create hindrance in the swift drug advancement. There has been a continuous upsurge in the expenses and the time invested for patient recruitment. Product development process is subject to a higher proportion of errors subsequently resulting in financial loss. Majorly due to the lack of funding, the evaluation of drug efficiency is not being accomplished as clinical testing is stopped prematurely. The above-described factors have been contributing significantly in the reduction of the accepted drugs. In fact, the upcoming integration and engagement of artificial intelligence and multiple machine learning companies with pharmaceutical labs will surely speed up the drug development path as they are computationally implemented and thus less susceptible to human-caused technical errors. Machine learning will significantly reduce the time and cost of the drug development process by discovering new understanding in the vast biological, medical or health-related data sets. The possible utilization of AI is to provide a platform and enable it to differ from the incompetence and unreliability which becomes apparent in the traditional advancement processes of drugs meanwhile reducing distortions and human interventions in the system. Experts firmly believe that AI is capable enough to bring about a permanent change in the medical field and the process by which drugs are developed, their interactions with patients and the possible side effects that may occur on the patients. However, to be proficient with the drug advancement using AI, one must obtain the domain expertise to have a clear understanding and familiarity with the method to train several algorithms. This would help creating an acceptable workspace such that AI and physicians can work in symposium, as artificial intelligence would be capable of analyzing the large datasets and the physicians would be proficient in training machines, setting procedures or optimizing the examined data for an efficient and precise drug development system. Besides the well-known benefits and advantages of artificial intelligence in accelerating the advancement process of drugs, effective real-time experiments are yet to be performed. One of the major factors driving the growth of this market is that AI and machine learning have allowed pharmaceutical companies to operate in a much more efficient manner and have improved the success rates substantially at the very initial phases of the drug development procedure. Machine learning is used throughout the drug development process which helps in increasing its efficiency and robustness, significantly reducing the time and cost of bringing new drugs to market. These improvements could save lives and reduce the patient distress by providing drugs more swiftly to those in need, and could also allow research workers to devote more resources in the areas which have neglected conditions and limited patient population (also called rare or orphan diseases). The AI and ML approaches have the potential to lead to a more effective and safer health care.

Resources

i) https://health.gov/
ii) http://sideeffects.embl.de/
iii) https://www.drugbank.ca/
iv) http://zinc.docking.org/

v) https://www.ebi.ac.uk/chembl/
vi) https://pubchem.ncbi.nlm.nih.gov/
vii) https://www.genome.jp/kegg/
viii) http://stitch.embl.de/
ix) http://www.bindingdb.org
x) http://bioinformatics.charite.de/supertarget
xi) http://www.rcsb.org/pdb/
xii) http://www.rcsb.org/
xiii) https://clinicaltrials.gov/

References

1. Munoz, A., *Machine learning and optimization*, Courant Institute of Mathematical Sciences, New York, NY, 2014, URL: https://www. cims.nyu.edu/~munoz/files/ml_optimization.pdf [accessed 2016-03-02][WebCite Cache ID 6fiLfZvnG].
2. Paul, D., Sanap, G., Shenoy, S., Kalyane, D., Kalia, K., Tekade, R.K., Artificial intelligence in drug discovery and development. *Drug Discovery Today*, 26, 80, 2021.
3. Gupta, R., Srivastava, D., Sahu, M., Tiwari, S., Ambasta, R.K., Kumar, P., Artificial intelligence to deep learning: Machine intelligence approach for drug discovery. *Mol. Diversity*, 25, 1315, 2021.
4. Saikin, S.K., Kreisbeck, C., Sheberla, D., Becker, J.S., Aspuru-Guzik, A., Closed-loop discovery platform integration is needed for artificial intelligence to make an impact in drug discovery. *Expert Opin. Drug Discovery*, 14, 1, 2019.
5. Réda, C., Kaufmann, E., Duriez, A.D., Machine learning applications in drug development. *Comput. Struct. Biotechnol. J.*, 18, 241, 2020.
6. Eliopoulos, H., Giranda, V., Carr, R., Tiehen, R., Leahy, T., Gordon, G., Phase 0 trials: An industry perspective. *Clin. Cancer Res.*, 14, 3683, 2008.
7. Xue, H., Li, J., Xie, H., Wang, Y., Review of drug repositioning approaches and resources. *Int. J. Biol. Sci.*, 14, 1232, 2018.
8. Matthews, H., Hanison, J., Nirmalan, N., Omics-informed drug and biomarker discovery: Opportunities, challenges and future perspectives. *Proteomes*, 4, 28, 2016.
9. Díaz, Ó., Dalton, J., Giraldo, J., Artificial intelligence: A novel approach for drug discovery. *Trends Pharmacol. Sci.*, 40, 550, 2019.
10. Zhavoronkov, A., Vanhaelen, Q., Oprea, T.I., Will artificial intelligence for drug discovery impact clinical pharmacology? *Clin. Pharmacol. Ther.*, 107, 780, 2020.
11. Pandey, A., *Drug Discovery and Development Process*, NorthEast BioLab, NorthEast Biolabs, 925, Sherman Ave, Hamden, CT 06514, United States, 2020.

12. Reed, J.Z., *AI Technologies Can Support Drug Safety Assessment*, Pharmaceutical Executive, 2 Clarke Dr Suite 100, Cranbury, NJ 08512, US, 2018.
13. Chan, H., Shan, H., Dahoun, T., Vogel, H., Yuan, S., Advancing drug discovery via artificial intelligence. *Trends Pharmacol. Sci.*, 40, 592, 2019.
14. Tripathi, M.K., Nath, A., Singh, T.P., Ethayathulla, A.S., Kaur, P., Evolving scenario of big data and Artificial Intelligence (AI) in drug discovery. *Mol. Diversity*, 25, 1439, 2021.
15. Freedman, D.H., *Hunting for New drugs with AI*, Scientific American, 2020.
16. Adam, G., Rampášek, L., Safikhani, Z. *et al.*, Machine learning approaches to drug response prediction: Challenges and recent progress. *NPJ Precis. Oncol.*, 4, 19, 2020.
17. Mohs, R.C. and Greig, N.H., Drug discovery and development: Role of basic biological research. *Alzheimers Dement (N Y)*, 3, 4, 651–657, 2017.
18. 4 Application Areas of Artificial Intelligence in Drug Discovery, 2020, https://www.wipro.com/holmes/4-application-areas-of-artificial-intelligence-in-drug-discovery/.
19. Lakdawala, A.S., Okafo, G., Baldoni, J., Palovich, M., Sikosek, T., Sahni, V., Adapting drug discovery to artificial intelligence. *Drug Target Rev.*, 1, 50, 2018.
20. Anderson, A.C., Structure-based functional design of drugs: From target to lead compound. *Methods Mol. Biol.*, 823, 359–366, 2012.
21. Hall, D.R., Ngan, C.H., Zerbe, B.S., Kozakov, D., Vajda, S., Hot spot analysis for driving the development of hits into leads in fragment-based drug discovery. *J. Chem. Inf. Model.*, 52, 199, 2012.
22. Reymond, J.L., Deursen, R.V., Blum, L.C., Ruddigkeit, L., Chemical space as a source for new drugs. *J. MedChemComm*, 1, 30, 2010.
23. Perez-Gracia, J.L., Sanmamed, M.F., Bosch, A., Patiño-Garcia, A., Schalper, K.A., Segura, V., Bellmunt, J., Tabernero, J., Sweeney, C.J., Choueiri, T.K., Martín, M., Fusco, J.P., Rodriguez-Ruiz, M.E., Calvo, A., Prior, C., Paz-Ares, L., Pio, R., Gonzalez-Billalabeitia, E., Gonzalez Hernandez, A., Páez, D., Melero, I., Strategies to design clinical studies to identify predictive biomarkers in cancer research. *Cancer Treat. Rev., 53*, 79, 2017.
24. Deliberato, R.O., Celi, L.A., Stone, D.J., Clinical note creation, binning, and artificial intelligence. *JMIR Med. Inf.*, *5*, e24, 2017.
25. Naggapan, P., Can artificial intelligence predict drug side effects. *J. MedShadow*, 2018.
26. Reddy, A.S. and Zhang, S., Polypharmacology: Drug discovery for the future. *Expert Rev. Clin. Pharmacol.*, 6, 41, 2013.
27. Dimasi, J.A., Risks in new drug development: Approval success rates for investigational drugs. *Clin. Pharmacol. Ther.*, 69, 297, 2001.
28. Shim, J.S. and Liu, O.J., Recent advances in drug repositioning for the discovery of new anticancer drugs. *Int. J. Biol. Sci.*, 10, 654, 2014.
29. Xue, H., Li, J., Xie, H., Wang, Y., Review of drug repositioning approaches and resources. *Int. J. Biol. Sci.*, 14, 1232, 2018.

30. Tanoli, Z., Vähä-Koskela, M., Aittokallio, T., Artificial intelligence, machine learning, and drug repurposing in cancer. *Expert Opin. Drug Discovery*, 16, 977, 2021.
31. Mak, K.K. and Pichika, M.R., Artificial intelligence in drug development: Present status and future prospects. *Drug Discovery Today*, 24, 773, 2019.
32. Wishart, D.S., Feunang, Y.D., Guo, A.C., Lo, E.J., Marcu, A., Grant, J.R., Sajed, T., Johnson, D., Li, C., Sayeeda, Z., Assempour, N., Iynkkaran, I., Liu, Y., Maciejewski, A., Gale, N., Wilson, A., Chin, L., Cummings, R., Le, D., Pon, A., Wilson, M., DrugBank 5.0: A major update to the DrugBank database for 2018. *Nucleic Acids Res.*, 46, D1074, 2018.
33. Law, V., Knox, C., Djoumbou, Y., Jewison, T., Guo, A.C., Liu, Y., Maciejewski, A., Arndt, D., Wilson, M., Neveu, V., Tang, A., Gabriel, G., Ly, C., Adamjee, S., Dame, Z.T., Han, B., Zhou, Y., Wishart, D.S., DrugBank 4.0: Shedding new light on drug metabolism. *Nucleic Acids Res.*, 42, D1091, 2014.
34. Irwin, J.J. and Shoichet, B.K., ZINC – a free database of commercially available compounds for virtual screening. *J. Chem. Inf. Model.*, 45, 177, 2005.
35. Gaulton, A., Hersey, A., Nowotka, M., Bento, A.P., Chambers, J., Mendez, D., Mutowo, P., Atkinson, F., Bellis, L.J., Cibrián-Uhalte, E., Davies, M., Dedman, N., Karlsson, A., Magariños, M.P., Overington, J.P., Papadatos, G., Smit, I., Leach, A.R., The ChEMBL database in 2017. *Nucleic Acids Res.*, 45, D945, 2017.
36. Gaulton, A., Bellis, L.J., Bento, A.P., Chambers, J., Davies, M., Hersey, A., Light, Y., McGlinchey, S., Michalovich, D., Al-Lazikani, B., Overington, J.P., ChEMBL: A large-scale bioactivity database for drug discovery. *Nucleic Acids Res.*, 40, D1100, 2012.
37. Kim, S., Chen, J., Cheng, T., Gindulyte, A., He, J., He, S., Li, Q., Shoemaker, B.A., Thiessen, P.A., Yu, B., Zaslavsky, L., Zhang, J., Bolton, E.E., PubChem 2019 Update: Improved access to chemical data. *Nucleic Acids Res.*, 47, D1102, 2019.
38. Kanehisa, M., Furumichi, M., Tanabe, M., Sato, Y., Morishima, K., Kegg: New perspectives on genomes, pathways, diseases and drugs. *Nucleic Acids Res.*, 45, D353, 2016.
39. Kuhn, M., von Mering, C., Campillos, M., Jensen, L.J., Bork, P., STITCH: Interaction networks of chemicals and proteins. *Nucleic Acids Res.*, 36, D684, 2008.
40. Liu, T., Lin, Y., Wen, X., Jorissen, R.N., Gilson, M.K., BindingDB: A web-accessible database of experimentally determined protein-ligand binding affinities. *Nucleic Acids Res.*, 35, D198, 2007.
41. Hecker, N., Ahmed, J., von Eichborn, J., Dunkel, M., Macha, K., Eckert, A., Gilson, M.K., Bourne, P.E., Preissner, R., SuperTarget goes quantitative: Update on drug-target interactions. *Nucleic Acids Res.*, 40, D1113, 2012.
42. Berman, H.M., Westbrook, J., Feng, Z., Gilliland, G., Bhat, T.N., Weissig, H., Shindyalov, I.N., Bourne, P.E., The protein Data Bank. *Nucleic Acids Res.*, 28, 235, 2000.

43. Rose, P.W., Bi, C., Bluhm, W.F., Christie, C.H., Dimitropoulos, D., Dutta, S., Green, R.K., Goodsell, D.S., Prlic, A., Quesada, M., Quinn, G.B., Ramos, A.G., Westbrook, J.D., Young, J., Zardecki, C., Berman, H.M., Bourne, P.E., The RCSB protein Data Bank: New resources for research and education. *Nucleic Acids Res.*, 41, D475, 2013.
44. Agarwal, H., *Drug Repurposing: Advantages and Key Approaches*, Technology Networks, Woodview Bull lane Industrial Estate Sudbury, C010 OFD, UK, 2021.
45. Fogel, D.B., Factors associated with clinical trials that fail and opportunities for improving the likelihood of success: A review. *Contemp. Clin. Trials Commun.*, 11, 156, 2018.
46. Basile, A.O., Yahi, A., Tatonetti, N.P., Artificial intelligence for drug toxicity and safety. *Trends Pharmacol. Sci.*, 40, 624, 2019.
47. Tannenbaum, C. and Day, D., Age and sex in drug development and testing for adults. *Pharmacol. Res.*, 121, 83, 2017.
48. Collins, F.S. and Varmus, H., A new initiative on precision medicine. *N. Engl. J. Med.*, 372, 793–795, 2015.
49. Onakpoya, I.J., Heneghan, C.J., Aronson, J.K., Worldwide withdrawal of medicinal products because of adverse drug reactions: A systematic review and analysis. *Crit. Rev. Toxicol.*, 46, 477, 2016.
50. Segall, M.D. and Barber, C., Addressing toxicity risk when designing and selecting compounds in early drug discovery. *Drug Discovery Today*, 19, 688, 2014.
51. Could AI Help Create New Medicines? US Government Accountability Office on Feb 06, 2020, https://blog.gao.gov/2020/02/06/could-ai-help-create-new-medicines/.

4

Deep Learning for the Selection of Multiple Analogs

C. Deepa[1], D. Balaji[2], V. Bhuvaneswari[2], L. Rajeshkumar[2], M. Ramesh[3]* and M. Priyadharshini[4]

[1]*Department of Artificial Intelligence and Data Science, KIT-Kalaignarkarunanidhi Institute of Technology, Coimbatore, Tamil Nadu, India*
[2]*Department of Mechanical Engineering, KPR Institute of Engineering and Technology, Coimbatore, Tamil Nadu, India*
[3]*Department of Mechanical Engineering, KIT-Kalaignarkarunanidhi Institute of Technology, Coimbatore, Tamil Nadu, India*
[4]*Department of Computer Science and Engineering, VIT-AP, Andhra Pradesh, India*

Abstract
Artificial intelligence (AI) is a field of computer science and engineering that works based on the principle and operation of human brain. Machine learning (ML) and deep learning (DL) are two subsets of AI where ML could develop models from the training data to which it is exposing and DL contains numerous layers with which the geometric transformations of the developed models run through. It was stated in various researches that the digitized data acquisition system in AI, ML, and DL has taken the computer infrastructure to newer heights which were formerly considered to be a pure human intervened systems. Current chapter elaborates the latest advancements in AI technologies along with their applications, enumerates the challenges faced by these technologies that retards their full scale implementation and also provides an overview about the social, legal and economic aspects. All these are discussed for various applications like drug delivery, health care, and medical systems.

***Keywords*:** Deep learning, machine learning, multiple analogs, artificial intelligence

**Corresponding author*: mramesh97@gmail.com

Inamuddin, Tariq Altalhi, Jorddy N. Cruz and Moamen Salah El-Deen Refat (eds.) Drug Design Using Machine Learning, (117–142) © 2022 Scrivener Publishing LLC

4.1 Introduction

Since 1791, the term analogy has been applied in natural science to refer to structural and functional similarity. It is resulting from the Latin and Greek analogia [1–3]. When applied to medicines, this description suggests that the analog of an established drug molecule is chemically and therapeutically identical to the original components. The biochemical strategy of analogs utilizes straightforward and established medicinal chemistry techniques such as homolog synthesis, vinylog synthesis, isostere synthesis, positional isomers synthesis, optical isomers synthesis, ring system transformation, and twin drug synthesis. The term "analog design" refers to the process of modifying a drug molecule or other variety of chemicals in order to create a new molecule with chemical and biological resemblance to the model compound. A structural analog, also called a biochemical analog or just an analog, is a complex that has a like construction to additional complex but differs in one or more components [4]. It can be distinguished by the substitution of more than one atom, dynamic areas, or substructures for extra particles, areas, or additional structures. A structural analog can be fictional being generated from another compound, at least theoretically. Despite their maximum biochemical resemblance, constructional analogs are not always functional analogs and can exhibit a wide range of physical, chemical, biochemical, and pharmacological characteristics. In the process of medicine detection, moreover a great number of organizational analogs of a preliminary main complex are evaluated and the results as portion of a construction–movement interaction investigation, or a database are filtered for organizational analogs of a main complex [5, 6]. Example for lead compound and its analog is presented in Figure 4.1 [6].

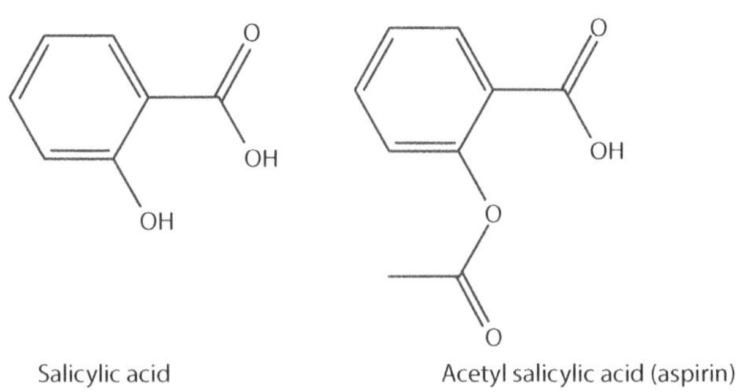

Figure 4.1 Example of a lead compound (salicylic acid) and its analog (acetyl salicylic acid) [6].

Many well-established fields, such as natural language processing, speech recognition, and machine vision, had witnessed enormous growth due to AI techniques. For drug industry and chemical scientists, drug design and development are a critical area of research. Reduced effectiveness, off-target shipment, time consumption, and increased price, on the other hand, impose a barrier and challenges on production of medicines. Additionally, complex and large data sets derived from branch of molecular biology, study of proteomes, DNA sequences analysis, and research that studies new tests and treatments obstruct the drug discovery pipeline. AI and ML technologies are critical in the discovery and development of new medications. In other words, DL methods and artificial neural network (ANN) have redesigned the field. A wide variety of drug discovery processes have benefited from the use of ML and DL algorithms, including the following: chemical methods, framework simulated vetting, alkene silico, toxic effects prognostication, narcotic tracking and discharge, structure-based model construction, quantifiable framework relation estimation, drug repositioning, poly pharmacognosy, and physiochemical activity. The historical evidence supports the application of AI and DL in this sector. Additionally, novel data mining, retrieval, and management techniques aided the development of newly established modeling procedures significantly. In description, developments in artificial intelligence and DL enable a more balanced medicine design and detection procedure, which will ultimately benefit humanity [7–9].

4.2 Goals of Analog Design

By modifying the chemical composition of the lead compound in order to maintain or enhance the desired pharmacologic effect while minimizing undesirable pharmacological, physical, and chemical properties, a superior therapeutic agent may be created. As a pharmacological probe, to achieve good understanding into the toxicology of the lead molecule and possibly uncover new knowledge of basic biology. Photonic ADCs powered by DL that concurrently leverages the benefits of electronics and photonics and overwhelms their bottlenecks, in that way avoiding the ADC trade-off between rapidity, band of frequencies and exactness is described in some works [10, 11]. According to the results, the proposed framework outstrips state-of-the-art ADCs with residential development maximum quantity, proving that DL works fine in photonic ADC systems. An architecture has been presented for building high-performance ADCs that takes benefit of data recovery via DL technology. A photonic front-end, electronic

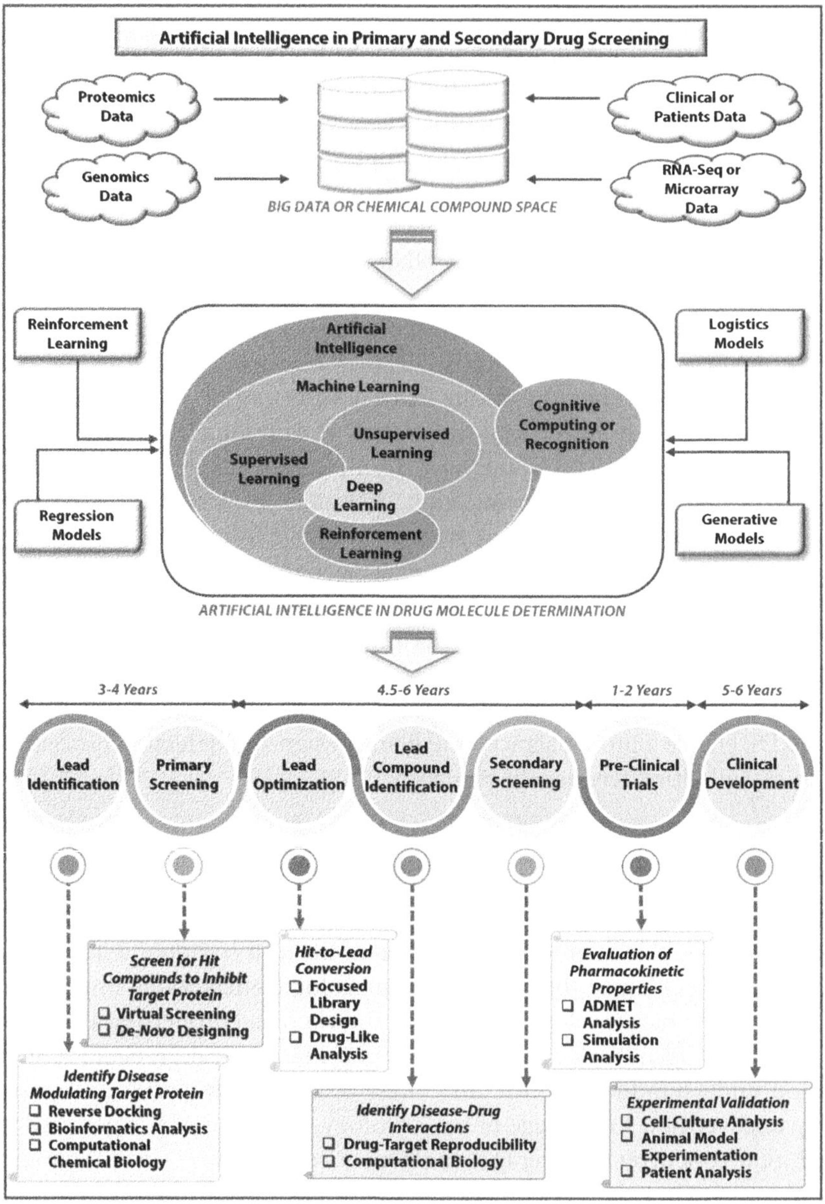

Figure 4.2 Artificial intelligence in drug screening [12].

quantization and DL data recovery comprise the DL-powered photonic analog-to-digital conversion (DL-PADC) architecture, as shown in Figure 4.2 [12].

Using analog recollection plans to construct systems in the human brain and nervous system computer hardware accelerator pedal for DL applications, few authors conducted a survey on recent progress in the field [13, 14]. In addition to a deep learning overview, they discussed the appealing feature for deep neural network (DNN) device accelerator pedal, as well as the research area of customized digital activators for DL. For their conclusion, they outlined what they believe are the next steps in the development of feasible analog-memory-based DNN hardware accelerators.

4.3 Deep Learning in Drug Discovery

In most of the recent studies, ML and DL was proved to have solved various common problems occurring in chemo informatics through novel concepts and approaches along with the predictive performance enhancement of the structure-property models, domain containing the model applicability, structure generation with customized and desirable characteristics and property of modeling of functional endpoint representations such as response curve and phase diagrams and aid in developing species with multiple molecules (Figure 4.3) [15]. Several artificial intelligence applications, including computer vision, diagnosis, and gaming, have benefited

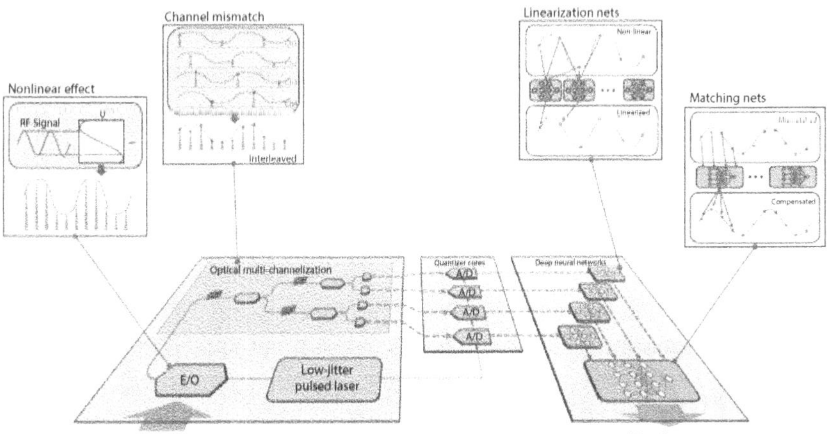

Figure 4.3 Schematic representations of the DL-PADC architecture [15].

from recent advances in DL technologies [16–20]. As a computer-aided drug discovery field, ML is one of the most essential and fastest-evolving topics [21]. Instead of relying on explicit formulae like significant interaction or molecular subtleties replications, ML techniques use design acknowledgement procedures to distinguish mathematical interactions among empirical observations of molecules and extrapolate them to anticipate the characteristics of new complexes. ML algorithms are also more efficient than physical models and can be easily scaled to large datasets even without extensive computing resources.

Using ML to help students recognize and utilize interactions among chemical structures and their bioactivities (SAR) is one of the primary applications of ML in pharmaceutical research [22]. An example of this would be if we had a successful drug candidate and wanted to optimize its selectivity, biological responses, or physiochemical properties. As recently as before fifty years, this type of error can only be solved by a series of expensive and labor-intensive phases of medicinal chemistry syntheses. It is now possible to model quantitative structure-property relationships (QSPR) using modern ML and create AI programs that correctly assess in silico how reactive species might influence biological 5n label [23, 24]. The relationship between the AI, ML and DL is presented in Figure 4.4 [24].

Just after introduction of ML, AI was perhaps the most browsed term on Google in September 2015. While some consider ML to be the major AI implementation, others see it as a subcategory of AI [25, 26]. While AI refers to computer programs that are able to deliberate and act like creatures, ML goes beyond that, allowing the machine to learn without being openly automated with algorithms such as Nave Bayes, decision trees, hidden Markov models, and others. AI advanced further with the evolution of social networks, which allowed machines to classify and organize inputted data much like the brain doe Igor Aizenberg and his co-workers introduced the term "deep learning" for the initial period in the early 20th century, while discussing artificial neural networks (ANN). Development of human efforts starts from AI which covers ML and DL. These three are hand in hand with each other [27]. ML either employs administered learning, in which the model is trained using 5n label data, in which the input is labeled with the desired production tags, or employs unsubstantiated learning, in which the prototypical is practiced using 5n label data and yet makes it look for recurring patterns in the input facts [28]. Remaining include half-supervised learning, which combines controlled and non-controlled learning; self-controlled having to learn, which is a subset of self-supervised learning, which employs a two-step process in which unattended having to learn creates labels for 5n label data and the final aim

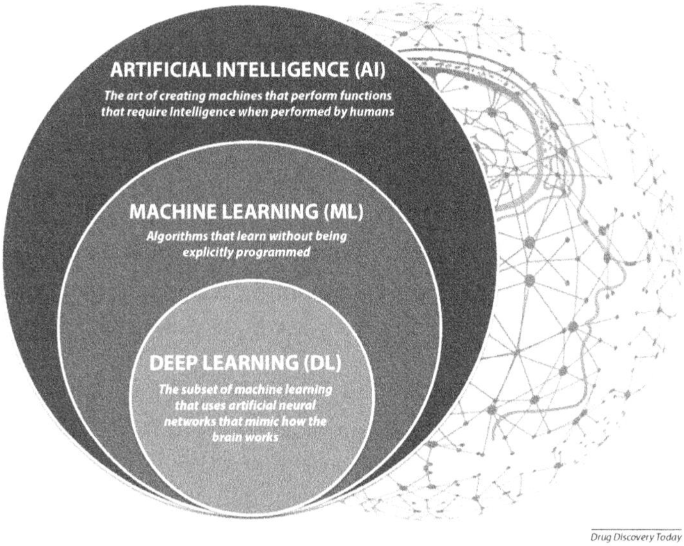

Figure 4.4 Relationship between AI, ML, and DL [24].

is to create a controlled learning prototypical; and strengthened learning, a subset of self-supervised learning [29, 30]. The first model of a neural network was created in 1940s, when McCulloch and Pitts established their article. The DL algorithm is a ML approach that utilizes ANNs with numbers of layers of nonlinear processing units to create a data representation. The advantage of DL in drug discovery will have significant benefit for the drug discovery industry. It takes time and money to discover new drugs, and DL may be used to both expedite and reduce costs. In the past decade, technological progress and the increasing adoption of automated processes have led to the creation and gathering of immense quantities of information and biomedical data [31].

4.4 Chloroquine Analogs

The global health community has struggled to address the worldwide epidemic of coronavirus illness 2019, known as COVID-19, and unfortunately, we do not have any treatment options to combat it. Among the current drugs, only symptomatic relief is provided; the successful use of chloroquine and its equivalents has been demonstrated for the diagnosis of COVID-19 related pneumonia. Chloroquine phosphate and hydroxychloroquine sulphate received FDA approval in March 2020 for the treatment of patients with severe pneumonia who are also infected with SARS-CoV-2. The mode of action of these drugs had been unclear due to a lack of understanding of the SARS-CoV-2, but positive findings have changed that. The global community of researchers has made numerous advances in the creation of chloroquine derivatives with a more effective response to SAR-CoV-2 aims. Due to the fact that computational modeling techniques (homology modeling, molecular docking, molecular dynamic simulation, QSAR, pharmacophore, etc.) are proving to be very much supportive for identifying new agent to slow down the chemical reaction opposite to SARS-CoV-2 targets, the present era has witnessed a substantial amount of progress in this field. Researchers are investigating the use of chloroquine phosphate and its analogs to treat SARS-CoV-2 by introducing various computational procedures. We have discussed recent research that looks at using computer models to develop and discover novel medications against SARS-CoV-2, following the *in-silico* design of chloroquine analogs. The chapter provides a general overview of the field of computational drug discovery and its successes [32, 33].

4.5 Deep Learning in Medical Field

4.5.1 Scientific Study of Skin Diseases

The field of dermatology and other specialties had promising results with DL applications. It is important for modern doctors to know the main elements of DL in order to employ new applications and determine their efficiency and limitations. We will review current and new medical potential of DL in dermatology in the next article of the dual portion series and discuss potential and limitations in the future. Section one of the section provides overview of fundamentals of DL to help medical and technical experts communicate more effectively. The clinical practice of dermatology is greatly enhanced by the advances, solutions, and support offered by DL. It has been proven that DL applications can accurately identify skin diseases that are common among dermatologists. Further refinements and rigorous validation are needed in prospective randomized controlled trials to make sure that patients receive proper care and are safe, to make dermatologists and dermato-pathologists more productive, and to ensure patients have access to dermatologic care of high quality [34, 35].

4.5.2 Anatomical Laparoscopy

The recent tendency in therapeutic audiovisual system enhancement is to use images of various modalities for analysis and visualization, like slender band pictures or fluorescent pictures. The technique of detecting positions in laparoscopic picture is proposed. It is dependent on DL technologies and utilizes extra details obtained since fluorescent pictures. The primary element is a minimal data set of images acquired in white light for CNN training and for retrieving extra details from high-resolution images acquired during ICG laparoscopy using traditional ML methods. When compared to methods based on CNN, the mixture of CNN strategy and ML strategy for fluorescent information use improves the quality of landmarks segmentation. On real laparoscopic images, the proposed method was evaluated [36].

4.5.3 Angiography

Clinical and vascular computed tomography (CT) imagery properties of affected role were studied to support clinicians in analyzing affected role with atherosclerosis, according to the study. Rapamycin (RAPA) was given to 316 affected roles with arteries disease that were hospitalized for urgency healing on a patient's coronary computed tomography angiography (CCTA), a set of delineated LVM was chosen as the area of interest for imaging. Eighty percent of the CCTA images were randomly selected for training, and the remaining 20% of the CCTA images were verified. Under different correlation thresholds, the correlation matrix method was utilized to detect small picture elements. About 40 times maximum than physically divided input, CCTA diagnostic parameters were used for validation. There was a 91.6% average similarity coefficient among the dice. With a segmentation time of 0.51 seconds, the anticipated technique also shaped very minor centroid distances and volume differences. Because of

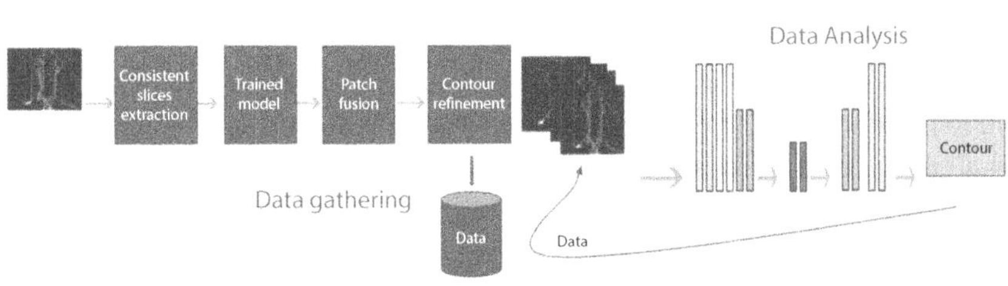

Figure 4.5 CT analysis [38].

this, the DL model was able to accurately identify a patient's atherosclerotic lesion area, as well as measure and assist in the diagnosis of long-term atherosclerosis clinical cases. Atherosclerosis diagnosis and treatment effect analysis could be greatly aided by it [37–39].

Despite this, some flaws in the research. Atherosclerosis affected role were added in this investigation, but only 100 CCTA images were randomly selected and continuously used for model training. For future myocardium segmentation on CCTA data captured by health facilities and CT scanning equipment, the outcomes would be further validated (Figure 4.5). Since each doctor has different expertise and experience, each doctor's left ventricular myocardium contour labeling will be different, and this DL algorithm will not be able to correct such differences. As a result, just symptoms suggestive or confirmed coronary artery disease is eligible to participate in this study. Further research is needed on the outcomes of the myocardial technique in sick people with other illnesses and at different developmental stages. Lastly, the model is still in its infancy, and it is not yet known how much it will reduce the requirement of dentists in clinical practice. The future of research must be enhanced [40].

4.5.4 Interpretation of Wound

While DL applications are considered revolutionary in a variety of medical specialties, notwithstanding the graphic nature of the field, forensic implementations have been scarce. For instance, a crime science diagnostician may gain after DL-based instruments for interpreting shooting wounds. Main objective of this proof-of-concept training was to determine whether trained neural network architectures are capable of predicting shooting distance class from a basic photo of a gunfire wound. Data for 204 gunshot wound images was collected from piglet carcasses shot with a 0.22 Long Rifle pistol. To accurately classify images based on their shooting distance, neural net architectures were trained, validated, and tested using a set of data. The AI developer software was used for in-depth learning. According to the investigation, the multilayer perceptron-based (MLP 24 16 24) prototype obtained a 98% testing accuracy. During testing, the trained model correctly identified all of the deleterious, communication, and close-range shots, but incorrectly identified one long-range shot. Our study proved that using DL-based tools to aid gunshot wound interpretation will be beneficial to medical examiners in the future. We anticipate that these findings will assist as a foundation for upcoming educations on wound interpretation classification schemes of greater scale [25, 41, 42]. The wound variants is presented in Figure 4.6 [40].

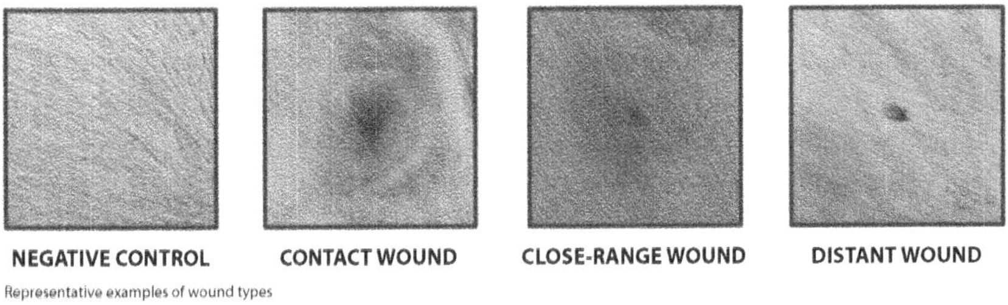

Figure 4.6 Wound variants [40].

In this experimental study, researchers were looking into the capability of DL algorithms to accurately determine gunshot range from photos of gunshot wounds. Among our 204-image data set, a multilayer perceptron-based deep network was most accurate, with a checking precision of 98 %. Such results suggest that we should conduct further research on larger-scale forensic wound interpretation algorithms. However, in medical specialties, like forensics, AI and DL submissions have been uncommon, and prior research has focused on subjects other than forensic pathology. The first study we are aware of that investigates DL when interpreting gunshot wounds. Data were collected from four types of gunshot wounds: contact shot, close-range shot, distant shot, and a control group with no bullet wounds. The DL approach had the distinct visual characteristics of each wound type as its foundation. The multilayer perceptron-based model, which is extremely well trained, got everything right in the independent testing set with its 100% accuracy for identifying negatives, contact shots, and close-range shots, but it incorrectly classified one faraway shot as a negative control (88.9 %) [43, 44].

The results of this research recommend that criminological diagnosticians may advantage from using DL procedures to analyze gunshot wounds. Although the study was small (only 204 photographs since 19 piggie remains) and restricted to individual kinds of gunfire wounds, the primary limitations of the study are not surprising. While this initial research used only one weapon type and caliber, more educations are required to see how DL handles a dataset with more variation. External validation sets were not used in this study, apart from those used for training and testing the algorithms. We also did not evaluate the algorithm's performance against the gold standard. Due to this, the current algorithm is extremely limited in its use in external settings. Because this study was only a proof-of-concept, and because the best-performing algorithm had high classification accuracy, it appears evident that more research is required to create stronger and broadly relevant algorithms for criminological use. The next step should be to implement efficient algorithms that use a broad range of images to train on human tissue. A better model for calculating shooting distance would be one that continuously adjusts, rather than being set at a discrete value. Other indices to be measured might include the type of weapon, the kind of bullet, and bullet trajectory, or, on a broader scale, virtually any relevant wound (such as missile injuries, blunt trauma, or virtually any forensically significant lesion). A fantastic environment for rigorous scientific research would be provided by huge, multi-facility image libraries. Due to legal limitations, ML is not yet widely used for generating evidence that is both reliable and understandable. While AI is capable of displaying bias in its application of datasets and evaluations of events, it is difficult to identify it as a witness in the courthouse [45]. We hope that in the future, DL algorithms will give forensic pathologists the means to reconstruct the events of the crime. This would be, for example, assisting the forensic pathologist with the screening of large datasets for a particular detail or showing sources of opportunity involvement. Notably, the forensic pathologist would always retain final interpretation authority. A DL algorithm, with a trained model, proved to be 98% accurate in predicting the type of gunshot wound (close-range shot, contact shot, or long-range shot) from a single photo of a gunshot wound. This study showed promising results for larger studies into the application of DL to forensic wound interpretation [46, 47].

4.5.5 Molecular Docking

While the severity of SARS CoV-2 has only recently been discovered, the disease has already proven to be a grave threat to global public health. At the moment, there is no available medication or vaccine to combat SARS-CoV-2. Drug repurposing, or the use of existing drugs to treat new diseases, represents a timely method to discover effective SARS-CoV-2 treatments in this pressing situation. Experiments are being performed to find new uses for drugs, and computational approaches are increasingly being used and become increasingly efficient. Here, we introduce a sound experimental approach that combines DL with molecular docking trials to recognize hopeful applicants for the treatment of COVID-19, all of which are currently FDA-approved drugs. Our team has developed a new DL method called deep DTA to identify drug-protein bonding attractions characterized as KIBA scores for 24 SARS-CoV-2 viral proteins. The docking simulations were done using FDA-recognized drugs with the top KIBA scores. It was simulated docking of 168 individual drugs, including those with both experimentally confirmed and predicted activity. Our group adopted a new, high-throughput virtual flow screening platform to significantly decrease the amount of time needed to run a total of 50,000 simulations. In that 49 FDA-approved drugs with AutoDockvina binding affinity values and highest consensus KIBA scores is created for use in the fight against SARS-CoV-2 [48].

4.5.6 Breast Cancer Detection

High-density breasts have received scrutiny for mammographic sensitivity. Also, a high density of breast tissue is associated with an increased chance of developing breast cancer. Despite its advantages, digital breast tomosynthesis (DBT) has not been widely accepted in screening for a variety of reasons. It remains to be seen how DL-based computer-aided detection systems are affected by the variations in breast density. A computer-aided detection program using DL techniques was used to grade the likelihood of cancer on a scale of 1 to 10. 13838 mammograms were taken. A BIRADS density score was available for each case. A total of 11, 51, 73, and 22 cancers were represented in the different BIRADS categories. A Kruskal-Wallis test for those with cancer diagnoses yielded $P=0.9225$, indicating no statistically significant differences. Similarly, in patients who did not have cancer, the density categories had a significant difference ($P<0.0001$). While some risk categories have uniformly high risk values across all density categories, cancer cases show the opposite trend. Even women with dense breasts can benefit from DL and improved screening sensitivity [49, 50].

4.5.7 Polycystic Organs

The assessment of disease progression and drug efficiency relies on volumetric. While accurate and rapid methods for volumetry have not yet been developed, this has hindered the development of PKLD therapies, as volumetry has not yet been widely implemented in clinical practice. This study uses AI-based volumetry for PKLD to be presented. In the first instance, AI performance was measured. We used deep CNN to learn from CT scans of ADPKD patients who were segmented into 175 areas, which were verified by three experts and agreed upon with images of 214 patients using volumetry. An interobserver correlation coefficient, Dice similarity coefficient, and Bland–Altman plots were created for 39 separations in the authentication set. Following this, DSC and ICC comparison of AI parting of 50 arbitrary CT imageries with significant outcome. The AI's DSC and ICC were 0.961 and 0.999729, respectively. Roughly 95% of CT scans had an error rate within 3 % (46.2% error <1 %, 48.7 % error 1 % ≤error<3 %). AI demonstrated a mixed level of success when compared to specialists. The AI-based volumetry for PKLD was both fast, accurate. This finding implies that AI could be applied in clinical settings, where human specialists perform similarly [46, 51, 52].

4.5.8 Bone Tissue

Using ML, imaging and analysis techniques can be transformed for healthcare applications, which will offer automation and improved accuracy and efficiency in diagnostics and treatment, as well as give insight into the mechanics of tissue deformation and fracture. We describe a novel investigation that uses CNNs, ResNet, and transfer learning to classify and predict motorized conditions of cortical and trabecular bone tissue from synchrotron-radiation microcomputed tomography pictures developed in uniaxial nonstop solidity in situ. To solve this challenge, we conducted an experiment on a dataset with more than three million samples. For the cortical and trabecular bone, with optimized CNN constructions, we gained skilled replicas those confidential new imageries among unsuccessful and unspoiled lessons with over 98% correctness. Our results attained 98% correctness on the dataset, after utilizing a pre-trained ResNet. This suggests that influential classifiers for synchrotron-radiation micro-computed tomography CT imageries can be established even with rare in imitable exercise trials and that doing so may help further development by incorporating more data and training methods [53, 54].

4.5.9 Interaction Drug-Target

The coronavirus (SARS-CoV-2) has been found in Wuhan, China, and it is rapidly spreading, with a rising incidence rate worldwide. This has a number of drug options because of the scarcity of effective treatment options, so China is testing various strategies, including drug repurposing. Despite the fact that blocks the ability of HIV, ritonavir, and darunavir are planned to attack virus-related proteinases, they are each unique. In forecast, however, it may also bind to replication complex SARS-CoV-2 components with Kd< 1000 nM inhibitor power. As well, we found that Kaletra (lopinavir/ritonavir) and other antiviral agents can be used to treat SARS-CoV-2 (Figure 4.7). We advise giving the MT-DTI model's list of antiviral drugs some consideration when devising effective SARS-CoV-2 treatment strategies [55].

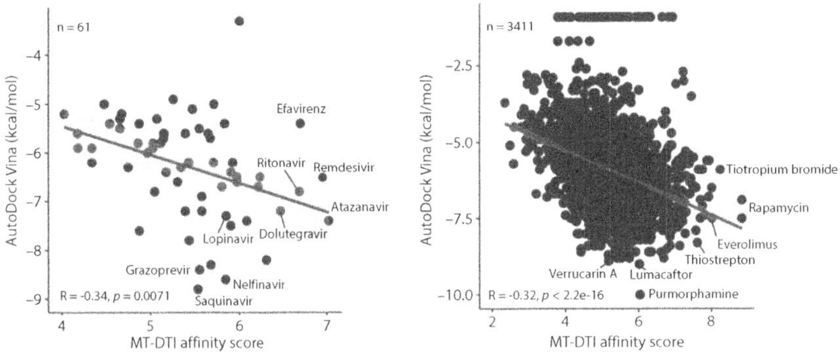

Figure 4.7 Drug target interaction score [32].

4.5.10 Pancreatic Issue Prediction

A model for the post-surgical recurrence of pancreatic neuroendocrine tumors (PNETs) by using preoperative CT images was modeled and authenticated. Our team gathered data on 74 people with pNENs by retrospectively reviewing the pathology of their tumors. The radiologists, radiomics, and DL radiomics (DLR) used a previously established internal group of models to train and evaluate CT findings to predict the 5-year pNEN recurrence. A, V, and AV arterial, venous, and arterial and venous contrast phases were established for radiomics and DLR models. The patients were divided and clinical information was added to the optimal model, which was then further developed. DLR-A model best reflected optimal function, which was improved from an AUC of 0.80 to 0.83 with additional clinical data. The AUC of the model used to gauge CT findings was 0.52. There was a significant difference in the DLR-A versus random models in the validation group. There was a significant difference in recurrence-free survival between high- and low-risk groups. The preoperative recurrence prediction model for pNEN patients after radical surgery was successfully created using DLR. This enables the assessment of pNEN recurrence risk and will help clinicians make better decisions [56–58].

4.5.11 Prediction of Carcinoma in Cells

KIRCC, a cancer that causes fatalities, can occur in those with kidney sickness. DeepSurv employs a depth feed-forward neural network and a Cox proportional threats occupation to deliver optimized existence consequences. The DeepSurv algorithm was improved to better identify the treatment candidates based on overall mortality for subjects with KIRCC. All of the KIRCC bodily alteration protein variants were retrieved from the TCGA-KIRC database. In DeepSurv+, an enhanced accuracy of 95.1 % was discovered, having found 610 high-risk variants related to mortality. In contrast, the initial DeepSurv model only found 485. The tRNA required to charge route, the D-myo-inositol-5-phosphate various metabolic passageway, the DNA double-strand disruption overhaul by non-homologous end-joining trail, the super pathway of phosphate substances, the 3-phosphoinositide environment is characterized, the manufacturing of nitric oxides and oxygen in phagocytes passageway, the synaptic long-term anxiety passageway, the semen movement trail, and the involvement of JAK2 in hormone-like cytokine up-regulation were all discovered. In this research, the biological findings imply that the KIRCC pathways related to cancer cell development, cancer cell variation, and resistant reply reserve are more likely to be linked to cancer. The project's findings indicated that the upgraded DeepSurv model could accurately identify high-risk variants linked to mortality and identify the candidate genes. High-risk variants that increase KIRCC mortality are well recognized by the proposed model in the context of KIRCC overall mortality [59].

Automatic analysis and visualization of medical images with multiple wavelengths are explored. This also includes a variety of methods for presenting multispectral images. The projected technique is dependent on the synthesis of an image from a white light source and an image from an image in the near infrared channel. One of the benefits is that the data are presented in the form of a special level map that takes into account the way the human eye works. The CIEDE2000 metric is used to calculate the quality of a visualization. The preprocessing and improvement of the white light image is a focal point. The article explores different approaches to the use of ML, DL, and a combination of the two for cancer diagnosis using medical multi-spectral imaging. DL's benefits can be fully realized in a constrained database through the combined approach. The methods and algorithms described in are each demonstrated by real-world applications [60, 61].

4.5.12 Determining Parkinson's

There are indications that adenosine receptors may be utilized as a method of treatment for Parkinson's disease (PD). For this project, the authors used DL, pharmacophore models, and docking to discover dual adenosine A1 and A2A receptor antagonists. Of the nineteen hits found in the ChemDiv library, the two compounds with the greatest strong bonding attraction and aggressive nature for A1/A2A ARs at the nanomolar level had a 1,2,4-triazole scaffold. Two more MD simulations provided strong evidence of bonding relations of the A1/A2A ARs with two compounds. Of particular interest are the 1,2,4-triazole by-products, which are the greatest strong dual A1/A2A AR rivals found in our education and might help as a foundation for future research. This new method of multistage screening can be used to identify strong drug binders for other targets [62, 63].

For the treatment of this disease, it was explored several in silico screening methods that incorporated DL, pharmacophore, and molecular docking to test over 1 million molecules in the ChemDiv library. At first, the cAMP functional assay showed five compounds with pIC50 values of 4.20 to 6.78, which were found to have antagonist activity toward A1/A2AAR. Six of the eight compounds, all of which displayed antagonistic activity for A1AR and A2AAR (pIC50s of 4.20–6.78), were also found to bind A1/A2A ARs (pKi values of 4.71–7.49). The bonding attraction and functional movement with pKi values at the nanomolar range were shown by C8 and C9, which have the highest Ki values (pKi of 7.16–7.49 and pIC50 of 6.31–6.78). New 1,2,4-triazole by-products C8 and C9 are a new dual A1/A2A AR antagonist (Figure 4.8). According to the MD simulations of the A1/A2A ARs with C8 and C9, the interaction is very strong. C8 and C9 both demonstrated promise for future development of anti-disease Parkinson's agents following optimization (Figure 4.9) [64–67].

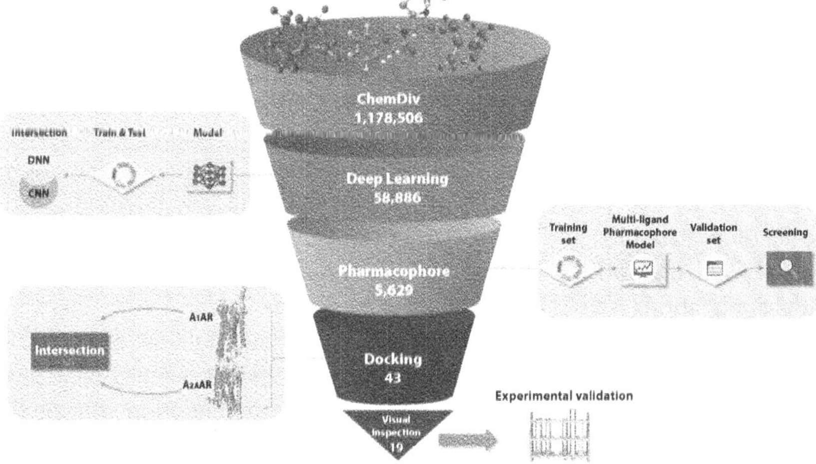

Figure 4.8 Process for Parkinson's [64].

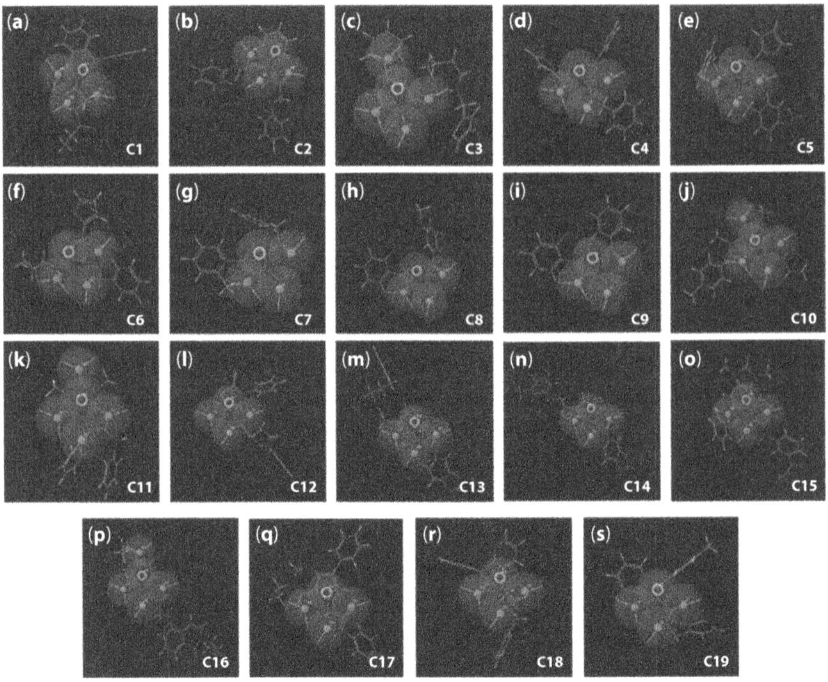

Figure 4.9 Parkinson's analysis [64].

4.5.13 Segregating Cells

The research for cell-based healing approaches for vital nervous scheme illnesses is hampered by challenge of predicting and detecting the diversity of neural stem cells (NSCs) into neurons. We conjecture that DL will be able to pull out minutiae from larger datasets, and that a deep neural network can be used to identify fate of NSCs with a greater degree of reliability. Furthermore, our method provides greater accuracy of the system when evaluated in numerous, self-reliant, intended situations that showcase innumerable persuaders, with neurotrophic factor, hormone, little molecular structures and small elements. We expect that our neural network-based method for finding NSCs will expedite the advancement of NSC applications [68–71].

Despite the tantalizing prospects of NSC transplantation, the difficult task of directing NSC differentiation to specific cell types presents a challenge. Biomarkers are commonly used to detect cell differentiation during the neurogenesis process. During the process, cell characteristics are evaluated. Although studies of various NSC fate factors are abundant, it is still unclear exactly how neurons are formed, especially because early cellular changes in the developmental process are hard to identify. An identification procedure that is applicable to any effective substance, regardless of what pathways they may follow, is necessary to support the advancement of effective agents in the treatment of neurodegenerative diseases and neurological injuries. Instrumentation for data collection is enhanced, but one of the greatest obstacles is that data gathered is often unintelligible due to current device limitations [72–76]. The stem cell analysis is presented in Figure 4.10 [73].

Existing approaches rely heavily on human cognition, but it is difficult for humans to see small changes in cellular morphologies or predict the results of drug interactions [77–80]. DL makes it possible to extract features automatically by using vast datasets to solve challenging problems in the biomedical field. To maximize the use of individual cells, we decided to make use of DL and identify NSC differentiation prospectively [81–84].

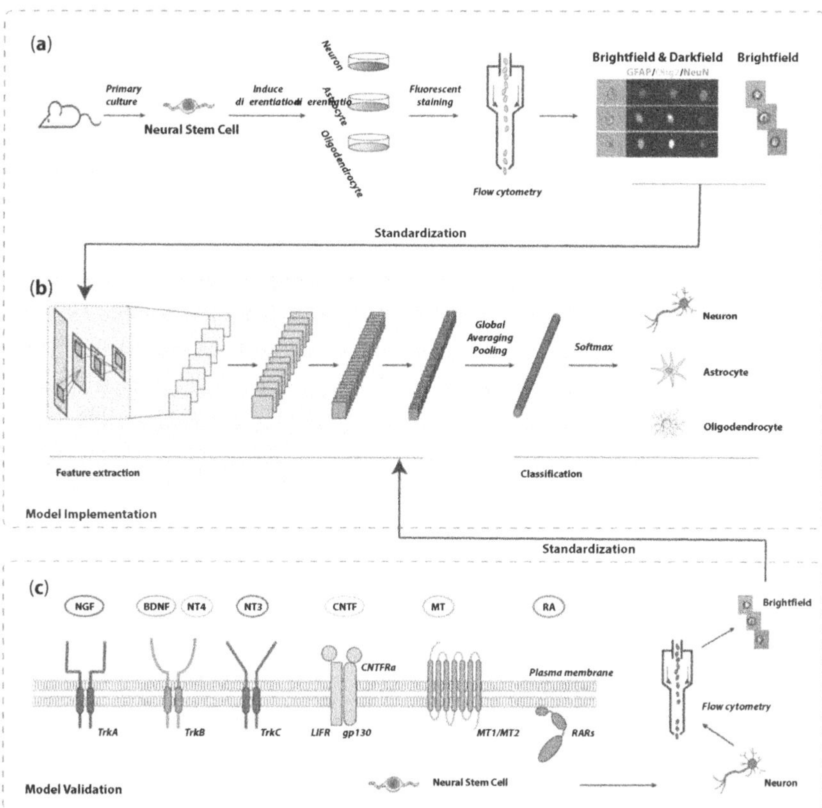

Figure 4.10 Stem cell analysis [73].

4.6 Conclusion

Recent researches pointed out that DL has penetrated into healthcare and drug delivery systems. ML techniques were characterized by the levels of modeling, statistical inference modes, various facets of data types, matching between input and outputs, duality of the models and their inference. From all the above discussions, it could be stated that the latest advancements in DL techniques had influenced the frontline fields like drug delivery and medicine. In drug discovery field, chemical structure data fusion, and evaluation of model efficiency progressing towards the relevant end points may fuel the advancements in AI technologies in that field. Quantum ML is the upcoming technique that is currently employed in drug delivery systems based on biochemical efforts. In order to improve the classical ML algorithms and quantum techniques, quantum physics are combined with the principles of ML so that this emerges as a most critical tool in drug delivery. AI techniques along with advanced DL may bring up new facets in computer industry through the reduction of work demand, time and cost during the early phase of the application. In the near future, scope for further expanding the applicability of these techniques can be made by generating novel finger-print reading systems and progressing towards the supplementary criteria development for the accurate chemical system presentation. Learned features and theory trained models can also be developed from the DL models which were readily available and plastic in nature which kindles the further developments. In the medical field, DL enhanced the process of clinical diagnosis and multiple analog decision making in majority of the medical domain. Yet, adaptation of the medical practitioners to evolve as interpreters, integrators of information, supporters of patients and being a part of medical education system has been a great challenge to them. If it is done, then DL serves as an excellent tool to provide them the required advanced methods for practicing.

References

1. Rey, A., *Dictionnaire historique de la langue française*, Dictionnaires Le Robert, Paris, 1992.
2. Varnek, A. and Baskin, I., Machine learning methods for property prediction in chemoinformatics: Quo Vadis? *J. Chem. Inf. Model.*, 52, 1413, 2012.
3. Ali, S.M., Hoemann, M.Z., Aubé, J., Georg, G.I., Mitscher, L.A., Jayasinghe, L.R., Butitaxel analogues: Synthesis and structure-activity relationships. *J. Med. Chem.*, 40, 236, 1997.

4. Saravana Kumar, A., MaivizhiSelvi, P., Rajeshkumar, L., Delamination in drilling of sisal/banana reinforced composites produced by hand lay-up process. *Appl. Mech. Mater.*, 867, 29, 2017.
5. Cherkasov, A., Muratov, E.N., Fourches, D., Varnek, A., Baskin, I.I., Cronin, M., Dearden, J., Gramatica, P., Martin, Y.C., Todeschini, R., Consonni, V., QSAR modeling: Where have you been? Where are you going to? *J. Med. Chem.*, 57, 4977, 2014.
6. Drug discovery and development, 2021, April 7, Retrieved June 24, 2021, from https://chem.libretexts.org/@go/page/227708.
7. Ramesh, M. and Rajeshkumar, L., Wood flour filled thermoset composites, in: *Thermoset composites: preparation, properties and applications*, vol. 38, p. 33, Materials Research Foundations, Millersville, PA 17551, United States, 2018.
8. Badillo, S., Banfai, B., Birzele, F., Davydov, I.I., Hutchinson, L., Kam-Thong, T., Siebourg-Polster, J., Steiert, B., Zhang, J.D., An introduction to machine learning. *Clin. Pharmacol. Ther.*, 107, 871, 2020, https://doi.org/10.1002/cpt.1796.
9. Majumdar, D., Trends in pattern recognition and machine learning. *Def. Sci. J.*, 1985, https://doi.org/10.14429/dsj.35.6027.
10. Ramesh, M. and Kumar, L.R., Bioadhesives, in: *Green adhesives*, Inamuddin, R., Boddula, M.I., Ahamed, Asiri, A.M. (Eds.), p. 1 46, 2020, ust be carefully dried [44, 45-167.
11. Aggarwal, M. and Murty, M.N., Deep Learning, in: *Springer Briefs in Applied Sciences and Technology*, 2021, https://doi.org/10.1007/978-981-33-4022-0_3.
12. Gupta, R., Srivastava, D., Sahu, M., Tiwari, S., Ambasta, R.K., Kumar, P., Artificial intelligence to deep learning: Machine intelligence approach for drug discovery. *Mol. Divers.*, 25, 1315, 2021, https://doi.org/10.1007/s11030-021-10217-3.
13. Schmidhuber, J., Deep learning in neural networks: an overview. *Neural Netw.*, 61, 85, 2015, https://doi.org/10.1016/j.neunet.2014.09.003.
14. Ramesh, M., Rajeshkumar, L., Bhuvaneshwari, V., Bamboo fiber reinforced composites, in: *Bamboo Fiber Composites. Composites Science and Technology*, M. Jawaid, S. Mavinkere Rangappa, S. Siengchin (Eds.), Springer, Singapore, 2021, https://doi.org/10.1007/978-981-15-8489-3_1.
15. Xu, S., Zou, X., Ma, B., Chen, J., Yu, L., Zou, W., Deep-learning-powered photonic analog-to-digital conversion. *Light Sci. Appl.*, l8, 66, 2019.
16. Hu, Y.H. and Hwang, J.N., Introduction to neural networks for signal processing, in: *Handbook of Neural Network Signal Processing*, pp. 12–41, CRC Press, Boca Raton, FL, 2001.
17. Angermueller, C., Pärnamaa, T., Parts, L., Stegle, O., Deep learning for computational biology. *Mol. Syst. Biol.*, 12, 878, 2016, https://doi.org/10.15252/msb.20156651.
18. McCulloch, W.S. and Pitts, W., A logical calculus of the ideas immanent in nervous activity. *Bull. Math. Biophys.*, 5, 115, 1943.

19. Ramesh, M., Deepa, C., Kumar, L.R., Sanjay, M.R., Siengchin, S., Life-cycle and environmental impact assessments on processing of plant fibres and its bio-composites: A critical review. *J. Ind. Text.*, 2020, https://doi.org/10.1177/1528083720924730.
20. Gawehn, E., Hiss, J.A., Schneider, G., Deep learning in drug discovery. *Mol. Inform.*, 35, 3, 2016.
21. Papadatos, G., Gaulton, A., Hersey, A., Overington, J.P., Activity, assay and target data curation and quality in the ChEMBL database. *J. Comput. Aided Mol. Des.*, 29, 885, 2015.
22. Kim, S., Thiessen, P.A., Bolton, E.E., Chen, J., Fu, G., Gindulyte, A., Han, L., He, J., He, S., Shoemaker, B.A., Wang, J., PubChem substance and compound databases. *Nucleic Acids Res.*, 44, D1202, 2016.
23. Balaji, D., Ramesh, M., Kannan, T., Deepan, S., Bhuvaneswari, V., Rajeshkumar, L., Experimental investigation on mechanical properties of banana/snake grass fiber reinforced hybrid composites. *Mater. Today: Proc.*, 42, 350, 2021.
24. Lavecchia, A., Deep learning in drug discovery: Opportunities, challenges and future prospects. *Drug Discovery Today*, 24, 2017, 2019.
25. Lecun, Y., Bengio, Y., Hinton, G., Deep learning. *Nature*, 521, 436, 2015.
26. Ramesh, M., Deepa, C., Tamil Selvan, M., Rajeshkumar, L., Balaji, D., Bhuvaneswari, V., Mechanical and water absorption properties of calotropis gigantea plant fibers reinforced polymer composites. *Mater. Today: Proc.*, 46, 3367, 2020.
27. Krizhevsky, A., Sutskever, I., Hinton, G.E., Image Net classification with deep convolutional neural networks. *Adv. Neural Inf. Process. Syst.*, 25, 1097, 2012.
28. Tompson, J.J., Jain, A., LeCun, Y., Bregler, C., Joint training of a convolutional network and a graphical model for human pose estimation. *Adv. Neural Inf. Process. Syst.*, 2, 1799, 2014.
29. Anthimopoulos, M., Christodoulidis, S., Ebner, L., Christe, A., Mougiakakou, S., Lung pattern classification for interstitial lung diseases using a deep convolutional neural network. *IEEE Trans. Med. Imaging*, 35, 1207, 2016.
30. Bhuvaneswari, V., Priyadharshini, M., Deepa, C., Balaji, D., Rajeshkumar, L., Ramesh, M., Deep learning for material synthesis and manufacturing systems: A review. *Mater. Today: Proc.*, 46, 3263, 2021.
31. Silver, D., Schrittwieser, J., Simonyan, K., Antonoglou, I., Huang, A., Guez, A., Hubert, T., Baker, L., Lai, M., Bolton, A., Chen, Y., Mastering the game of Go without human knowledge. *Nature*, 550, 354, 2017.
32. Beck, B.R., Shin, B., Choi, Y., Park, S., Kang, K., Predicting commercially available antiviral drugs that may act on the novel coronavirus (SARS-CoV-2) through a drug-target interaction deep learning model. *Comput. Struct. Biotechnol. J.*, 18, 784, 2020.
33. Tsai, H., Ambrogio, S., Narayanan, P., Shelby, R.M., Burr, G.W., Recent progress in analog memory-based accelerators for deep learning. *J. Phys. D: Appl. Phys.*, 51, 283001, 2018.

34. Kumar, V. and Roy, K., Computational modeling of chloroquine analogues for development of drugs against novel coronavirus (nCoV), in: *Silico Modeling of Drugs Against Coronaviruses. Methods in Pharmacology and Toxicology*, K. Roy (Ed.), Humana, New York, NY, 2021, https://doi.org/10.1007/7653_2020_55.
35. Ramesh, M., Maniraj, J., Rajeshkumar, L., Biocomposites for energy storage, in: *Biobased Composites: Processing, Characterization, Properties, and Applications*, A. Khan, S.M. Rangappa, S. Siengchin, A.M. Asiri (Eds.), pp. 123–142, Wiley Online Library, Hoboken, NJ, USA, 2021.
36. Puri, P., Comfere, N., Drage, L.A., Shamim, H., Bezalel, S.A., Pittelkow, M.R., Davis, M.D., Wang, M., Mangold, A.R., Tollefson, M.M., Lehman, J.S., Deep learning for dermatologists: Part II. Current applications. *J. Am. Acad. Dermatol.*, 2021, https://doi.org/10.1016/j.jaad.2020.05.053.
37. Pozdeev, A.A., Obukhova, N.A., Motyko, A.A., Anatomical landmarks detection for laparoscopic surgery based on deep learning technology, in: *2021 IEEE Conference of Russian Young Researchers in Electrical and Electronic Engineering (ElConRus)*, pp. 1668–1672, 2021.
38. Ji, F., Zhou, S., Bi, Z., Computed tomography angiography under deep learning in the treatment of atherosclerosis with rapamycin. *J. Healthc. Eng.*, 4543702, 2021, https://doi.org/10.1155/2021/4543702.
39. Ramesh, M., Rajeshkumar, L., Balaji, D., Bhuvaneswari, V., Green composite using agricultural waste reinforcement, in: *Green Composites. Materials Horizons: From Nature to Nanomaterials*, S. Thomas and P. Balakrishnan (Eds.), pp. 21–34, Springer, Singapore, 2021.
40. Oura, P., Junno, A., Junno, J.A., Deep learning in forensic gunshot wound interpretation—A proof-of-concept study. *Int. J. Legal Med.*, 135, 2101, 2021.
41. Hosny, A., Parmar, C., Quackenbush, J., Schwartz, L.H., Aerts, H.J., Artificial intelligence in radiology. *Nat. Rev. Cancer*, 18, 500, 2018.
42. Frykberg, R.G. and Banks, J., Challenges in the treatment of chronic wounds. *Adv. Wound Care (New Rochelle)*, 4, 560, 2015.
43. Ramesh, M. and Rajeshkumar, L., Technological advances in analyzing of soil chemistry, in: *Applied Soil Chemistry*, Inamuddin, M.I. Ahamed, R. Boddula, T. Altalhi (Eds.), pp. 61–78, Wiley-Scrivener Publishing LLC, USA, 2021.
44. Yu, K.H., Beam, A.L., Kohane, I.S., Artificial intelligence in healthcare. *Nat. Biomed. Eng.*, 2, 719, 2018.
45. Rajkomar, A., Dean, J., Kohane, I., Machine learning in medicine. *N. Engl. J. Med.*, 380, 1347, 2019.
46. Margagliotti, G. and Bollé, T., Machine learning & forensic science. *Forensic Sci. Int.*, 298, 138, 2019.
47. Ramesh, M., Rajeshkumar, L., Balaji, D., Aerogels for insulation applications, in: *Aerogels II: Preparation, Properties and Applications*, vol. 98, Inamuddin (Ed.), pp. 57–76, Materials Research Foundations, United states, 2021.
48. Nikita, E. and Nikitas, P., On the use of machine learning algorithms in forensic anthropology. *Legal Med.*, 47, 101771, 2020.

49. Fan, F., Ke, W., Wu, W., Tian, X., Lyu, T., Liu, Y., Liao, P., Dai, X., Chen, H., Deng, Z., Automatic human identification from panoramic dental radiographs using the convolutional neural network. *Forensic Sci. Int.*, 314, 110416, 2020.
50. Ramesh, M., Rajeshkumar, L., Deepa, C., Tamil Selvan, M., Kushvaha, V., Asrofi, M., Impact of silane treatment on characterization of Ipomoea Staphylina plant fiber reinforced epoxy composites. *J. Nat. Fibers*, 2021, https://doi.org/10.1080/15440478.2021.1902896.
51. Ramesh, M., Rajeshkumar, L., Balaji, D., Influence of process parameters on the properties of additively manufactured fiber-reinforced polymer composite materials: A review. *J. Mater. Eng. Perform.*, 30, 4792, 2021.
52. Peña-Solórzano, C.A., Albrecht, D.W., Bassed, R.B., Burke, M.D., Dimmock, M.R., Findings from machine learning in clinical medical imaging applications–Lessons for translation to the forensic setting. *Forensic Sci. Int.*, 110538, 2020.
53. Porto, L.F., Lima, L.N.C., Franco, A., Pianto, D., Machado, C.E.P., de Barros Vidal, F., Estimating sex and age from a face: A forensic approach using machine learning based on photo-anthropometric indexes of the Brazilian population. *Int. J. Legal Med.*, 134, 2239, 2020.
54. Ramesh, M., Rajeshkumar, L., Balaji, D., Mechanical and dynamic properties of ramie fiber reinforced composites, in: *Mechanical and Dynamic Properties of Biocomposites*, R. Nagarajan, S.M.K. Thiagamani, S. Krishnasamy, S. Siengchin (Eds.), pp. 275–322, Wiley, Germany, 2021.
55. Saukko, P. and Knight, B., *Knight's forensic pathology*, CRC Press, Boca Raton, FL, 2015.
56. Dolinak, D., Matshes, E., Lew, E.O., *Forensic pathology: Principles and practice*, Elsevier, Amsterdam, Boston, 2005.
57. Ramesh, M., Rajeshkumar, L., Balaji, D., Bhuvaneswari, V., Sivalingam, S., Self-healable conductive materials, in: *Self-Healing Smart Materials*, Inamuddin, M.I. Ahamed, R. Boddula, T.A. Altalhi (Eds.), pp. 297–320, Wiley, United States, 2021.
58. Ramesh, M., Rajeshkumar, L., Saravanakumar, R., Mechanically-induced self-healable materials, in: *Self-Healing Smart Materials*, Inamuddin, M.I. Ahamed, R. Boddula, T.A. Altalhi (Eds.), pp. 379–404, Wiley, United States, 2021.
59. Denton, J.S., Segovia, A., Filkins, J.A., Practical pathology of gunshot wounds. *Arch. Pathol. Lab. Med.*, 130, 1283, 2006.
60. Gless, S., AI in the courtroom: A comparative analysis of machine evidence in criminal trials. *Geo. J. Int'l L.*, 51, 195, 2019.
61. Anwar, M.U., Adnan, F., Abro, A., Khan, M.R., Rehman, A.U., Osama, M., Javed, S., Baig, A., Shabbir, M.R., Assir, M.Z., *Combined deep learning and molecular docking simulations approach identifies potentially effective FDA approved drugs for repurposing against SARS-CoV-2, ChemRxiv*, Cambridge Open Engage, Cambridge, 2020.

62. Ramesh, M., Deepa, C., Niranjana, K., Rajeshkumar, L., Bhoopathi, R., Balaji, D., Influence of Haritaki (Terminalia chebula) nano-powder on thermo-mechanical, water absorption and morphological properties of Tindora (Coccinia grandis) tendrils fiber reinforced epoxy composites. *J. Nat. Fibers*, 2021, https://doi.org/10.1080/15440478.2021.1921660.
63. Dustler, M., Dahlblom, V., Tingberg, A., Zackrisson, S., The effect of breast density on the performance of deep learning-based breast cancer detection methods for mammography, in: *15th International Workshop on Breast Imaging (IWBI2020)*, vol. 11513, p. 1151324, 2020.
64. Wang, M., Hou, S., Wei, Y., Li, D., Lin, J., Discovery of novel dual adenosine A1/A2A receptor antagonists using deep learning, pharmacophore modeling and molecular docking. *PLoS Comput. Biol.*, 17, e1008821, 2021.
65. Shin, T.Y., Kim, H., Lee, J.H., Choi, J.S., Min, H.S., Cho, H., Kim, K., Kang, G., Kim, J., Yoon, S., Park, H., Expert-level segmentation using deep learning for volumetry of polycystic kidney and liver. *Investig. Clin. Urol.*, 61, 555, 2020.
66. Shen, S.C.Y., Fernández, M.P., Tozzi, G., Buehler, M.J., Deep learning approach to assess damage mechanics of bone tissue. *J. Mech. Behav. Biomed. Mater.*, 104761, 2021.
67. Ramesh, M., Deepa, C., Rajeshkumar, L., Tamilselvan, M., Balaji, D., Influence of fiber surface treatment on the tribological properties of calotropis gigantea plant fiber reinforced polymer composites. *Polym. Compos.*, 42, 4308, 2021, https://doi.org/10.1002/pc.26149.
68. Song, C., Wang, M., Luo, Y., Chen, J., Peng, Z., Wang, Y., Zhang, H., Li, Z.P., Shen, J., Huang, B., Feng, S.T., Predicting the recurrence risk of pancreatic neuroendocrine neoplasms after radical resection using deep learning radiomics with preoperative computed tomography images. *Ann. Transl. Med.*, 9, 833, 2021.
69. Chen, J.B., Yang, H.S., Moi, S.H., Chuang, L.Y., Yang, C.H., Identification of mortality-risk-related missense variant for renal clear cell carcinoma using deep learning. *Ther. Adv. Chronic. Dis.*, 12, 2040622321992624, 2021.
70. Ramesh, M., Rajeshkumar, L., Bhoopathi, R., Carbon substrates: A review on fabrication, properties and applications. *Carbon Lett.*, 31, 557, 2021.
71. Obukhova, N.A., Motyko, A.A., Pozdeev, A.A., Learning from multiple modalities of imaging data for cancer detection/diagnosis, in: *Advanced Machine Learning Approaches in Cancer Prognosis*, pp. 75–109, Springer, Cham, 2020.
72. Devarajan, B., Saravanakumar, R., Sivalingam, S., Bhuvaneswari, V., Karimi, F., Rajeshkumar, L., Catalyst derived from wastes for biofuel production: A critical review and patent landscape analysis. *Appl. Nanosci.*, 2021, https://doi.org/10.1007/s13204-021-01948-8.
73. Zhu, Y., Huang, R., Wu, Z., Song, S., Cheng, L., Zhu, R., Deep learning-based predictive identification of neural stem cell differentiation. *Nat. Commun.*, 12, 1, 2021.

74. Zhang, J. and Jiao, J., Molecular biomarkers for embryonic and adult neural stem cell and neurogenesis. *BioMed. Res. Int.*, 727842, 2015.
75. Melo-Braga, M.N., Schulz, M., Liu, Q., Swistowski, A., Palmisano, G., Engholm-Keller, K., Jakobsen, L., Zeng, X., Larsen, M.R., Comprehensive quantitative comparison of the membrane proteome, phosphoproteome, and sialiome of human embryonic and neural stem cells. *Mol. Cell. Proteomics*, 13, 311, 2014.
76. Ramesh, M., Balaji, D., Rajeshkumar, L., Bhuvaneswari, V., Saravanakumar, R., Khan, A., Asiri, A.M., Tribological behavior of glass/sisal fiber reinforced polyester composites, in: *Vegetable Fiber Composites and their Technological Applications*, Composites Science and Technology, M. Jawaid and A. Khan (Eds.), pp. 445–459, Springer, Singapore, 2021.
77. Wang, S., Li, Z., Shen, H., Zhang, Z., Yin, Y., Wang, Q., Zhao, X., Quantitative phosphoproteomic study reveals that protein kinase a regulates neural stem cell differentiation through phosphorylation of catenin beta1 and glycogen synthase kinase 3β. *Stem Cells*, 34, 2090, 2016.
78. Bao, Y., Zhao, X., Wang, L., Qian, W., Sun, J., Morphology-based classification of mycobacteria-infected macrophages with convolutional neural network: Reveal EsxA-induced morphologic changes indistinguishable by naked eyes. *Transl. Res.*, 212, 1, 2019.
79. Mohankumar, D., Amarnath, V., Bhuvaneswari, V., Saran, S.P., Saravanaraj, K., Gogul, M.S., Sridhar, S., Kathiresan, G., Rajeshkumar, L., Extraction of plant based natural fibers – A mini review. *IOP Conf. Ser.: Mater. Sci. Eng.*, 1145, 012023, 2021.
80. Ragoza, M., Hochuli, J., Idrobo, E., Sunseri, J., Koes, D.R., Protein–ligand scoring with convolutional neural networks. *J. Chem. Inf. Model.*, 57, 942, 2017.
81. Sacile, R., Montaldo, E., Ruggiero, C., Nieburgs, H.E., Nicolò, G., A decision support system to detect morphologic changes of chromatin arrangement in normal-appearing cells. *IEEE Trans. Nanobiosci.*, 2, 118, 2003.
82. Balaji, D., Bhuvaneswari, V., Priya, A.K., Nambirajan, G., Joenas, J., Nishanth, P., Rajeshkumar, L., Kathiresan, G., Amarnath, V., Renewable Energy Resources: Case Studies. *IOP Conf. Ser.: Mater. Sci. Eng.*, 1145, 012026, 2021.
83. Mamoshina, P., Vieira, A., Putin, E., Zhavoronkov, A., Applications of deep learning in biomedicine. *Mol. Pharm.*, 13, 1445, 2016.
84. Wainberg, M., Merico, D., Delong, A., Frey, B.J., Deep learning in biomedicine. *Nat. Biotechnol.*, 36, 829, 2018.

5

Drug Repurposing Based on Machine Learning

Laxmi Tripathi[1], Praveen Kumar[2], Kalpana Swain[3] and Satyanarayan Pattnaik[3*]

[1]*Department of Pharmaceutical Chemistry, Agra Public Pharmacy College, Agra, Uttar Pradesh, India*
[2]*Department of Pharmaceutical Chemistry, Faculty of Pharmacy, Uttar Pradesh University of Medical Sciences, Saifai, Etawah, Uttar Pradesh, India*
[3]*Division of Advanced Drug Delivery, Talla Padmavathi College of Pharmacy, Warangal, India*

Abstract

Drug repurposing identifies new pharmacological indications for existing drugs. It is a promising approach due to the possibility of reduced development timelines and overall costs. The growth of substantial and publicly available electronic health-related and biomedical data leads the path of computer aided drug repurposing strategies. They repurpose drugs via drug-based strategies and disease-based strategies. Machine learning is a state-of-the-art screening approach. Databases widely used for drug repurposing included chemical, medical, pharmacological, and biological databases. This chapter compiles various data resources mentioned under various heads. The limitations of classical statistical approaches proved them ineffectual in drug repurposing and lead to inconsistent findings. Drug repurposing through machine learning algorithms could overcome the limitations of conventional statistical approaches and their unreliable interpretations. Further, case studies of drug examples repurposed through machine learning programs are also discussed in this chapter.

Keywords: Drug repurposing, machine learning, data resources, network-based approach, text mining, semantics-based approaches

**Corresponding author*: drsatyapharma@gmail.com

Inamuddin, Tariq Altalhi, Jorddy N. Cruz and Moamen Salah El-Deen Refat (eds.) Drug Design Using Machine Learning, (143–164) © 2022 Scrivener Publishing LLC

5.1 Introduction

The traditional drug discovery approaches for development of new drug candidates for treatment of diseases is not only a very time-consuming process, but also an expensive affair with a very low success rate. In this scenario, exploring newer indications for the approved therapeutics with time-tested safety profiles for the treatment of off-label indications is a very appealing strategy in drug development. Repositioning, reprofiling, retasking, recycling, rescuing, therapeutic switching, and redirection are the most common synonyms to explain the drug repositioning.

Table 5.1 Comparison between conventional drug discovery & development strategies with drug repurposing strategies.

Conventional drug discovery & development	Drug repurposing
Time-consuming	Shorter duration of development
Laborious	Relatively simpler
Highly expensive	Low monetary cost
High failure ratio	Low failure ratio
Large regulatory requirements for drug approval	Regulatory support has already been established
Methods of synthesis and assays need to be established	Established methods of synthesis and assays
Toxicological parameters need to be established	Established toxicological parameters
The pharmaceutical supply chain needs to be developed	Existing pharmaceutical supply chains
Unknown possibility of combining with other drugs for effective treatment	Known possibility of combining with other drugs for effective treatment
A dosing regimen needs to be established	Well-established dose regimen
Pharmacokinetics (PK) and pharmacodynamics (PD) properties need to be ascertained	Favorable pharmacokinetics (PK) and pharmacodynamics (PD) properties

Repurposing employs the integrated efforts of experimental or activity-based and computational or *in silico-based* techniques to arrive at new indications of therapeutic entities. Thus, repurposing has emerged as an innovative approach to reprofile suitable, already approved and safe drugs for the treatment of challenging, rare, and orphan disease conditions [1]. The drug repurposing technique transcends the conventional drug discovery and development process in many ways (Table 5.1).

The Johns Hopkins Drug Library (JHDL), a library of existing drugs, contains 2,200 repurposed drug molecules approved by US-FDA or its foreign counterparts for use in new therapeutic indications. It also mentions about 800 non-approved repurposed drug candidates that have entered various phases of human clinical trials. NIH Chemical Genomics Centre (NCGC) has prepared a list of existing drugs known as NCGC Pharmaceutical Collection (NPC) containing 2,400 repurposed molecular entities approved for clinical application in the US (FDA), Japan (NHI), Canada (HC), and EU (EMA) [2]. A recent study estimated a pharmaceutical industry market of $24.4 billion for repurposed drugs in 2015 that rose to $31.3 billion in 2020 [1].

Conventional drug repurposing studies focus on discovering similarities in drug effect and mode of action (MoA) [3], exploring new clinical usages through assessing the existing drug molecule for novice drug-targets [4], exploring common features among drugs for example chemistry and adverse events [5], or uncovering drug-disease correlation [6]. The development of computational drug repurposing approaches has been empowered by the massive development of extensive and publicly available electronic health-related and biomedical data and was integrated with the help of high-performance computing [7, 8].

5.2 Computational Drug Repositioning Strategies

Computational drug repurposing approach explores the potential interconnections among drug-related and disease-related expression signatures (Figure 5.1). Intriguingly, this approach has resulted in the confirmation of novel therapeutic indications for the many existing drugs [9]. Generally, there are two basic drug repurposing hypotheses. According to the first hypothesis, there exists interconnections among various disease and hence, a drug candidate for a particular disease may find applications for treatment of other interrelated diseases. The second hypothesis believes in the confounding nature of drugs, which may have different target sites and act in different paths. Hence, based on the origination of findings, drug

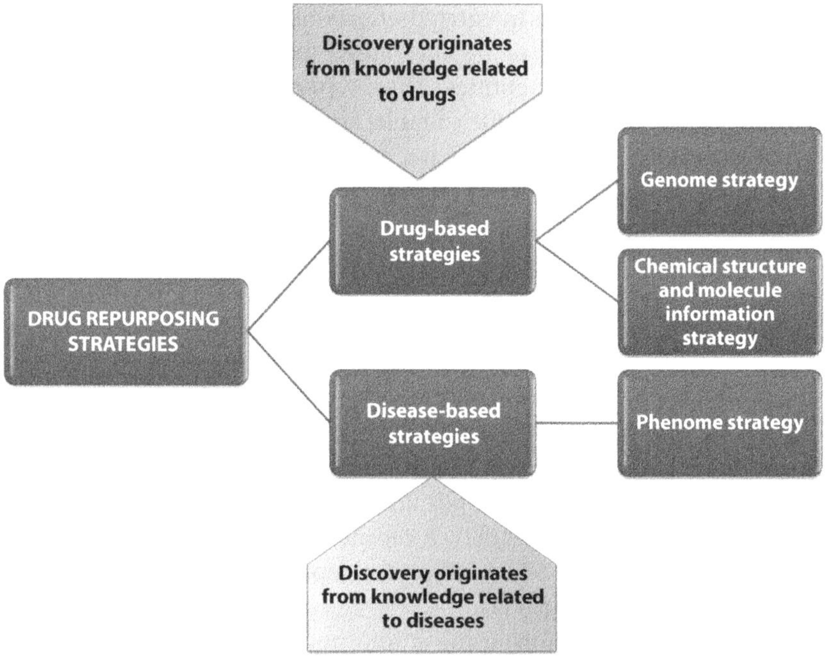

Figure 5.1 Drug repurposing strategies.

repurposing studies can be classified into two categories, i.e., (i) drug-based approach and (ii) disease-based approach [8, 10].

5.2.1 Drug-Based Strategies

If considerable drug-related data like chemical, biomedical, molecular, genomics, pharmaceutical, etc., is available and detailed pharmacology is established for the candidate drug, drug-based strategies are employed for repurposing. The research under this category is based on the speculation that if for two drugs R1 and R2, the pharmacology and mechanism is similar and if drug R1 is effective in treating Dt (target disease), then R2 has potential in treatment of Dt. Approaches under the strategy include are the genome approach [11, 12], and the molecular chemistry information approach [13].

The genome drug-based approach presumes that common indications are due to alike genetic profiles. Drug-drug and drug-disease interrelationships are investigated under gene expression profiles datasets for finding novel clinical indications for old molecules. Such studies use microRNAs (miRNAs) [14].

The molecular chemistry information approach utilize the information related to the chemistry of the candidate drugs for repurposing possibilities owing to the fact that there often exist a close association of structure-activity of chemical substances [15]. Chemical structure similarity is measured by various computational structural similarity search algorithms tools like ChemMine, etc [16].

5.2.2 Disease-Based Strategies

This strategy depends on reviewing and analysing information related to the target disease which may include the symptoms, clinical pathology, and phenotype traits to predict new indications. If the drug-related data are inadequately insufficient, then disease-based strategies are employed. The research under this category is based on the speculation that if alike profiles and indications are present for two diseases, D1 and D2, and drug *Rt* is used to treat D1, then *Rt* has the strong candidature for treating disease D2. Phenome strategy comes under this category [6].

The phenome is explained as a comprehensive set of phenotypic traits details and include all phenotypes expressed by a cell, tissue, organ or organism. For drug repurposing, it connects drugs with clinical responses since it considers the incognizant influences of the bioactivities on the physiology of the body [6].

5.3 Machine Learning

Machine learning (ML) is the process to train machines so as to allow them to learn in the absence of any significant adoption of programs. It is a branch of artificial intelligence based on the idea that systems can learn from data, identify patterns, and make decisions with minimal human intervention. The mainstay of intelligent software used to develop machine intelligence is statistical learning methods. There must be a connection between the discipline of database and machine learning algorithms because they require data to learn [16]. The machine learning methods include (i) supervised machine learning, (ii) unsupervised machine learning, (iii) semi-supervised machine learning, and (iv) reinforcement machine learning methods (Figure 5.2).

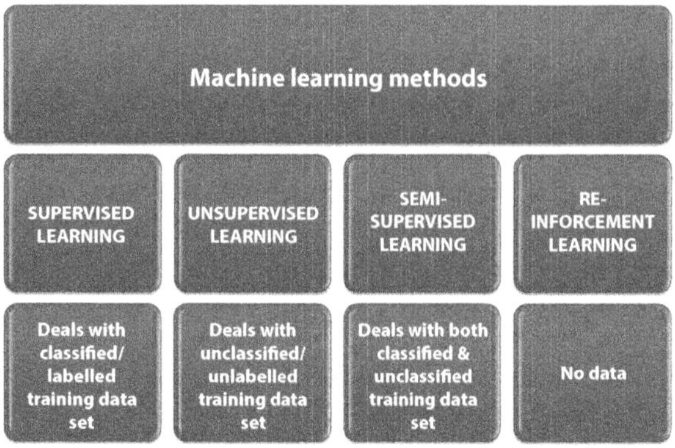

Figure 5.2 Types of machine learning methods.

Supervised machine learning methods infer a function or mapping from a classified or labelled training dataset. Algorithms used to map training data set in supervised machine learning are regression and classification. Unsupervised machine learning methods deal with unclassified/unlabeled datasets. The two main branches of unsupervised learning comprise clustering and dimensionality reduction.

After a model is generated from any of the above-discussed machine learning methods, the same should be validated and evaluated to ascertain its performance. For this, the data are divided into training data set and testing data set. A training set is employed to construct the model and a testing set is employed to validate the constructed model. Many methods are available for validation of machine learning models like train-test split, cross-validation, Wilcoxon signed-rank test, McNemar's test, etc [17–19].

Machine learning has proved itself as an excellent screening approach that has captivated recognition for detecting potential indications for already existing drugs. Drug repurposing has been treated as an ML problem, which in turn has predicted potential association of diverse group of drugs and diseases.

5.4 Data Resources Used for Computational Drug Repositioning Through Machine Learning Techniques

The massive amount of data produced nowadays has given support to the development of amazing drug repurposing strategies. Databases widely used for drug repurposing include chemical, medical, pharmacological, and biological databases (Figure 5.3) [20]. The other varieties of data sources for repurposing are genomics and proteomics databases [21, 22]. The chemical databases contain a tremendous volume of helpful information related to the chemical structures of drugs such as two-/three-dimensional topological information. These data are generally used for foretelling new clinical applications for drugs with identical structural properties [23]. Many drug-repurposing strategies are based on a large volume of biomedical articles containing published data pertaining to biological activities. Generally speaking, more than one database works in combination to conclude meaningful drug repurposing predictions [24]. Table 5.2 consists of data resources classified according to the type of data they contain for use in drug repurposing studies.

Data resources can also be classified on the behalf of objectives that they aim to meet through machine learning programs (Figure 5.4, Table 5.3). They include (i) resources predicting drug–target activity, (ii) cell-based pharmacogenomic data resources and, (iii) biological pathway information resources.

The drug–target activity resources are employed in priming machine learning models for computational forecasting and drug-repositioning [25]. They are divided into three categories, i.e., quantitative bioactivity

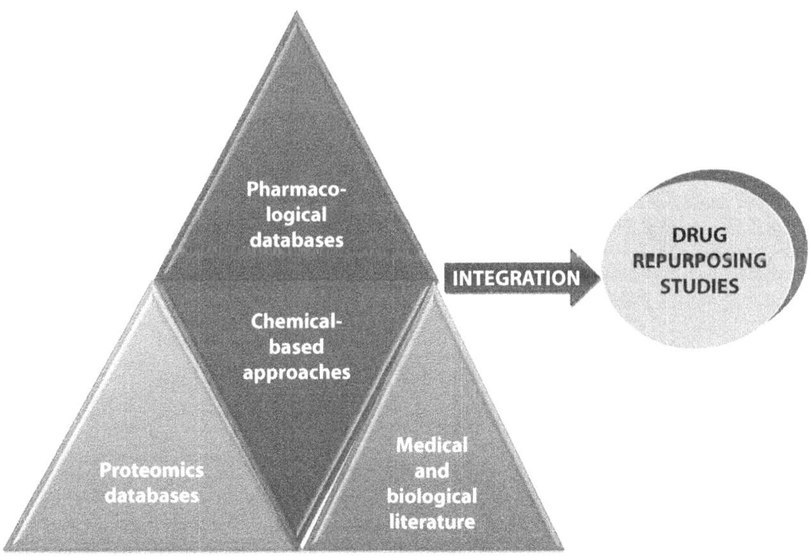

Figure 5.3 Classification of data resources based on the type of data they contain for use in drug repurposing.

Table 5.2 Data resources used for drug repurposing studies.

S. no.	Data type	Data resource
1.	Genome	Array Express, Expression Atlas, Gene Expression Omnibus (GEO), Gene Set Enrichment Analysis (GSEA), Gene Signature Database (GeneSigDB), Gene Ontology (GO), International Cancer Genome Consortium, Kyoto Encyclopaedia of Genes and Genomes (KEGG)
2.	Phenome	ClinicalTrials.gov, Side Effect Resource (SIDER)
3.	Chemical structure	ChEMBL, Chemicalize, Drug Bank, Drug Central, PubChem, Protein Data Bank (PDB), SWEET LEAD, The NCGC Pharmaceutical Collection (NPC), Therapeutic Target Database (TTD)
4.	Phenome/ genome	repoDB, Online Mendelian Inheritance in Man (OMIM), The Pharmacogenetics and Pharmacogenomics Knowledge Base (Pharm GKB)
5.	Phenome/ chemical structure	Drugs @FDA Database

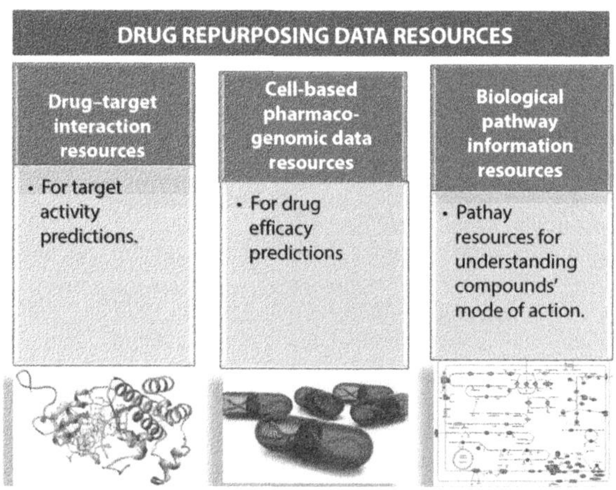

Figure 5.4 Classification of data resources based on the objectives they aim to meet for drug repurposing.

Table 5.3 Data resources based on the objectives of drug repurposing.

S. no.	Objectives	Data resources
1	Drug–target interaction	Binding DB, ChEMBL, Chemical Checker, Drug Central, Drug Target Commons (DTC), Drug Target Profiler (DTP), Gtop DB, PDSP Ki, Probes & Drugs Portal, STITCH, Drug Central, Drug Target Profiler (DTP), Drug Bank, DGIdb, GLIDA, Pharm GKB, Super Target, Swiss Target Prediction, STITCH, ChEMBL, Drug Target Commons (DTC), PubChem.
2.	Cell-based pharmacogenomic data	CellMiner CDB, Dependency Map (DepMap), Genomics of Drug Sensitivity in Cancer (GDSC), gCSI, LINCS, NCATS, Open Data Portal, Pharmaco DB.
3.	Biological pathway information	Pathway Common, Kyoto Encyclopaedia of Genes and Genomes (KEGG), Reactome, MetaCyc, SIGNOR 2.0, PathBan.

data, binary interactions, and unary interactions. They are employed for target activity predictions and provides the probability of forecasting if the candidate molecule be effective. Pharmacogenomics deals with genetic influence of subjective response to drugs including *ex-vivo* models and cell-culture information [26].

5.5 Machine Learning Approaches Used for Drug Repurposing

We deal with data such as drug-target interactions, gene expression, protein networks, clinical trial reports, drug adverse event reports, and electronic health records while computational drug repurposing. Nevertheless, these data are complex, high-dimensional, and noisy, and put forward new challenges for the development of computational techniques that can comprehend these information so as to foretell new clinical usages of old and approved drugs. Among the vast amount of genomic, phenomic, and chemical databases, classical statistical approaches are ineffectual in discovering molecular targets of a drug. These approaches are more interpretative for the development of such drug repurposing strategies that can get better off the limitations of classical statistical approaches and their unreliable interpretations [24]. Databases have promoted the swift development of various novel machine learning programs that employ these data for drug repurposing. Based on the core methodologies of machine learning, the approaches are divided into three major categories and are discussed in the following sub-sections.

5.5.1 Network-Based Approaches

These are vital for repurposing of drugs because of their associated potential to consolidate multiple data sources. These approaches are broadly classified into two types i.e., (i) network-based cluster approaches and, (ii) network-based propagation approaches [27].

The former approaches focus on novice drug-disease/target associations and aspire to detect various sub-networks utilizing cluster algorithms [24, 28–31].

Preliminary information transmits from the source node to all network nodes and few sub-network nodes. Based on propagation strategies, these approaches are classified into local approaches and global approaches. Local propagation approaches work on only limited information of the network and can go wrong in making accurate predictions [32] in some cases. Many recent research works are concentrated on global approaches to accomplish superlative performance. Examples of network-based propagation approaches include PROSPECTR, PRINCE, etc.

The networks may further be classified into homogeneous and heterogeneous classes. Homogeneous networks employ a single source of information to sketch out a disease pathway and recognize drug targets associated with multiple pathways. Heterogeneous networks are usually incorporated with various biological entities and hence, aid in upgraded efficiency of earlier models and propose tools to design more efficient and stable approaches [33, 34].

Cluster algorithms are employed to detect captivating elements for recognizing biological modules. But the lacuna with this method is the lack of existence of standards to assess correlation among biological modules [30, 35].

5.5.2 Text Mining-Based Approaches

Text mining is a computer aided process that uses natural language processing to extract valuable insights from unstructured text and has been extensively utilized to extract new worthwhile biological entity relationships from a huge volume of biological and medical literature [36]. The schematic process channels of text mining are presented in Figure 5.5.

In the information retrieval process, suitable information is screened out from the literature. The information is filtered due to the presence of some futile concepts in the literature. Subsequently, the goal of biological name entity recognition process is to identify concepts of biological interest in the text by mapping all relevant words and phrases to a set of predefined categories. Later, in the biological information extraction and the biological knowledge discovery steps, the relevant information is drawn out to discover knowledge regarding biological concepts and construct a knowledge graph [37–42].

5.5.3 Semantics-Based Approaches

Semantics-based approaches are lately applied to drug repurposing. The steps in these methods are depicted in Figure 5.6. Firstly, biological entity relationships are extracted from preliminary information in huge medical databases such as a chemical, pharmacological, biological, genomics, and biomedical database to construct the semantic network [43].

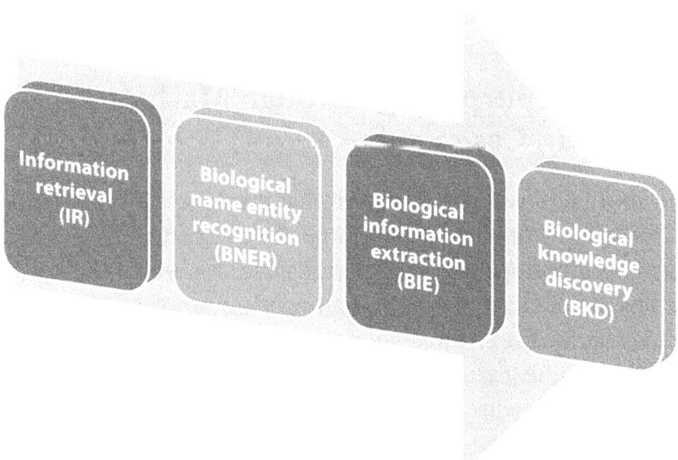

Figure 5.5 Channel for text mining (TM) technique.

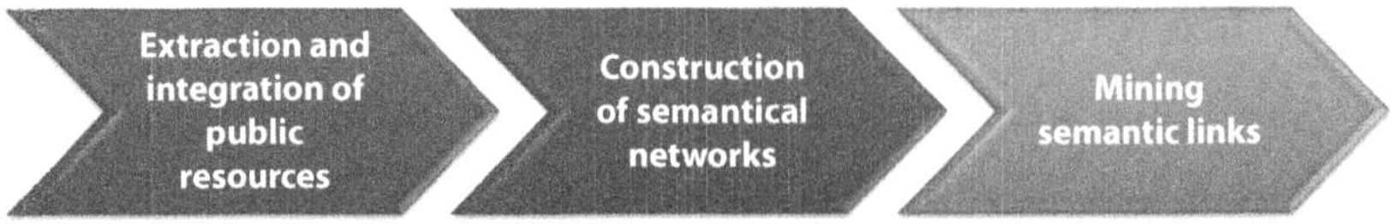
Extraction and integration of public resources
Construction of semantical networks
Mining semantic links

Figure 5.6 Workflow of semantics-based approaches.

Table 5.4 Drug repurposing approaches.

S. no.	Approach	Method/class	Examples of tools
1.	Networks-based drug repositioning	Cluster	RNSC, RRW, ClusterONE, MBiRW
		Propagation	MBiRW, PRINCE, DrugNet
2.	Text mining	Static	Biovista, BioWisdom, FACTA+, EDGAR, EXTRACT2, Anni 2.0, DrugQuest
		Dynamic	PolySearch, TextFlow, MaNER, BEST, Alibaba

The biggest obstacle in building a semantic network is the consolidation of multi-source data. Hence, there is an urgent need to build semantic networks that carry profuse medical data [44, 45]. Various semantics-based approaches have been reported as far as drug repurposing is concerned [46–48]. The tools used for drug repurposing approaches are summarized in Table 5.4.

5.6 Drugs Repurposing Through Machine Learning-Case Studies

From the above discussion, it is advent that machine-learning method masticates large volume of data to determine which existing drug molecule can be employed for therapeutic benefit in diseases for which they are not prescribed thus accelerating the drug repurposing process [49–53]. In literature, we may find many examples of drugs that have found newer indications through the machine learning program. All the approaches discussed above whether concerned with supervised machine learning or unsupervised machine learning or semi-supervised machine learning are largely contributing to drug repurposing studies [54–56]. Table 5.5 discusses some examples of drugs repurposed through machine learning approaches.

Table 5.5 Drug examples repurposed through machine learning.

S. no.	Drug	Earlier indication	New indication	Ref.
1.	Nitrendipine	Calcium channel blocker	Treat hypokalemic periodic paralysis	[46]
2.	Barbiturate	Treatment of migraines	Insomnia	[49]
3.	Tamoxifen	Treatment of breast cancer	Ovarian cancer	[50]
4.	Amprenavir	Antiretroviral protease inhibitor - AIDS	COVID-19	[51]
5.	Topiramate	Antiepileptic	Inflammatory bowel disease (IBD)	[52]
6.	Carbamazepine	Antiepileptics	Cardiac therapy	[9]
7.	Cyproheptadine	5-HT2 receptor antagonist	Depression/ anxiety	[53]
8.	Chlorcyclizine	Antipsychotic	Depression/ anxiety	
9.	Pizotifen	5-HT2A/2C antagonist	Depression/ anxiety	
10.	Metformin	Anti-diabetic	Depression/ anxiety	
11.	Valproate	Anticonvulsant	Schizophrenia	
12.	Pioglitazone	Anti-diabetic	Schizophrenia	
13.	Felodipine	Anti-hypertensive	Schizophrenia	
14.	Aspirin	NSAIDs	Schizophrenia	

(Continued)

Table 5.5 Drug examples repurposed through machine learning. (*Continued*)

S. no.	Drug	Earlier indication	New indication	Ref.
15.	Mefuparib	Poly-ADP-ribose polymerase 1 inhibitor	COVID-19	[54]
16.	Toremifene	Selective estrogenic receptor modulator for the treatment of breast cancer	COVID-19	
17.	Dexamethasone	Glucocorticoid	COVID-19	

5.6.1 Psychiatric Disorders

Prediction of novel indications with a focus on psychiatric disorders has been made feasible with various advanced ML approaches including deep neural networks, support vector machine, random forest, gradient boosted machine with trees, and logistic regression with elastic net regularization [54]. Top repurposed candidates predicted for depression/anxiety disorders include trifluoperazine, perphenazine, fluphenazine, and thioridazine. Few others to mention include cyproheptadine, chlorcyclizine, pizotifen, trichostatin A, vorinostat, and tetrandrine. Top repurposed candidates predicted for schizophrenia include protriptyline, maprotiline, clomipramine, raloxifene, nordihydroguaiaretic acid, pioglitazone, tretinoin, and felodipine.

5.6.2 Alzheimer's Disease

Rodriguez *et al.* reported Drug Repurposing in Alzheimer's Disease (DRIAD), an ML framework that enumerated the relation between the pathology of the severity of Alzheimer's disease and molecular mechanisms [55]. The researchers developed a repurposing approach that integrated omics database pertaining to drug-induced perturbation of nerve cells and disease caused modifications in the patients' brains. The analysis yielded a ranked list of candidates, with several anti-inflammatory drugs used to treat rheumatoid arthritis and blood cancers emerging as top contenders (e.g., Olumiant). These drugs belong to a class of medications known as Janus kinase inhibitors.

5.6.3 Drug Repurposing for Cancer

Advanced "omics" coupled with machine learning and artificial intelligence (deep learning) methods have elucidated targets and pathways critical to identify potential candidates for therapeutic benefit in cancer [57]. Machine learning helped identify novel inhibitors of Indoleamine 2,3-dioxygenase (IDO) and adenosine A2A receptor (A2AR) that served as potential candidates for cancer treatment [57]. Lee *et al.* developed an ML method for identification of molecular markers for acute myeloid leukemia [58]. In another intriguing study, ML method was adopted within a bioinformatics pipeline to identify promising multi-target drugs for treatment of breast cancer [59]. Further, the findings were confirmed by *in vitro* experiments to validate the ML method.

5.6.4 COVID-19

A COVID-19 disease map was utilized to construct a model of COVID 19 infection and all subsequent functional consequences that occurred in the host cells [60]. The potential drugs that were predicted include sirolimus, ciclosporin, and hydroxychloroquine.

Cheng *et al.* demonstrated that a network-based methodology can identify the relative network configuration of drug–target modules for the disease module. They prioritized potentially efficacious pair-wise drug combinations for both hypertension and cancer [61]. Zhou *et al.* used a network-based methodology designed by Cheng *et al.* to identified three potential drug combinations for COVID-19, including sirolimus + dactinomycin, mercaptopurine + melatonin, and toremifene + emodin [62].

In another study, Mohapatra *et al.* demonstrated an ML model based on the Naive Bayes algorithm with a 73% accuracy rate to predict the molecules that might treat SARS-VoV-2 infection [51]. Researchers initially trained their model with the SARS-VoV-2 protease inhibitors. These novel investigational drug candidates were then subjected to validation employing molecular docking approaches. They predicted around ten FDA-approved commercial drugs namely amprenavir, fosamprenavir, indinavir, saquinavir, darunavir, ritonavir, paritaprevir, lopinavir, atazanavir, and tipranavir that could be employed as repurposed drugs for the treatment of novel SARS Coronavirus. Among all, three of the drugs, fosamprenavir, indinavir, and amprenavir, fulfilled the criteria well among which the antiretroviral drug amprenavir came out to be the most effective drug based on the selected criteria [51].

Table 5.6 Some herbal drugs repurposed through the machine learning program.

S. no.	Drug	Original indication	Predicted indication
1.	Bromocriptine	Treat symptoms of hyperprolactinemia & hypogonadism	Parkinson disease
2.	Methylprednisolone	treat inflammatory disorders of the skin, blood, kidney, eye, thyroid, and intestinal disorders	Osteoarthritis, Autoimmune hemolytic anemia, Acute myeloid leukemia
3.	Triamcinolone	Treat inflammation, and discomfort of various skin conditions, including psoriasis	Osteoarthritis
4.	Testosterone	Clinical hypogonadism in men and osteoporosis in women	Calcification Polycystic ovary syndrome Hyperplasia
5.	Cortisol	Diagnose disorders of the adrenal gland	Edema Alopecia
6.	Ephedrine	Treatment of allergic disorders	Headache Cough
7.	Podophyllotoxin	Anti-viral drug	Leukemia
8.	(−)-Prostaglandin E1	Used in neonates with ductal-dependent cardiac lesions.	Hypertension
9.	Irinotecan	Treatment of skin, gastric, pancreatic cancer	Neuroblastoma
10.	Salicylic acid	Psoriasis, ichthyoses	Hypertension

5.6.5 Herbal Drugs

In addition to chemical drugs, some herbal drugs are also finding their new indications through machine learning programs [63]. Machine learning tools like classification algorithms, logistic regression and random forest were utilized to in the development of ML model. The key findings are presented in Table 5.6.

5.7 Conclusion

Drug repurposing or repositioning is a technique utilizing which existing drugs are used for therapeutic benefit in emerging and challenging diseases. The global health community has realized that cutting down the timeline of the conventional new drug development process is of utmost importance in the current time. The excessive cost and long-time duration involved with traditional drug discovery process has triggered researchers to explore repurposing of drugs for newer indications. Repurposed drugs share a huge market in the pharmaceutical sector with about $31.3 billion. ML technology has captivated recognition for detecting potential indications for already existing drugs. Databases widely used for drug repurposing included chemical, medical, pharmacological, and biological databases. Among the huge amount of genomic, phenomic, and chemical databases, classical statistical approaches proved ineffectual in discovering molecular targets of a drug. Drug repurposing through machine learning algorithms could overcome the limitations of traditional drug discovery process. Thus, machine learning (ML) algorithms are one of the promising approaches to drug repurposing that learns patterns in biological data related to drugs and then links them up to their potential of treating specific diseases, thus predicting novel indications of already existing drugs.

References

1. Rudrapal, M., Khairnar, S.J., Jadhav, A.G., Drug Repurposing (DR): An emerging approach in drug discovery, in: *Drug Repurposing—Hypothesis, Molecular Aspects and Therapeutic Applications*, F.A. Badria (Ed.), IntechOpen, London, United Kingdom, 2020. Available from: https://www.intechopen.com/chapters/727.
2. Shim, J.S. and Liu, J.O., Recent advances in drug repositioning for the discovery of new anticancer drugs. *Int. J. Biol. Sci.*, 10, 654, 2014.

3. Parvathaneni, V., Kulkarni, N.S., Muth, A., Gupta, V., Drug repurposing: A promising tool to accelerate the drug discovery process. *Drug Discovery Today*, 24, 2076, 2019.
4. Gloeckner, C., Garner, A.L., Mersha, F., Oksov, Y., Tricoche, N., Eubanks, L.M., Lustigman, S., Kaufmann, G.F., Janda, K.D., Repositioning of an existing drug for the neglected tropical disease onchocerciasis. *Proc. Natl. Acad. Sci.*, 107, 3424, 2010.
5. Kort, E. and Jovinge, S., Drug repurposing: Claiming the full benefit from drug development. *Curr. Cardiol. Rep.*, 23, 62, 2021.
6. Dudley, J.T., Deshpande, T., Butte, A.J., Exploiting drug–disease relationships for computational drug repositioning. *Brief. Bioinf.*, 12, 303, 2011.
7. Li, J., Zheng, S., Chen, B., Butte, A.J., Swamidass, S.J., Lu, Z., A survey of current trends in computational drug repositioning. *Brief. Bioinf.*, 17, 2, 2015.
8. Jarada, T.N., Rokne, J.G., Alhajj, R., A review of computational drug repositioning: Strategies, approaches, opportunities, challenges, and directions. *J. Cheminform.*, 12, 46, 2020.
9. Napolitano, F., Zhao, Y., Moreira, V., Tagliaferri, R., Kere, J., D'Amato, M., Greco, D., Drug repositioning: A machine-learning approach through data integration. *J. Cheminform.*, 5, 30, 2013.
10. Ashburn, T.T. and Thor, K.B., Drug repositioning: Identifying and developing new uses for existing drugs. *Nat. Rev. Drug Discovery*, 3, 673, 2004.
11. Iorio, F., Bosotti, R., Scacheri, E., Belcastro, V., Mithbaokar, P., Ferriero, R., Murino, L., Tagliaferri, R., Brunetti-Pierri, N., Isacchi, A. *et al.*, Discovery of drug mode of action and drug repositioning from transcriptional responses. *Proc. Natl. Acad. Sci.*, 107, 621, 2010.
12. Lamb, J., Crawford, E.D., Peck, D., Modell, J.W., Blat, I.C., Wrobel, M.J., Lerner, J., Brunet, J.P., Subramanian, A., Ross, K.N. *et al.*, The connectivity map: Using gene-expression signatures to connect small molecules, genes, and disease. *Science*, 313, 1929, 2006.
13. Keiser, M.J., Setola, V., Irwin, J.J., Laggner, C., Abbas, A.I., Hufeisen, S.J., Jensen, N.H., Kuijer, M.B., Matos, R.C., Tran, T.B. *et al.*, Predicting new molecular targets for known drugs. *Nature*, 462, 175, 2009.
14. Iorio, F., Rittman, T., Ge, H., Menden, M., Saez-Rodriguez, J., Transcriptional data: A new gateway to drug repositioning? *Drug Discovery Today*, 18, 350, 2013.
15. Swamidass, S.J., Mining small-molecule screens to repurpose drugs. *Brief. Bioinf.*, 12, 327, 2011.
16. Rognan, D., Chemogenomic approaches to rational drug design. *Br. J. Pharmacol.*, 152, 38, 2007.
17. Mohammed, M., Khan, M., Bashier, E., *Machine Learning: Algorithms and Applications*, CRC Press, Florida, United States, 2016, 10.1201/9781315371658.
18. Nasteski, V., An overview of the supervised machine learning methods. *Horizons*, 4, 51, 2017.

19. Muhamedyev, R., Machine learning methods: An overview. *Comput. Model. New Technol.*, 19, 14, 2015.
20. Wishart, D.S., Knox, C., Guo, A.C. *et al.*, DrugBank: A comprehensive resource for *in silico* drug discovery and exploration. *Nucleic Acids Res.*, 34, 668, 2006.
21. Mewes, H.W., Hani, J., Pfeiffer, F., Frishman, D., MIPS: A database for protein sequences and complete genomes. *Nucleic Acids Res.*, 26, 33, 1998.
22. Bernstein, F.C., Koetzle, T.F., Williams, G.J. *et al.*, The protein data bank: A computer-based archival file for macromolecular structures. *J. Mol. Biol.*, 112, 535, 1977.
23. Seiler, K.P., George, G.A., Happ, M.P. *et al.*, ChemBank: A small-molecule screening and cheminformatics resource database. *Nucleic Acids Res.*, 36, 351, 2008.
24. Xue, H., Li, J., Xie, H., Wang, Y., Review of drug repositioning approaches and resources. *Int. J. Biol. Sci.*, 14, 1232, 2018.
25. Pemovska, T., Johnson, E., Kontro, M. *et al.*, Axitinib effectively inhibits BCR-ABL1 (T315I) with a distinct binding conformation. *Nature*, 519, 102, 2015.
26. Tanoli, Z., Vähä-Koskela, M., Aittokallio, T., Artificial intelligence, machine learning and drug repurposing in cancer. *Expert Opin. Drug Discovery*, 16, 977, 2021.
27. Wu, H., Gao, L., Dong, J., Yang, X., Detecting overlapping protein complexes by rough-fuzzy clustering in protein-protein interaction networks. *PLoS One*, 9, e91856, 2014.
28. Yu, L., Huang, J., Ma, Z., Zhang, J., Zou, Y., Gao, L., Inferring drug-disease associations based on known protein complexes. *BMC Med. Genomics*, 8, S2, 2015.
29. Wu, C., Gudivada, R.C., Aronow, B.J., Jegga, A.G., Computational drug repositioning through heterogeneous network clustering. *BMC Syst. Biol.*, 7, Suppl 5, S6, 2013.
30. Subelj, L. and Bajec, M., Unfolding communities in large complex networks: Combining defensive and offensive label propagation for core extraction. *Phys. Rev. E. Stat. Nonlin. Soft. Matter Phys.*, 83, 036103, 2011.
31. Emig, D., Ivliev, A., Pustovalova, O. *et al.*, Drug target prediction and repositioning using an integrated network-based approach. *PLoS One*, 8, e60618, 2013.
32. Mei, J.P., Kwoh, C.K., Yang, P. *et al.*, Drug–target interaction prediction by learning from local information and neighbors. *Bioinformatics*, 29, 238, 2012.
33. Ai, N., Wood, R.D., Welsh, W.J., Identification of nitazoxanide as a group metabotropic glutamate receptor negative modulator for the treatment of neuropathic pain: An *in silico* drug repositioning study. *Pharm. Res.*, 32, 2798, 2015.

34. Wu, Z., Wang, Y., Chen, L., Network-based drug repositioning. *Mol. Biosyst.*, 9, 1268, 2013.
35. Frey, B.J. and Dueck, D., Clustering by passing messages between data points. *Science*, 315, 972, 2007.
36. Li, J., Zhu, X., Chen, J.Y., Building disease-specific drug-protein connectivity maps from molecular interaction networks and PubMed abstracts. *PLoS Comput. Biol.*, 5, e1000450, 2009.
37. Gramatica, R., Di Matteo, T., Giorgetti, S., Barbiani, M., Bevec, D., Aste, T., Graph theory enables drug repurposing–how a mathematical model can drive the discovery of hidden mechanisms of action. *PLoS One*, 9, e84912, 2014.
38. Weeber, M. *et al.*, Using concepts in literature-based discovery: Simulating Swanson's Raynaud–fish oil and migraine–magnesium discoveries. *J. Am. Soc. Inf. Sci. Technol.*, 52, 972, 2001.
39. Cheng, D., Knox, C., Young, N. *et al.*, PolySearch: A web-based text mining system for extracting relationships between human diseases, genes, mutations, drugs and metabolites. *Nucleic Acids Res.*, 36, W399, 2008.
40. Perovšek, M., Kranjc, J., Erjavec, T., Cestnik, B., Lavrač, N., TextFlows: A visual programming platform for text mining and natural language processing. *Sci. Comput. Program.*, 121, 128, 2016.
41. Moreno, I., Moreda, P., Romá-Ferri, M.T., MaNER: A MedicAl named entity recogniser. *Applications of Natural Language to Information Systems*, p. 418, 2015.
42. Lee, S., Kim, D., Lee, K., Choi, J., Kim, S., Jeon, M. *et al.*, BEST: Next-generation biomedical entity search tool for knowledge discovery from biomedical literature. *PLoS One*, 11, e0164680, 2016.
43. Palma, G., Vidal, M.E., Raschid, L., Drug-target interaction prediction using semantic similarity and edge partitioning. *ISWC*, 1, 131, 2014.
44. Mullen, J., Cockell, S.J., Woollard, P., Wipat, A., An integrated data driven approach to drug repositioning using gene-disease associations. *PLoS One*, 11, e0155811, 2016.
45. Chen, B., Ding, Y., Wild, D.J., Assessing drug target association using semantic linked data. *PLoS Comput. Biol.*, 8, e1002574, 2012.
46. Mullen, J., Cockell, S.J., Tipney, H., Woollard, P.M., Wipat, A., Mining integrated semantic networks for drug repositioning opportunities. *Peer J.*, 19, 4, e1558, 2016.
47. Zhu, Q., Tao, C., Shen, F., Chute, C.G., Exploring the pharmacogenomics knowledge base (PharmGKB) for repositioning breast cancer drugs by leveraging web ontology language (OWL) and cheminformatics approaches. *Pac. Symp. Biocomput.*, 19, 172, 2014.
48. Wild, D.J., Ding, Y., Sheth, A.P., Harland, L., Gifford, E.M., Lajiness, M. S. Systems chemical biology and the semantic web: What they mean for the future of drug discovery research. *Drug Discovery Today*, 17, 469, 2012.

49. Cichonska, A., Rousu, J., Aittokallio, T., Identification of drug candidates and repurposing opportunities through compound-target interaction networks. *Expert Opin. Drug Discovery*, 10, 1333, 2015.
50. Lee, J.Y., Shin, J.Y., Kim, H.S. *et al.*, Effect of combined treatment with progesterone and tamoxifen on the growth and apoptosis of human ovarian cancer cells. *Oncol. Rep.*, 27, 87, 2012.
51. Mohapatra, S., Nath, P., Chatterjee, M., Das, N., Kalita, D. *et al.*, Repurposing therapeutics for COVID-19: Rapid prediction of commercially available drugs through machine learning and docking. *PLoS One*, 15, e0241543, 2020.
52. Dudley, J.T., Sirota, M., Shenoy, M., Pai, R.K., Roedder, S., Chiang, A.P., Morgan, A.A., Sarwal, M.M., Pasricha, P.J., Butte, A.J., Computational repositioning of the anticonvulsant topiramate for inflammatory bowel disease. *Sci. Transl. Med.*, 3, 96ra76, 2011.
53. Zhao, K. and So, H.C., Drug repositioning for schizophrenia and depression/anxiety disorders: A machine learning approach leveraging expression data. *IEEE J. Biomed. Health Inform.*, 23, 1304, 2019.
54. Zhou, Y., Wang, F., Tang, J., Nussinov, R., Cheng, F., Artificial intelligence in COVID-19 drug repurposing. *Lancet Digit. Health*, 2, e667, 2020.
55. Rodriguez, S., Hug, C., Todorov, P., Moret, N., Boswell, S., Evans, K., Zhou, G., Johnson, N., Hyman, B., Sorger, P., Albers, M., Sokolov, A., Machine learning identifies candidates for drug repurposing in Alzheimer's disease. *Nat. Commun.*, 12, 1033, 2021.
56. Hannun, A.Y., Rajpurkar, P., Haghpanahi, M., Tison, G.H., Bourn, C., Turakhia, M.P., Ng, A.Y., Cardiologist-level arrhythmia detection and classification in ambulatory electrocardiograms using a deep neural network. *Nat. Med.*, 25, 65, 2019.
57. Issa, N.T., Stathias, V., Schürer, S., Dakshanamurthy, S., Machine and deep learning approaches for cancer drug repurposing. *Semin. Cancer Biol.*, 68, 132, 2021.
58. Lee, S.I., Celik, S., Logsdon, B.A., Lundberg, S.M., Martins, T.J., Oehler, V.G., Estey, E.H., Miller, C.P., Chien, S., Dai, J., Saxena, A., Blau, C.A., Becker, P.S., A machine learning approach to integrate big data for precision medicine in acute myeloid leukemia. *Nat. Commun.*, 9, 42, 2018.
59. Vitali, F., Cohen, L.D., Demartini, A., Amato, A., Eterno, V., Zambelli, A., Bellazzi, R.A., Network-based data integration approach to support drug repurposing and multi-target therapies in triple negative breast cancer. *PLoS One*, 11, e0162407, 2016.
60. Loucera, C., Esteban-Medina, M., Rian, K., Falco, M.M., Dopazo, J., Peña-Chilet, M., Drug repurposing for COVID-19 using machine learning and mechanistic models of signal transduction circuits related to SARS-CoV-2 infection. *Signal Transduction Target Ther.*, 11, 290, 2020.
61. Cheng., F., Kovács, I.A., Barabási, A.L., Network-based prediction of drug combinations. *Nat. Commun.*, 10, 1197, 2019.

62. Zhou, Y., Hou, Y., Shen, J., Huang, Y., Martin, W., Cheng, F., Network-based drug repurposing for novel coronavirus 2019-nCoV/SARS-CoV-2. *Cell Discovery*, 6, 14, 2020.
63. Kim, E., Choi, A., Nam, H., Drug repositioning of herbal compounds via a machine-learning approach. *BMC Bioinf.*, 20, 247, 2019.

6

Recent Advances in Drug Design With Machine Learning

Muhammad Faisal[1,2]

[1]*Division of Bio-Medical Science & Technology, KIST School, University of Science and Technology (UST), Seoul, Republic of Korea*
[2]*Department of Chemistry, Quaid-i-Azam University, Islamabad, Pakistan*

Abstract

Machine learning (ML) methods have been of special attention, since they can be utilized in numerous steps of the drug discovery process, for example, investigating biological activity of new candidates through construction of model, prediction of target structure, optimization or discovery of hits, and development of models that predict the pharmacokinetic and toxicological (ADMET) aspect of compounds. In this book chapter, ML algorithms applied in drug discovery and associated techniques are summarized. Further, the applications that generate promising results and methods are also discussed. The chapter focuses on how these powerful tools are being used in recent years of research. Additionally, an in-depth analysis of the remaining limitations and challenges and suggestions for promising future directions for research are provided. Hopefully, this chapter will offer insight to the researchers working in the area of computational drug discovery in terms of comprehending and developing novel bioprediction approaches.

Keywords: Machine learning, artificial intelligence, drug discovery, deep learning, drug design, docking, chemoinformatics

Email: mfaisal4646@gmail.com

Inamuddin, Tariq Altalhi, Jorddy N. Cruz and Moamen Salah El-Deen Refat (eds.) Drug Design Using Machine Learning, (165–194) © 2022 Scrivener Publishing LLC

6.1 Introduction

Artificial intelligence (AI) can be defined as the capability for a machine to learn, reason, and correct itself just like human intelligence. Machine learning (aka. computational statistics, or statistical learning) is a subset of AI and can be thought of as the process of creating a computational algorithm to study the embedded structure from data. Data can be prices, images, gene expression data, costs of goods, or any data, which may have hidden patterns [1, 2]. These methods do not require the user to explicitly code the solution to the problem; instead algorithms are coded, which will identify trends in the data and use these to make those predictions. ML is classified into regulated, unaided, and support learning [3, 4]. Deep learning (DL), in particular, being a subdiscipline of ML, works on extracting higher-level information from raw data in multiple layers/steps. The strategy is that each subsequent layers/steps learns a more abstract and composite representation of the raw data compared with the previous layer [5].

Drug discovery is very significant for pharmaceutical industries. Currently, discovery of new medicine is still a very costly and time-taken course, which requires Phases I, II, and III for clinical trials. In the recent years, ML methods in AI, have been broadly utilized and attained state-of-the-art achievement in diverse areas, for instance, bioinformatics, image processing, automatic speech recognition (ASR), etc. One very vital utility of these AI methods is in the area of drug discovery, making this process cheaper and faster [2, 6, 7]. That is to say, ML-based methodologies are extremely effective tools that can assist in numerous steps of the process of drug discovery, such as construction of models to estimate and/ or classify bioactivity of new ligands, prediction of target structure, optimization or discovery of hit candidates, as well as creation of models that classify and/ or predict pharmacokinetic and toxicological (ADMET) aspects of candidates to avoid molecules with undesirable profiles [8]. Further, in the process of drug development, the creation of models using ML methods can aid the screening and optimization of molecules that will experience preclinical and clinical trials. As a result, various pharmaceutical industries have started to invest in resources, services, and technologies to produce and curate data sets to assist research in this field. Moreover, technology giants, like Google, IBM, biotechnology start-ups, and academic centers, are not only offering cloud-mediated computation facilities but also working in the healthcare and pharmaceutical space with industry partners [9–11].

The current drug discovery approaches include structure-based drug design (SBDD) and ligand-based drug design (LBDD) protocols to develop/find a lead or hit molecule as drug candidate. In the 1990s, high-throughput screening approaches were extensively utilized in the pharmaceutical industry, but it needs a lot of investment and time to screen and choose promising candidates [12, 13]. The application of computational methods in the early drug discovery process improved during recent decades attributed to various reasons, such as the demand to carry out trials for toxic and inactive candidates along with the possibility of recognizing potential compounds by virtual screenings (VS), a process that is both more costly effective and faster in comparison with experimental trials. Figure 6.1 demonstrates some drug design methods employed in hit/lead investigation [14, 15].

This book chapter delivers a comprehensive, organized summary of the recent research developments in the AI-mediated drug discovery process. To be more precise, ML algorithms used for drug discovery, bioactivity prediction using DL, and application of ML in docking and chemoinformatics are reviewed. Finally, the current state of the area, containing the existing issues and suggestions for promising future perspectives for research are discussed.

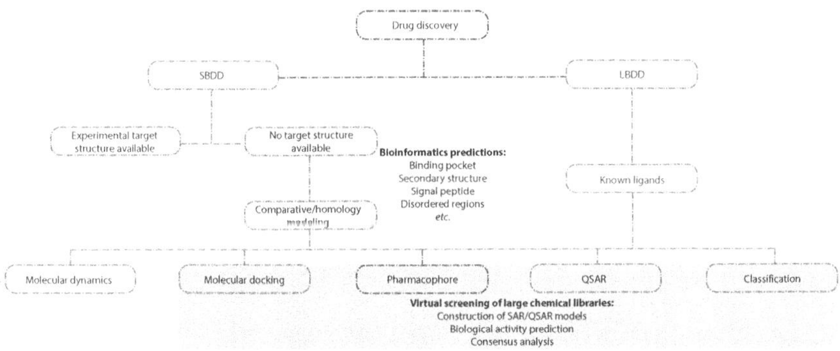

Figure 6.1 Approaches utilized in the process of drug discovery and two key fields where ML is adopted (LBDD and SBDD). In LBDD analyses, diverse methodologies can be applied, such as QSAR techniques, pharmacophore model and classification methods. In SBDD analyses, numerous approaches can be utilized, like molecular dynamics, molecular docking, and homology modeling.

6.2 Categorization of Machine Learning Tasks

The machine learning (ML) problems can be usually divided into four subcategories, which include supervised learning, unsupervised learning, reinforcement learning and semisupervised learning, as displayed in Figure 6.2, and all are explained in the upcoming section [16].

6.2.1 Supervised Learning

Supervised learning is a learning, which has well-labeled data that means correct output of the data is associated with them. This labeled dataset is utilized to train the models and is shown in Figure 6.3 [17]. The new dataset is provided to this trained model to generate predictions. Mainly, in supervised learning models, the dependency and relationship between the input features and the target outputs are examined. These learned relationships facilitate the model to predict new data. Frequently used supervised models include neural networks, random forest (aka. random decision forest) support vector machine, decision tree, etc. [18].

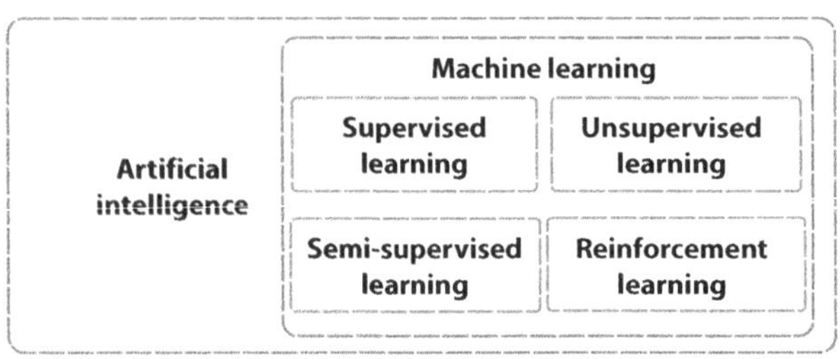

Figure 6.2 Categorization of machine learning tasks.

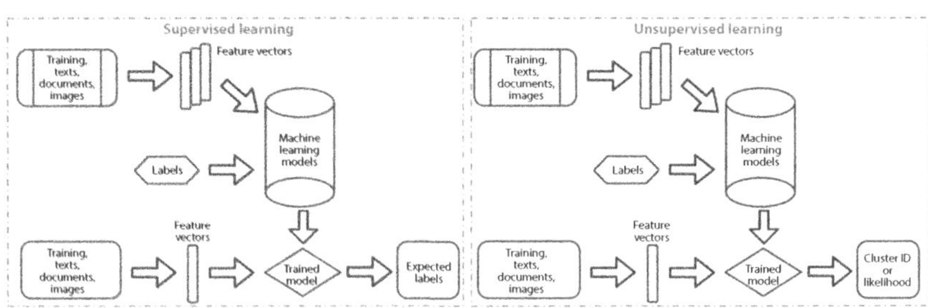

Figure 6.3 Supervised learning (left) and unsupervised learning (right).

6.2.2 Unsupervised Learning

Unsupervised learning means train the model with dataset, which is not labeled or classified, and allow the model to investigate it without any guidance and is illustrated in Figure 6.3. In this learning process, model needs to group shuffled information mediated upon their patterns, dissimilarities and similarities without knowing any training data in advance [18–20]. Here, the dataset is in unstructured form, which contains unknown data, missing values, noisy data, etc. In contrast to supervised learning, no instructor is available in unsupervised learning which means the model will not get any labeled training dataset. Therefore, models have to determine out the hidden pattern within the unlabeled data by its own. When model finds the hidden pattern in the dataset, it produces clusters of them. Once the clusters are produced, a new dataset or unknown data are provided to the model to figure out its cluster. The unsupervised models are precisely employed in the scenario where the human expert has not any prior knowledge of what to determine in the data [16]. Frequently used unsupervised models contain k-means clustering and association rules.

6.2.3 Semisupervised Learning

In the aforementioned two kinds of learning, either whole the records of dataset are labeled or not labeled. The semisupervised learning comes between unsupervised learning (labels in dataset do not exist) and supervised learning (labels in dataset exist) as displayed in Figure 6.4. Typically, it is expensive to do labeling of each record in the dataset and needs human expert to do this role [17–20]. Semisupervised learning is the effective methodology to build the models when some of the records are labeled in the dataset. Many researchers have examined that when unlabeled and

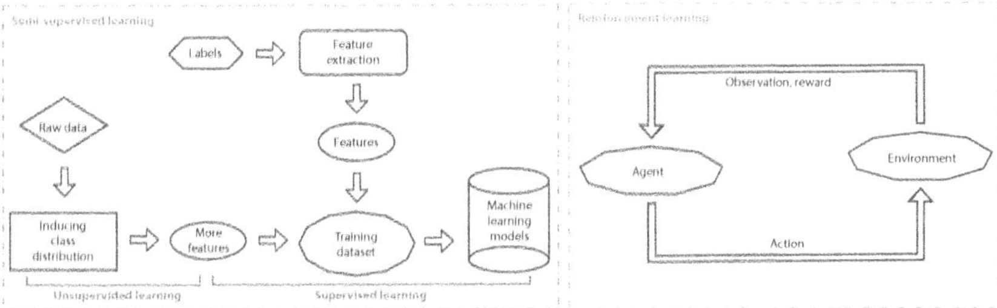

Figure 6.4 Semisupervised learning (left) and reinforcement learning (right).

labeled data are employed together, it can deliver improved learning with less human efforts and costs in comparison to unsupervised learning and supervised learning. This learning methodology implies that without knowing the group membership of unlabeled data, such data has vital information about the group features.

6.2.4 Reinforcement Learning

Reinforcement learning algorithm examines the environment repetitively before taking the actions. It facilitates the machines and software agents to automatically choose the best action to take within a specific situation. This methodology goals at using experiences, which are gathered by interacting with the environment that would minimize the risk or maximize the benefits. The agent demands reward as a feedback to examine its actions, this process is called as reinforcement signal as depicted in Figure 6.4 [16]. The agent has the authority to choose the perfect action to take in his current state, and uses hit and trial approach. The agent has the count of his correct and wrong answers, which is necessary to reward or penalize him. The frequently employed reinforced algorithms are deep adversarial networks, temporal difference (TD), and Q-Learning [21–23].

6.3 Machine Language-Mediated Predictive Models in Drug Design

The essential ML-mediated predictive models in drug design include the following four classifications.

6.3.1 Quantitative Structure-Activity Relationship Models (QSAR)

The biological activities which are typically modeled are half-maximal effective (EC_{50}) concentration, minimum inhibitory concentration (MIC), and half-maximal inhibitory concentration (IC_{50}) evaluated by implementing different biological assays [24]. The most frequently used statistical approaches in QSAR-based investigations are Kohonen neural network, principal component analysis, artificial neural network, etc. [25].

6.3.2 Quantitative Structure-Property Relationship Models (QSPR)

To correlate some valuable characteristics of the molecules such as melting point (MP), boiling point (B.P), λ max solubility, etc. the QSPR models are commonly employed [26]. Applications of the QSAR and QSPR models are discussed in detail in the next sections.

6.3.3 Quantitative Structure Toxicity Relationship Models (QSTR)

For medicinal purposes, the median of toxic and lethal dose parameters TD_{50} and LD_{50} is crucial. Numerous efforts have been done to construct predictive models for the prediction of these properties. For the molecular structure to be considered as a drug candidate, toxicity is an significant parameter that should be assessed [27].

6.3.4 Quantitative Structure Biodegradability Relationship Models (QSBR)

The biodegradability of a molecule in environmental conditions is also associated with its molecular structure. Therefore, QSBR models are valuable in investigating the biodegradability of a compound in the context of growing environmental legislation [28].

6.4 Machine Learning Models

Many computational methods have been found useful to establish QSAR relationships, for example multiple linear regression (MLR) and partial least squares (PLS). In recent years, interest is grown in the use of artificial neural networks (ANNs; aka. neural networks (NNs)) and support vector machines (SVM; aka. support vector networks) for QSAR studies [29, 30]. The most frequently used ML methods are categorized as unsupervised (such as self-organizing maps), supervised (for instance, SVMs, multilayer perceptrons and Bayesian neural network) and hybrid models, for example, counterpropagation neural networks (CPNNs), having the benefits of both unsupervised and supervised learning methods [31]. Some recent promising algorithms are discussed in the section.

6.4.1 Artificial Neural Networks (ANNs)

In soft computing, ANNs are very famous and deeply analyzed techniques. ANNs have many important applications; for instance, primary VS of molecules, QSAR investigations, molecule classification, identification of potential drug targets, and localization of functional and structural features of biopolymers [29–31]. Some other areas in which ANN techniques have been used are biology, computer science, physics, psychology, robotics, pattern identification, and others [32, 33]. In QSAR approaches that employ regression investigation, it is crucial to formerly suppose output-input relation (e.g., quadratic or linear function), but in the case of ANNs, there is no prior input-output relationship as a prior requirement. ANNs have the exclusive capability to adapt to highly complex nonlinear relations. Since 1988, ANN methods are being progressively employed in QSAR investigation and are often utilized for analysis of data with growing attention in chemistry and associated areas of research [34]. ANNs are a set of computational algorithms that are mediated on the neuronal interconnections like that found in natural organisms [24]. One of the chief benefits of ANNs over classical statistical models is that in data, they provide flexibility to determine relationships that are more complex. The significant features of ANNs entail nonlinearity, fault tolerance, and universality, modeling assumptions, and independence of statistical, making them predominantly appropriate for tremendously complex data [35]. In medicinal chemistry, numerous ANN-based models have been disclosed and applied to solve several issues. Such models are self-organizing maps, counter propagation networks, multi-layer perceptrons (MLPs), probabilistic neural networks, and others [35].

6.4.2 Self-Organizing Map (SOM)

It is an approach that keeps the topology of the data set by using visualization, extrapolation, and clustering. A data of high-dimensional spaces can be investigated by utilizing a SOM network by protruding it into a 2D plane. In this methodology, as per a prearranged topological approach, all the neurons in the array are associated with their closest neighbors only. The result is under input data projections, such that the points, which are contiguous in the high dimensional space, will also be contiguous in the Kohonen network (aka. Kohonen map) [36]. The chief advantage of the SOM to that of other projection approaches is that the algorithm is easy for implementation, very straightforward, and fast to compute. A SOM contains the subsequent steps: (i) in the active layer, all the neurons achieve the similar multidimensional input; (ii) a training pattern is offered to the network to investigate the winning neuron; (iii) the weights of winner neuron were updated *via* the present learning rate, although for the neighbors the rate of learning is scaled-down relative to its distance to the winner [24]. Thus, the information of that pattern will be confined to the winner neuron only; and (iv) as per the cluster linked with the respective winner neuron, a fresh pattern is classified in the grid [36].

6.4.3 Multilayer Perceptrons (MLPs)

Multilayer perceptrons (MLPs) are the feed-forward neural networks because all of the information of the data flows in only one direction, from the input unit to the output unit, and are most commonly employed in supervised ML investigations. MLP is very fast and easy to use, however its training is known a highly delicate process as it is sluggish, and there is no assurance that the attained minimum is global. The problem faced during the training of the MLP is the assignment of the architecture of the proper network, i.e., the number of neurons in each layer and number of hidden layers [37, 38]. For the training of MLP network, numerous algorithms can be employed, such as Levenberg-Marquardt, quasi-Newton, delta-bar-delta, quick propagation, conjugate gradient descent, backpropagation, etc. [39].

6.4.4 Counter Propagation Neural Networks (CPNN)

These are the hybrid models which consist of three layers: a hidden competitive layer (designated by SOM), an input layer, and a Grossberg layer (aka. output linear layer), which is exclusively associated to the competitive layer and therefore, it delivers a platform to couples supervised and unsupervised learning features [40, 41]. In CPNN, the training process includes two important stages: (i) for clustering of input data in discrete groups with the help of SOM layer, an unsupervised learning algorithm is employed, and (ii) Grossberg layer (output layer) is fed by the hidden layer output by using a supervised learning scheme for adjusting the weights between the Grossberg layer and hidden one [24]. The successful application of this method was used to construct a model that predicts the inhibitors for the active site of human thrombin [42]. Some other valuable application was in predicting the enhanced antimicrobial potency of 3-hydroxy pyridine-4-one against *Staphylococcus aureus* [43].

6.4.5 Bayesian Neural Networks (BNNs)

A neural network model is believed to be as Bayesian neural network, which uses Bayesian methods in its learning process, and these have been effectively applied in numerous chemical studies. In one of the previous reports by Bishop, it was proposed that this methodology is much better than the classical ANNs on account of its better capability on minimization of errors, capability to consider finest input data and for matching models, only training sets are employed, which is an significant aspect when the sample contains small number of data sets, and these small data sets can make the ANNs learning process very challenging [44].

6.4.6 Support Vector Machines (SVMs)

It is a supervised ML methodology, which was developed by Vapnik and coworkers, and is also called as VC theory (Vapnik Chervonenkis theory), which facilitates the property value prediction on the basis of ranking, regression and classification of compounds [45]. Frequently, for binary properties or activity prediction, SVMs are utilized; for instance, to discriminate between drugs and nondrugs, the aqueous solubility of synthetic accessibility, or to distinguish between the compound's specific activity [46, 47]. The classifier in the data set uses the mathematical functions whose complexity can be decreased by using SVM. For reducing complexity, it is required to regulate the dimension of VC (a scalar index of measure of complexity) [24]. By using the SVM protocol, a separate hyperplane can be constructed to reduce the distance between the nearest sample of each class and the classifier, and lies on the margins of the hyperplane, which is recognized as the margin of separation. The hyperplanes which are there to classify such margin are called as support hyperplanes, and the data points on these hyperplanes are recognized as support vectors [48]. In the area of chemoinformatics recently, some new methods identical to SVMs have also been established; for example, RVMs (relevance vector machines) introduced by tipping, which is a machine-learning method mediated on Bayesian inference and delivers probabilistic classification [49]. The SVM-mediated approaches are also applied for purposes of ligand-mediated virtual screening [50].

6.4.7 Naive Bayesian Classifier

The probabilistic models which use Bayes' rule are called Naive Bayes classifiers and are commonly employed in chemoinformatics for calculating biological properties instead of physicochemical features. The practical application of this technique was not only restricted up to virtual screening fields but also beneficial in phospholipidosis mechanism, compounds toxicity estimation, and for potential drug-like molecules classification of the protein target and bioactivity [51, 52]. Bayesian classifier approaches are mediated on Bayes' theorem, offering an approach for unfolding the probability (abbreviated as *P*) of an incident which may have been resulted due to any of two or more reasons as per equation (6.1) [53].

$$P\,(A/B) = \mathrm{P}(A/B)\mathrm{P(A)/P(B)} \tag{6.1}$$

In the above formula, the probability P for state *A* existing for a given state *B* was described. One of the critical features of this theorem is that if the knowledge of P(*A*), P(*B*/*A*), and P(*B*) is accessible, probabilities can be obtained without specific information about P(*A*/*B*). The motive of the Bayesian method is to offer an equation elucidating how a hypothesis alters in presence of new information.

6.4.8 K Nearest Neighbors (KNN)

The K nearest neighbors (KNN) algorithm is the uncomplicated and very intuitive method which is beneficial to predict the rank, class or property of a molecule mediated on nearest training examples in the feature space [54, 55]. It is a type of lazy learning or instance-mediated learning in which the approximation of function is made locally, and until classification, all the calculations are postponed. KNN is one of the straightforward algorithms for ML and can also be utilized for regression. The majority vote of neighbors can classify a molecule, and the molecule which is assigned to the class must be among the most common k nearest neighbors [24]. K is normally small and is a positive digit. The molecule is just allotted to the family of its nearest neighbor, if the value of k = 1. It is beneficial to select k as an odd number to circumvent tied votes in binary classification issues. For regression, the same technique can be used by just allocating the property value of the object to be the average of the values of its k nearest neighbors [56, 57]. The molecules set for which precise classification is known (the value of the property in the case of regression) is taken as neighbors and can be considered as a training set for the algorithm. To identify neighbors, position vectors do representation of the objects in multi-dimensional feature space. Typically, Euclidean distance (aka. L2 norm) is used; some other classical tools, for instance Mahalanobis distance (MD) Manhattan distance could be employed. The square root of the sum of squares differences among descriptor values is known as the L2 norm. MD takes the distribution of the points into consideration and is a valuable technique of finding the resemblance of a set of values calculated from a collection of unknown samples to a set of values from a known sample. The KNN is sensitive to the local structure of the data. Therefore, it is perfect for determining various parameters with the healthy locality, as is the case with prediction of protein function [56]. KNN has been successfully implicated for predicting the potency of the inhibition of protein kinases, dopamine D1 antagonists and anticonvulsants the psychoactivity of d compounds, such as cannabinoid, the biological profile of steroid, estrogen receptor agonists and of anti-inflammatory and anticancer drugs [58, 59].

6.4.9 Ensemble Methods

Ensemble methods make use of the aggregation of multiple weak learning algorithm outputs to yield a stronger ensemble consensus output. The chief purpose of employing ensemble models is to enhance model predictive performance [60]. The key element to the success of an ensemble algorithm is that the errors between the weak learners are uncorrelated; that is to say, the weak learners are as diverse as possible. One way to train diverse weak learners is to implement a series of diverse algorithms on the same training set and produce the ensemble from aggregating the resultant predictions. Other famous ensemble methods include bagging and boosting.

6.4.9.1 Boosting

Boosting is a technique of sequentially merging weak learners into one stronger ensemble learner. Each new predictor goals to correct the error from the previous predictor in the sequence [61]. The most famous approaches of boosting are adaptive boosting (AdaBoost) and gradient boosting. AdaBoost alters the sample distribution by updating the weights assigned to each instance to prioritize the instances that the previous predictor underfitted for the subsequent predictor, while gradient boosting objectives fit the next predictor in the sequence to the residual error from the previous predictor [60].

6.4.9.2 Bagging

Bagging refers to the utilization of the same algorithm on different subsets of the training set where the training set for each predictor is nominated by a sampling with replacement (bootstrapping) procedure [62]. The predictions for a new instance are then aggregated across all predictors; in classification, a majority voting aggregator often achieves this.

6.4.10 Random Forest

Random forests (RF) are famous algorithms in ML in the life sciences domain, attributed to their excellent performance together with comparatively simple interpretability and implementation [63]. The RF algorithm is an ensemble of weak learning decision trees implemented using bagging [64]. The difference between RFs and classical bagging methods is the additional randomization, which permits the construction of diverse, independent decision trees to diminish the correlation between the weak learners in the ensemble [65]. Each tree is grown as designated in decision trees, with the difference that extra randomization is presented by limiting the features from which the best feature (mediated on Gini impurity metrics or entropy) to split on for each node is selected to a subset of the total possible features [60]. By restricting to a random subspace of features, it is possible to enhance the tree diversity by preventing the condition where a few features always form the first splitting features and therefore dominate for all trees. This enhances the bias of the model and reduces the variance, which result in less overfitting than deep decision trees. Ultimately, all trees output the classification prediction for an instance, which are aggregated by majority voting to yield the final class. The proportion of trees voting for each class gives an indication of a class probability value, for instance if a RF model has one hundred trees and seventy trees have predicted class 1, the probability would be 0.7; this is not a true likelihood of the class prediction; nonetheless, as this does not take into account the distribution between classes [66]. RFs model nonlinear relationships between output data and features, are comparatively rapid to train, are less likely to overfit compared with decision trees, allow the interpretation of feature significance to the model, and do not need extensive tuning of model parameters. Compared to other approaches, RFs do not need strict feature scaling. On the other hand, their weaknesses lie in the fact that they cannot find error estimates for models and are less easily interpreted than some humbler algorithms [67, 68].

6.4.11 Deep Learning

Deep learning (DL) is a discipline of ML that goals to model data abstraction by constructing a complex structure composed of several processing layers.

The DL may discover the information structures within the large datasets by building distributed representation for the data [69, 70]. DL proved to improve in some cases the performance in different applications mediated on large datasets, such as image processing and speech recognition.

6.4.12 Synthetic Minority Oversampling Technique

When working with most supervised learning methods, it is of utmost importance that there is an even distribution of categories in the training set; this might otherwise cause bias in the predictions [71, 72]. The synthetic minority oversampling technique (SMOTE) is a technique that utilizes random oversampling to even the distribution of categories, but with some synthetic modification. It produces the synthetic examples *via* the below equation (6.2).

$$\text{Synthetic sample} = X + u.(XR - X), \quad 0 \leq u \leq 1 \tag{6.2}$$

X specifies the targeted sample from the minority class and X^R the classified nearest neighbor.

6.5 Machine Learning and Docking

The process of docking can be divided into two major steps: i) conformal search, and ii) free energy estimation. The latter phase is mostly error-prone and computationally extensive. The free energy estimation in a docking process is usually approximated by a much-simplified scoring function. The good scoring function is expected to have three properties: i) scoring power, i.e. the capability to properly predict the binding affinity for different binding poses, ii) ranking power or capability to rank the binding poses from a set of ligands with known poses against the same target, and iii) docking power—the capability to recognize the best binding pose of a particular ligand amongst different generated conformers [73]. To investigate cavities/pockets/poses on a single conformation of a biological receptor, numerous programs have been established, such as PRANK, DoGSiteScorer, SCREEN, SitePredict, Fpockt, etc. Some of these programs utilize machine learning algorithms [74] and are demonstrated in Table 6.1. In the next section, different statistical and ML methods are discussed in the context of the above-mentioned three properties.

Table 6.1 Algorithms/programs using ML methods for predicting druggability and/or binding site.

Algorithms/ programs	SBDD task	Description	ML method	Ref.
Nnscore 2.0	Scoring function	Rescoring docking solutions	ANNs	[75]
Nnscore 1.0	Scoring function	Rescoring and categorizing docking solutions	ANNs	[76]
PRANK	Prediction of binding site	Re-ranking/ rescoring predicted pockets	RF	[77]
DoGSiteScorer	Prediction of binding site	Druggability and pocket predicting	SVM	[78]
SCREEN	Prediction of binding site	Pocket predicting and characterizing	RF	[79]
SitePredict	Prediction of binding site	Predicting binding sites for small molecules and metal ions	RF	[74]

6.5.1 Scoring Power

Scoring power is defined as the capability of a scoring function to predict binding energy for a ligand-protein complex with known 3D coordinates. Ideally, the corresponding predicted scores should be linearly associated with binding affinities measured from experiments [80]. There are three categories of scoring functions: i) force field-mediated, ii) empirical, and iii) knowledge-mediated. All three are parametric approaches that involve approximating the fixed number of parameters mediated on the available experimental data. Therefore, the force field- techniques estimate the parameters of molecular mechanics energies approximated from ab initio simulations and/or experimental data [81, 82]. For empirical scoring functions, the complete energy term is composed of individual weighted energy terms, where the weight coefficients are attained from a regression on experimental binding energies. Ultimately, knowledge-mediated functions are the weakest predictors and are mediated on the concept that a huge database of ligand-protein complexes can be statistically mined for deducing rules and models implicitly enclosed in data [83, 84]. Numerous ML approaches are actively used for building VS scoring functions. Therefore, Kinnings *et al.* used Support Vector Machine (SVM) to derive individual weight terms of different protein families for the empirical scoring function [85]. The same technique can be utilized for deriving different parameter coefficients for force-field–mediated scoring function. Some ML approaches used ligand-protein features accessible in the literature (geometric features, pharmacophore attributes) for predicting the binding affinities. Few other nonparametric models tried to study nonlinear dependency of the structure of the ligand-protein complex with the binding affinity [86]. In this approximation, each parameter signifies the number of occurrences of a specific ligand-protein atom type pair interacting within a certain range of distance. The researchers used the random decision forest to model the correlation between binding affinity and these features. Overall, the features can be divided into (i) physical features (e.g., energy terms), (ii) chemical features (fingerprints), and (iii) geometric features (mediated on the structure of ligand-protein complex). The work by Li *et al.* used RF with a combination of different energy, as well as geometric features and showed that incorporating more features and training with more data can enhance the efficiency of the model [87]. In the work by Ballester *et al.*, the researchers utilized chemical descriptors to represent complex and revealed that having more precise chemical descriptors does not always lead to a more accurate model [88]. Recently, there had been a number of similar publications on scoring functions and ML [73, 80].

6.5.2 Ranking Power

Ranking power is defined as the capability of a scoring function to properly rank ligands for their binding affinity to the same protein. There are two traditional methodologies for assessing the ranking power: (i) high-level ranking and (ii) low-level ranking. The PDBbind v2013 database contains complexes with three different ligands against the same protein target [89]. The high-level ranking is defined by appropriately ordering the three ligands mediated on the binding affinity towards the protein target. On the other hand, the low-level ranking just needs to correctly recognize the best binding ligand out of the three. For any protein target, one point is awarded if the scoring function succeeds for low-level ranking/high-level ranking [80]. In an interesting study, authors evaluated a library of twenty conventional scoring functions and revealed that the approaches called the "S-score" ranked the ligands with the highest accuracy in both low-level and high-level ranking exercises [90]. The research work demonstrated by Ashtawy *et al.* assessed the ranking power of ML-mediated function on PDBbind 2007 and 2010 benchmark datasets [82]. The authors also employed a very diverse set of molecule features: RF-score, AffiScore, and X-score. For ML models they used boosting regression trees (BRT), SVM, RF, k-nearest neighbors (KNN), multivariate adaptive regression splines (MARS), and multivariate linear regression (MLR) [80]. Out of all these, they found ensemble-mediated approaches like RF and BRT worked the best, with RF having the best results for high-level ranking (62.5%) as well as low-level ranking (78.1%). Some of the other research works involved using nonparametric ML models, such as inductive logic programming (ILP) combined with SVM; and SVR-mediated scoring functions: i) SVR-empirical descriptor mediated, and ii) SVR-knowledge mediated [91, 92].

6.5.3 Docking Power

The docking power is defined as the capability of a scoring function to recognize the native binding pose among the generated ones. In other words, it should score the native pose as the best among all possibilities. The traditional method of testing a scoring function is to produce some decoy binding poses (usually few 100s) and include the native binding poses in them to see it gets scored on the top and whether the RMSD between the poses is low (<2.0A or so) [90]. Out of twenty scoring functions investigated by the authors of a review, ChemPLP@GOLD and Chemscore@GOLD resulted in a success rate above 80% [93].

Finding the right conformation is usually done using: genetic algorithms, molecular dynamics (MD), simulated annealing, Monte Carlo simulation, steepest descent optimization, and geometry methods. The significance of docking power of any scoring function has been widely reported in the literature [94]; there is a variety of ML-mediated scoring functions that are in-sensitive to accuracy of docking pose. Therefore, in an interesting study, the docking power of linear and ML-mediated scoring functions was compared and shown that the docking power of linear scoring functions is significantly higher than those of ML-mediated scoring functions [95]. In another investigation, researchers had employed DL approximation to predict the binding affinity values by extracting features from the poses obtained from two docking programs [96].

6.5.4 Predicting Docking Score Using Machine Learning

Progressive docking (PD) was the first disclosed technique that employed traditional QSAR methodology to simulate docking scores and further use them for decreasing the number of remaining docking jobs in a CADD pipeline [80]. The original idea of PD was to construct a model specific to the protein target site by means of a subset of docked molecules and to predict the scores for all the remaining molecules using the QSAR model with 3D descriptors. The predicted docking scores are then utilized to iteratively removing less promising molecules from an undocked database. In the last few years, there have been few similar investigations aimed to approximate docking scores using techniques, such as SVM, RF enhanced with conformal prediction statistics [97, 98]. These approaches used the same idea of PD, i.e., of progressive removal of undocked molecules mediated on some classification (instead of quantitative regression, as in the case of PD).

6.6 Machine Learning in Chemoinformatics

In the past decades, the amount of data produced in the area of chemistry has experienced an exponential growth. Breakthroughs in different domains, spanning from array-mediated technologies to liquid-handling ones and robotics, permitted the miniaturization of common procedures, which were commonly performed by operators. This development made it conceivable to address the throughput of past technologies, making them compatible with ultra-high throughput screening (uHTS) approaches and opening this area to computational techniques and ML methods [99]. Cheminformatics or chemoinformatics are the most common names employed to refer to the application of these approaches on chemical data. General data used in chemoinformatic workflows involve SMILES (simplified molecular input line entry specification), WLN (Wiswesser line notation), or SDF file (structure data format), which are representations of 2D or 3D chemical structures. In the past years, the SMILES notation has become more and more popular owing to the simplified rules utilized in comparison with the WLN ones [100]. In chemoinformatics, the application of ML approaches has become especially significant since their use for the inference of molecules' properties or their potencies in bioassays. The first uses of these techniques for these purposes, which are presently defined as QSAR and QSPR respectively, are dated back to the 1935 [101], and 1964 [101]. Initially, only simple linear regression model on compounds with few descriptors and covering small chemical spaces could be applied owing to the lack of computational power and data, but nowadays, these restrictions are being overcome and new techniques extending the applicability of QSAR and QSPR to nonlinear classification and regression tasks have been implemented and exhaustively analyzed. Repositories like ChEMBL, PubChem, etc., have been created to allow storage and retrieval of chemical information performing a crucial role in the evolution of chemoinformatics (Figure 6.5). The general workflow of QSAR and QSPR follows two steps: an encoding step and a mapping one as described in equation 6.3 [102].

$$\text{Activity or property} = \text{f(structure)} = \mathcal{M}(\mathcal{E}(\text{structure})) \tag{6.3}$$

During the encoding process, molecules are normally encoded into vectors of chemical descriptors, which are "numerical values that characterize molecular properties," as defined in [99], predicated from the 2D or 3D structure and mutual-orientation and time-dependent dynamics of molecules, which were, respectively, named 2D, 3D, and 4D chemical descriptors [103]. More than 5000 descriptors have been defined [104], and among them, molecular refractivity, ClogP, topological indices like the Wiener index, and 2D fingerprints are some examples, which can be calculated through closed-source software as DRAGON 7.0 [100] or open-source ones like PaDEL [105]. During

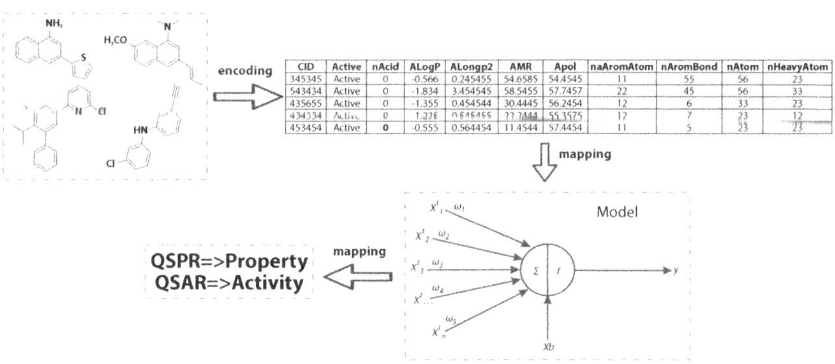

Figure 6.5 Workflows for QSAR and QSPR. Data are encoded in chemical descriptors and fingerprints and labeled with activities or properties. These data are then used to train a model, which will learn to predict properties or activities of features chemical compounds.

the second step, these vectors are mapped to an activity or property class through a function, which is commonly what most of ML techniques try to optimize. Other methodologies were proposed, to directly extract features from molecular structures, decreasing problems concerning descriptors definition, their computation and feature selection. An example of these approaches was reported by Lusci and colleagues, in which they used a Recursive neural network to encode undirected molecular graphs into vectors retaining, in this way, both structural and chemical information and managing to obtain, with this model, state-of-the-art performances in the investigation of aqueous solubility [102]. QSAR and QSPR techniques are playing an important part in drug discovery and particularly in "*de novo*" drug design. Certainly, the prediction of molecular properties can be highly valuable for the evaluation of those chemical compounds, which may pass all the phases of the drug development life cycle. An example of this is the solubility of drugs in water. Indeed, it defines the body absorption efficiency of the chemical compounds being examined, permitting the rejection of active compounds that, otherwise, would be discarded in successive stages. In recent years, other measures as drug toxicity highlight the usefulness of these models for the rejection of toxic molecules in the early phases of drug development, growing so the quality of selected candidates. Recently, many efforts were made to apply techniques mediated on deep learning models and generative ones in chemoinformatics. The work performed at the Bioinformatics Institute of the Johannes Kepler University of Linz is an illustrative example of the power of DL approaches, multitask and ensemble learning in toxicity prediction. During the Tox21 data challenge, this model (DeepTox) attained the best performances among all computational approaches in many assays [106]. The work performed by Bombarelli and coworkers, instead, is an exemplificative example of generative models in cheminformatics. Indeed, they used a RNN-variational autoencoder to encode SMILES strings into latent chemical space and decode them back, allowing so the use of this latent space for the generation of new molecules having specific properties [107]. The use of a three-stacked-LSTM for the generation of molecules was reported by Seglar *et al.* in their article [108], where they revealed the capability of their model to yield both data-sets of general molecules and data sets enriched in molecules with specific molecular properties, which they used to implement an *in-silico* "*de novo*" drug design cycle.

6.7 Challenges and Limitations for Machine Learning in Drug Discovery

There are numerous challenges for ML in drug discovery, spanning all domains, including data, algorithmic, practical, and political. Here, I will touch on each briefly. The first is the dependency on expensive (both in cost and time) experimental data for validation and training. This contrasts with the successes of DL in games such as Go [109] or chess [110], where training data can be perfectly created in simulations. This motivates the development of approaches that can learn from small quantities of data (e.g., few-shot learning or effectively utilize other available data (e.g., meta-learning, transfer learning) [111]. Further algorithmic challenges arise from the nature of chemical and biological data, both in terms of the format of such data as well as the inherent noise. A crucial challenge is how we quantify success. Prevailing human-led processes are far from infallible, but it is not presently possible to quantify medicinal chemistry success. In light of this, what is the bar for algorithmic success? Numerous have cautioned not to set the barrier for computational methodologies too high [112]. Ultimately, realizing the full impact of ML approaches will need significant resources to be invested. Experimental validation on real-world drug discovery projects is a critical next step to assess the contribution of ML in medicinal chemistry and identify fields requiring improvement.

6.8 Conclusion and Future Perspectives

The purpose of this book chapter is to summarize the present status of ML methods in the area of drug discovery within both industrial and academic contexts, and highlight its potential future utilizations. Numerous useful models for ML methods in drug discovery are reviewed. The chief benefit of using several AI approaches is their potentiality to accomplish complex tasks and reduce cycle time and labor demands during the early steps of drug discovery through leveraging *in silico* techniques for molecule design, assessment of synthetic pathway, and modeling ADMET. In the last years, the utilization of ML methods to advance some aspects of drug designing projects has become more usual, for instance prediction of secondary structures, investigating binding sites, docking simulations, and others.

It is also observed that RF and SVM are those algorithms which are extensively employed owing to high efficiency and accuracy; therefore, have the potential to revolutionize the field of drug designing. Presently, a significant application of ML methods is related to the prediction of scoring functions employed in docking and VS assays from a consensus, linking classical and ML approaches in order to enhance the prediction of docking solutions and binding sites. Due to more powerful supercomputers, more precise algorithms, and substantial public and private investment into the area, these applications are becoming more accurate, smart, time-efficient and cost-effective while improving efficacy.

The broadly used AI algorithms, mainly DL-mediated algorithms, were mainly established in the area of acoustic signal processing, natural language processing (NLP), and computer vision. However, on account of the reasons here, implementing fancy AI methods to the drug discovery process is relatively challenging. Primarily, the process of the drug discovery is very complex, and it includes expertise in a variety of area (medicine, chemistry, and biology; among others.). Also, for decision making, the process of drug discovery demands compelling evidence since it straightaway influences health of public and net profit of pharmaceutical industries. Nonetheless, many experts proved the fact that the future of drug discovery with machine learning technology is noticeably promising by their excellent struggles. The discrepancy between the two fields is still a big hurdle. Thus, ML researchers and other area researchers will need to work together closely to establish "drug-discovery-specific" ML technology for real advancements in the present drug discovery. ML researchers will need to recognize the properties of drug discovery data and make an effort to establish interpretable and appropriate algorithms that can elucidate the modes of action, to deliver evidence for making further decision. Researchers from other domain will need to produce chemical and biological data with negligible experimental errors and save them in unified platforms and innovative reporting tools for further developments to the ML systems. Having said that, the most significant thing for both research groups is to be open to working together to make a promising skeleton for a new revolution in the field of drug development. Hopefully, this chapter offers a nice starting point to close this gap.

References

1. Mak, K.-K. and Pichika, M.R., Artificial intelligence in drug development: Present status and future prospects. *Drug Discovery Today*, 24, 773, 2019.

2. Keshavarzi Arshadi, A., Webb, J., Salem, M., Cruz, E., Calad-Thomson, S., Ghadirian, N., Collins, J., Diez-Cecilia, E., Kelly, B., Goodarzi, H., Artificial intelligence for COVID-19 drug discovery and vaccine development. *Front. Artif. Intell.*, 3, 65, 2020.
3. Lake, F., Artificial intelligence in drug discovery: What is new, and what is next? *Future Drug Discovery*, 1, 1, 2019.
4. Cavasotto, C.N. and Di Filippo, J.I., Artificial intelligence in the early stages of drug discovery. *Arch. Biochem. Biophys.*, 108730, 12, 2020.
5. Álvarez-Machancoses, Ó. and Fernández-Martínez, J.L., Using artificial intelligence methods to speed up drug discovery. *Expert Opin. Drug Discovery*, 14, 769, 2019.
6. Bender, A. and Cortes-Ciriano, I., Artificial intelligence in drug discovery: What is realistic, what are illusions? Part 1: Ways to make an impact, and why we are not there yet. *Drug Discovery Today*, 26, 511, 2020.
7. Agrawal, P., Artificial intelligence in drug discovery and development. *J. Pharmacovigil.*, 6, 2, 2018.
8. Bender, A. and Cortes-Ciriano, I., Artificial intelligence in drug discovery: What is realistic, what are illusions? Part 2: A discussion of chemical and biological data used for AI in drug discovery. *Drug Discovery Today*, 26, 511, 2021.
9. Jiménez-Luna, J., Grisoni, F., Weskamp, N., Schneider, G., Artificial intelligence in drug discovery: Recent advances and future perspectives. *Expert Opin. Drug Discovery*, 16, 1, 2021.
10. Nagarajan, N., Yapp, E.K.Y., Le, N.Q.K., Kamaraj, B., Al-Subaie, A.M., Yeh, H.-Y., Application of computational biology and artificial intelligence technologies in cancer precision drug discovery. *BioMed. Res. Int.*, 2019, 1, 2019.
11. Zhu, H., Big data and artificial intelligence modeling for drug discovery. *Annu. Rev. Pharmacol. Toxicol.*, 60, 573, 2020.
12. Díaz, Ó., Dalton, J.A.R., Giraldo, J., Artificial intelligence: A novel approach for drug discovery. *Trends Pharmacol. Sci.*, 40, 550, 2019.
13. Bajorath, J., Kearnes, S., Walters, W.P., Meanwell, N.A., Georg, G.I., Wang, S., Artificial intelligence in drug discovery: Into the great wide open. *J. Med. Chem.*, 63, 8651, 2020.
14. Paul, D., Sanap, G., Shenoy, S., Kalyane, D., Kalia, K., Tekade, R.K., Artificial intelligence in drug discovery and development. *Drug Discovery Today*, 26, 80, 2020.
15. Zhavoronkov, A., Vanhaelen, Q., Oprea, T.I., Will artificial intelligence for drug discovery impact clinical pharmacology? *Clin. Pharmacol. Ther.*, 107, 780, 2020.
16. Khanna, D. and Rana, P.S., Ensemble approach for antigenic epitopes prediction using physicochemical properties, 2020, http://hdl.handle.net/10266/6050.

17. Chu, X., Lin, Y., Wang, Y., Wang, L., Wang, J., Gao, J., Mlrda: A multi-task semi-supervised learning framework for drug-drug interaction prediction. *Proc. 28th Int. Jt. Conf. Artif. Intell*, p. 4518, 2019.
18. Lo, Y.-C., Rensi, S.E., Torng, W., Altman, R.B., Machine learning in chemoinformatics and drug discovery. *Drug Discovery Today*, 23, 1538, 2018.
19. Sellwood, M.A., Ahmed, M., Segler, M.H.S., Brown, N., Artificial intelligence in drug discovery. *Future Med. Sci.*, 10, 17, 2018.
20. Jing, Y., Bian, Y., Hu, Z., Wang, L., Xie, X.-Q.S., Deep learning for drug design: An artificial intelligence paradigm for drug discovery in the big data era. *AAPS J.*, 20, 1, 2018.
21. Zhou, Z., Kearnes, S., Li, L., Zare, R.N., Riley, P., Optimization of molecules via deep reinforcement learning. *Sci. Rep.*, 9, 1, 2019.
22. Popova, M., Isayev, O., Tropsha, A., Deep reinforcement learning for *de novo* drug design. *Sci. Adv.*, 4, eaap7885, 2018.
23. Olivecrona, M., Blaschke, T., Engkvist, O., Chen, H., Molecular *de-novo* design through deep reinforcement learning. *J. Cheminform.*, 9, 1, 2017.
24. Pankaj, V., Development of machine learning tool for drug class prediction, 2020, http://hdl.handle.net/10603/300968.
25. Muhammad, U., Uzairu, A., Ebuka Arthur, D., Review on: Quantitative structure activity relationship (QSAR) modeling. *J. Anal. Pharm. Res.*, 7, 240, 2018.
26. Tropsha, A., Gramatica, P., Gombar, V.K., The importance of being earnest: validation is the absolute essential for successful application and interpretation of QSPR models. *QSAR Comb. Sci.*, 22, 69, 2003.
27. Devillers, J., Prediction of mammalian toxicity of organophosphorus pesticides from QSTR modeling. *SAR QSAR Environ. Res.*, 15, 501, 2004.
28. Lin, X., Li, X., Lin, X., A review on applications of computational methods in drug screening and design. *Molecules*, 25, 1375, 2020.
29. Nandi, S. and Bagchi, M.C., Activity prediction of some nontested anticancer compounds using GA-based PLS regression models. *Chem. Biol. Drug Des.*, 78, 587, 2011.
30. Goudarzi, N., Goodarzi, M., Chen, T., QSAR prediction of HIV inhibition activity of styrylquinoline derivatives by genetic algorithm coupled with multiple linear regressions. *Med. Chem. Res.*, 21, 437, 2012.
31. Gertrudes, J.C., Maltarollo, V.G., Silva, R.A., Oliveira, P.R., Honorio, K.M., Da Silva, A.B.F., Machine learning techniques and drug design. *Curr. Med. Chem.*, 19, 4289, 2012.
32. Abiodun, O.I., Jantan, A., Omolara, A.E., Dada, K.V., Mohamed, N.A., Arshad, H., State-of-the-art in artificial neural network applications: A survey. *Heliyon*, 4, e00938, 2018.
33. Kappen, H.J., An overview of neural network applications, 1996, http://hdl.handle.net/10603/300968.

34. Hoskins, J.C. and Himmelblau, D.M., Artificial neural network models of knowledge representation in chemical engineering. *Comput. Chem. Eng.*, 12, 881, 1988.
35. Milac, A.-L., Avram, S., Petrescu, A.-J., Evaluation of a neural networks QSAR method based on ligand representation using substituent descriptors: Application to HIV-1 protease inhibitors. *J. Mol. Graph. Model.*, 25, 37, 2006.
36. Schneider, P., Tanrikulu, Y., Schneider, G., Self-organizing maps in drug discovery: Compound library design, scaffold-hopping, repurposing. *Curr. Med. Chem.*, 16, 258, 2009.
37. Stokes, A., Hum, W., Zaslavsky, J., A minimal-input multilayer perceptron for predicting drug-drug interactions without knowledge of drug structure. *arXiv Prepr. arXiv2005.10644*. 1, 1, 2020.
38. Khan, S.R., Al Rijjal, D., Piro, A., Wheeler, M.B., AI-integration and plant-based traditional medicine for drug discovery. *Drug Discovery Today*, 26, 982, 2021.
39. Dara, S., Dhamercherla, S., Jadav, S.S., Babu, C.H., Ahsan, M.J., Machine learning in drug discovery: A review. *Artif. Intell. Rev.*, 1, 53, 2021.
40. Mather, P. and Tso, B., *Classification methods for remotely sensed data*, pp. 1–200, CRC Press, 2016.
41. Kuzmanovski, I. and Novič, M., Counter-propagation neural networks in Matlab. *Chemom. Intell. Lab. Syst.*, 90, 84, 2008.
42. Mlinsek, G., Novic, M., Hodoscek, M., Solmajer, T., Prediction of enzyme binding: Human thrombin inhibition study by quantum chemical and artificial intelligence methods based on X-ray structures. *J. Chem. Inf. Comput. Sci.*, 41, 1286, 2001.
43. Sabet, R., Fassihi, A., Hemmateenejad, B., Saghaei, L., Miri, R., Gholami, M., Computer-aided design of novel antibacterial 3-hydroxypyridine-4-ones: Application of QSAR methods based on the MOLMAP approach. *J. Comput. Aided Mol. Des.*, 26, 349, 2012.
44. Carreira-Perpinan, M.A., Mode-finding for mixtures of Gaussian distributions. *IEEE Trans. Pattern Anal. Mach. Intell.*, 22, 1318, 2000.
45. Zernov, V.V., Balakin, K.V., Ivaschenko, A.A., Savchuk, N.P., Pletnev, I.V., Drug discovery using support vector machines. The case studies of drug likeness, agrochemical-likeness, and enzyme inhibition predictions. *J. Chem. Inf. Comput. Sci.*, 43, 2048, 2003.
46. Podolyan, Y., Walters, M.A., Karypis, G., Assessing synthetic accessibility of chemical compounds using machine learning methods. *J. Chem. Inf. Model.*, 50, 979, 2010.
47. Jorissen, R.N. and Gilson, M.K., Virtual screening of molecular databases using a support vector machine. *J. Chem. Inf. Model.*, 45, 549, 2005.
48. Asif, A., Abbasi, W.A., Munir, F., Ben-Hur, A., pyLEMMINGS: Large margin multiple instance classification and ranking for bioinformatics applications. *arXiv Prepr. arXiv1711.04913*. 1, 1, 2017.

49. Tipping, M.E., Sparse Bayesian learning and the relevance vector machine. *J. Mach. Learn. Res.*, 1, 211, 2001.
50. Lowe, R., Mussa, H.Y., Mitchell, J.B.O., Glen, R.C., Classifying molecules using a sparse probabilistic kernel binary classifier. *J. Chem. Inf. Model.*, 51, 1539, 2011.
51. Koutsoukas, A., Lowe, R., KalantarMotamedi, Y., Mussa, H.Y., Klaffke, W., Mitchell, J.B.O., Glen, R.C., Bender, A., *In silico* target predictions: Defining a benchmarking data set and comparison of performance of the multiclass Naïve Bayes and Parzen-Rosenblatt window. *J. Chem. Inf. Model.*, 53, 1957, 2013.
52. Hert, J., Willett, P., Wilton, D.J., Acklin, P., Azzaoui, K., Jacoby, E., Schuffenhauer, A., New methods for ligand-based virtual screening: Use of data fusion and machine learning to enhance the effectiveness of similarity searching. *J. Chem. Inf. Model.*, 46, 462, 2006.
53. Gámez, J.A., Moral, S., Cerdan, A.S., *Advances in Bayesian networks*, pp. 1–300, Springer, 2013.
54. Konovalov, D.A., Coomans, D., Deconinck, E., Vander Heyden, Y., Benchmarking of QSAR models for blood-brain barrier permeation. *J. Chem. Inf. Model.*, 47, 1648, 2007.
55. Votano, J.R., Parham, M., Hall, L.H., Kier, L.B., Oloff, S., Tropsha, A., Xie, Q., Tong, W., Three new consensus QSAR models for the prediction of Ames genotoxicity. *Mutagenesis*, 19, 365, 2004.
56. De Ferrari, L., Aitken, S., van Hemert, J., Goryanin, I., EnzML: Multi-label prediction of enzyme classes using InterPro signatures. *BMC Bioinf.*, 13, 1, 2012.
57. Lowe, R., Mussa, H.Y., Nigsch, F., Glen, R.C., Mitchell, J.B.O., Predicting the mechanism of phospholipidosis. *J. Cheminform.*, 4, 1, 2012.
58. Singh, A. and Lakshmiganthan, R., Impact of different data types on classifier performance of random forest, naive bayes, and k-nearest neighbors algorithms, 2018, https://minerva-access.unimelb.edu.au/bitstream/handle/11343/216910/2017_Asmita_Different_Data.pdf.
59. Lavecchia, A., Machine-learning approaches in drug discovery: Methods and applications. *Drug Discovery Today*, 20, 318, 2015.
60. Giblin, K.A., *Predictive Modelling of the Primary and Secondary Pharmacology of Compounds in Drug Discovery*, 2020, https://www.repository.cam.ac.uk/handle/1810/303012.
61. Dietterich, T.G., An experimental comparison of three methods for constructing ensembles of decision trees: Bagging, boosting, and randomization. *Mach. Learn.*, 40, 139, 2000.
62. Breiman, L., *Bagging predictors (Technical Report 421)*, vol. 1, p. 4, Univ. California, Berkeley, 1994.
63. Touw, W.G., Bayjanov, J.R., Overmars, L., Backus, L., Boekhorst, J., Wels, M., van Hijum, S.A.F.T., Data mining in the Life Sciences with random forest: A walk in the park or lost in the jungle? *Brief. Bioinform.*, 14, 315, 2013.

64. Athey, S., Tibshirani, J., Wager, S., Generalized random forests. *Ann. Stat.*, 47, 1148, 2019.
65. Ho, T.K., The random subspace method for constructing decision forests. *IEEE Trans. Pattern Anal. Mach. Intell.*, 20, 832, 1998.
66. Niculescu-Mizil, A. and Caruana, R., Predicting good probabilities with supervised learning. *Proc. 22nd Int. Conf. Mach. Learn.*, vol. 1, p. 625, 2005.
67. Cortés-Ciriano, I., Ain, Q.U., Subramanian, V., Lenselink, E.B., Méndez-Lucio, O., IJzerman, A.P., Wohlfahrt, G., Prusis, P., Malliavin, T.E., van Westen, G.J.P., Polypharmacology modelling using proteochemometrics (PCM): Recent methodological developments, applications to target families, and future prospects. *Medchemcomm*, 6, 24, 2015.
68. Géron, A., *Hands-on machine learning with Scikit-Learn, Keras, and TensorFlow: Concepts, tools, and techniques to build intelligent systems*, pp. 100–260, O'Reilly Media, 2019.
69. Deng, L. and Yu, D., Deep learning: Methods and applications. *Found. Trends Signal Process.*, 7, 197, 2014.
70. Khamis, A.M., *Machine Learning Identification of Protein Properties Useful for Specific Applications*, 2016, https://repository.kaust.edu.sa/handle/10754/606030.
71. Lusa, L., Evaluation of smote for high-dimensional class-imbalanced microarray data. *2012 11th Int. Conf. Mach. Learn. Appl.*, vol. 2, p. 89, 2012.
72. Brunnsåker, D., Prediction of Liver Toxicity using Machine Learning to aid Drug Discovery, 2020, https://odr.chalmers.se/handle/20.500.12380/302109.
73. Khamis, M.A., Gomaa, W., Ahmed, W.F., Machine learning in computational docking. *Artif. Intell. Med.*, 63, 135, 2015.
74. Bordner, A.J., Predicting small ligand binding sites in proteins using backbone structure. *Bioinformatics*, 24, 2865, 2008.
75. Durrant, J.D. and McCammon, J.A., NNScore 2.0: A neural-network receptor–ligand scoring function. *J. Chem. Inf. Model.*, 51, 2897, 2011.
76. Durrant, J.D. and McCammon, J.A., NNScore: a neural-network-based scoring function for the characterization of protein–ligand complexes. *J. Chem. Inf. Model.*, 50, 1865, 2010.
77. Krivák, R. and Hoksza, D., Improving protein-ligand binding site prediction accuracy by classification of inner pocket points using local features. *J. Cheminform.*, 7, 1, 2015.
78. Volkamer, A., Kuhn, D., Rippmann, F., Rarey, M., DoGSiteScorer: A web server for automatic binding site prediction, analysis and druggability assessment. *Bioinformatics*, 28, 2074, 2012.
79. Nayal, M. and Honig, B., On the nature of cavities on protein surfaces: Application to the identification of drug-binding sites. *Proteins Struct. Funct. Bioinf.*, 63, 892, 2006.
80. Agrawal, V., *The discovery of small molecule inhibitors for TOX1 and ERG oncotargets with the development and use of progressive docking PD2. 0 approach*, 2019, http://hdl.handle.net/2429/71946.

81. Moustakas, D.T., Lang, P.T., Pegg, S., Pettersen, E., Kuntz, I.D., Brooijmans, N., Rizzo, R.C., Development and validation of a modular, extensible docking program: DOCK 5. *J. Comput. Aided Mol. Des.*, 20, 601, 2006.
82. Ashtawy, H.M. and Mahapatra, N.R., A comparative assessment of ranking accuracies of conventional and machine-learning-based scoring functions for protein-ligand binding affinity prediction. *IEEE/ACM Trans. Comput. Biol. Bioinform.*, 9, 1301, 2012.
83. Muegge, I., PMF scoring revisited. *J. Med. Chem.*, 49, 5895, 2006.
84. Wang, R., Lai, L., Wang, S., Further development and validation of empirical scoring functions for structure-based binding affinity prediction. *J. Comput. Aided Mol. Des.*, 16, 11, 2002.
85. Kinnings, S.L., Liu, N., Tonge, P.J., Jackson, R.M., Xie, L., Bourne, P.E., A machine learning-based method to improve docking scoring functions and its application to drug repurposing. *J. Chem. Inf. Model.*, 51, 408, 2011.
86. Ballester, P.J. and Mitchell, J.B.O., A machine learning approach to predicting protein–ligand binding affinity with applications to molecular docking. *Bioinformatics*, 26, 1169, 2010.
87. Li, H., Leung, K.-S., Wong, M.-H., Ballester, P.J., Substituting random forest for multiple linear regression improves binding affinity prediction of scoring functions: Cyscore as a case study. *BMC Bioinf.*, 15, 1, 2014.
88. Ballester, P.J., Schreyer, A., Blundell, T.L., Does a more precise chemical description of protein–ligand complexes lead to more accurate prediction of binding affinity? *J. Chem. Inf. Model.*, 54, 944, 2014.
89. Wang, R., Fang, X., Lu, Y., Yang, C.-Y., Wang, S., The PDBbind database: methodologies and updates. *J. Med. Chem.*, 48, 4111, 2005.
90. Li, Y., Han, L., Liu, Z., Wang, R., Comparative assessment of scoring functions on an updated benchmark: 2. Evaluation methods and general results. *J. Chem. Inf. Model.*, 54, 1717, 2014.
91. Amini, A., Shrimpton, P.J., Muggleton, S.H., Sternberg, M.J.E., A general approach for developing system-specific functions to score protein–ligand docked complexes using support vector inductive logic programming. *Proteins Struct. Funct. Bioinf.*, 69, 823, 2007.
92. Li, L., Wang, B., Meroueh, S.O., Support vector regression scoring of receptor–ligand complexes for rank-ordering and virtual screening of chemical libraries. *J. Chem. Inf. Model.*, 51, 2132, 2011.
93. Korb, O., Stutzle, T., Exner, T.E., Empirical scoring functions for advanced protein–ligand docking with PLANTS. *J. Chem. Inf. Model.*, 49, 84, 2009.
94. Gabel, J., Desaphy, J., Rognan, D., Beware of machine learning-based scoring functions on the danger of developing black boxes. *J. Chem. Inf. Model.*, 54, 2807, 2014.
95. Khamis, M.A. and Gomaa, W., Comparative assessment of machine-learning scoring functions on PDBbind 2013. *Eng. Appl. Artif. Intell.*, 45, 136, 2015.

96. Pereira, J.C., Caffarena, E.R., Dos Santos, C.N., Boosting docking-based virtual screening with deep learning. *J. Chem. Inf. Model.*, 56, 2495, 2016.
97. Ahmed, L., Georgiev, V., Capuccini, M., Toor, S., Schaal, W., Laure, E., Spjuth, O., Efficient iterative virtual screening with Apache Spark and conformal prediction. *J. Cheminform.*, 10, 1, 2018.
98. Svensson, F., Norinder, U., Bender, A., Improving screening efficiency through iterative screening using docking and conformal prediction. *J. Chem. Inf. Model.*, 57, 439, 2017.
99. Leach, A.R. and Gillet, V.J., *An introduction to chemoinformatics*, pp. 50–90, Springer, 2007.
100. Lazzeri, I., *Artificial intelligence in drug design: Generative adversarial network for molecules generation/submitted by Isaac Lazzeri*, 2018, https://epub.jku.at/obvulihs/content/titleinfo/2581902.
101. Hammett, L.P., Reaction Rates and Indicator Acidities. *Chem. Rev.*, 16, 67, 1935.
102. Lusci, A., Pollastri, G., Baldi, P., Deep architectures and deep learning in chemoinformatics: The prediction of aqueous solubility for drug-like molecules. *J. Chem. Inf. Model.*, 53, 1563, 2013.
103. Cherkasov, A., Muratov, E.N., Fourches, D., Varnek, A., Baskin, I.I., Cronin, M., Dearden, J., Gramatica, P., Martin, Y.C., Todeschini, R., QSAR modeling: Where have you been? Where are you going to? *J. Med. Chem.*, 57, 4977, 2014.
104. Sawada, R., Kotera, M., Yamanishi, Y., Benchmarking a Wide Range of chemical descriptors for drug-target interaction prediction using a chemogenomic approach. *Mol. Inform.*, 33, 719, 2014.
105. Yap, C.W., PaDEL-descriptor: An open source software to calculate molecular descriptors and fingerprints. *J. Comput. Chem.*, 32, 1466, 2011.
106. Mayr, A., Klambauer, G., Unterthiner, T., Hochreiter, S., DeepTox: Toxicity prediction using deep learning. *Front. Environ. Sci.*, 3, 80, 2016.
107. Gómez-Bombarelli, R., Wei, J.N., Duvenaud, D., Hernández-Lobato, J.M., Sánchez-Lengeling, B., Sheberla, D., Aguilera-Iparraguirre, J., Hirzel, T.D., Adams, R.P., Aspuru-Guzik, A., Automatic chemical design using a data-driven continuous representation of molecules. *ACS Cent. Sci.*, 4, 268, 2018.
108. Segler, M.H.S., Kogej, T., Tyrchan, C., Waller, M.P., Generating focused molecule libraries for drug discovery with recurrent neural networks. *ACS Cent. Sci.*, 4, 120, 2018.
109. Silver, D., Huang, A., Maddison, C.J., Guez, A., Sifre, L., Van Den Driessche, G., Schrittwieser, J., Antonoglou, I., Panneershelvam, V., Lanctot, M., Mastering the game of Go with deep neural networks and tree search. *Nature*, 529, 484, 2016.
110. Silver, D., Hubert, T., Schrittwieser, J., Antonoglou, I., Lai, M., Guez, A., Lanctot, M., Sifre, L., Kumaran, D., Graepel, T., A general reinforcement learning algorithm that masters chess, shogi, and Go through self-play. *Sci. (80-.)*, 362, 1140, 2018.

111. Imrie, F.M., *Deep learning approaches for pre-clinical drug discovery*, PhD thesis, University of Oxford, 2021.
112. Green, C.P., Engkvist, O., Pairaudeau, G., The convergence of artificial intelligence and chemistry for improved drug discovery. *Future Sci.*, 10, 22, 2018.

7

Loading of Drugs in Biodegradable Polymers Using Supercritical Fluid Technology

Janet de los Angeles Chinellato Díaz[1], Santiago Fernandez Bordín[2], Facundo Mattea[1] and Marcelo Ricardo Romero[1]*

[1]National University of Córdoba, Faculty of Chemical Sciences, Department of Organic Chemistry, Córdoba, Argentina, National Council for Scientific and Technical Research (CONICET), Institute for Research and Development in Process Engineering and Applied Chemistry (IPQA), Science Building II, Haya de la Torre and Medina Allende, Córdoba, Argentina
[2]Enrique Gaviola Physics Institute (IFEG), CONICET, Córdoba, Argentina, National University of Córdoba, Faculty of Mathematics, Astronomy, Physics and Computing (FAMAF), Córdoba, Argentina

Abstract

Biodegradable polymers are relevant materials for medical applications due to their similarity with biological tissues. The incorporation of drugs in biopolymers expands their functionalities and makes them very attractive in applications that involve oral, transdermal delivery and active food packaging. However, many biomolecules used as drugs are labile, and few methods allow incorporating these substances into polymers without degrading their structure. Supercritical fluid technology (SCF) is an environmentally friendly technique that allows efficient drug loading under mild conditions without leaving residues. With these characteristics in mind, this chapter has been structured with the aim to describe the main SCF techniques, biopolymer properties, and the types of drugs. Finally, a bibliographic summary is described in detail that summarizes the more relevant advances of drug loading optimization in biopolymers using SCF.

***Keywords*:** Polymers, supercritical, biodegradable, drug loading

**Corresponding author*: marceloricardoromero@gmail.com

Inamuddin, Tariq Altalhi, Jorddy N. Cruz and Moamen Salah El-Deen Refat (eds.) Drug Design Using Machine Learning, (195–224) © 2022 Scrivener Publishing LLC

This chapter describes the supercritical fluid techniques and the best-selected conditions for drug loading in the more relevant biodegradable biopolymers. A complete discussion based on bibliographic findings will allow readers to learn about the most recent discoveries of this technology.

7.1 Introduction

Advances in polymer science have a growing impact on drug delivery systems due to the manufacture of materials with well-defined structures and the ability to adjust their physicochemical and mechanical properties. In general, polymers interact with active substances, either by covalent bonds or by entrapment in a matrix, fulfilling a function of drug carrier, allowing their loading, the charge, and transporting the drug to the affected area. Drug carriers can be developed with different structures, such as nano and microparticles, microcapsules, lipoproteins, liposomes, micelles, among others [1].

For adequate drug administration, the polymeric structure needs to have the following main properties: (i) biodegradable but in the absence of premature degradation of the active substance; (ii) absence of the secondary effects of cytotoxic drugs on organs, tissues, or cells; (iii) increase in the bioavailability of the drug and its fraction on the area to be treated [1]. In the case of nonbiodegradable polymers, they must be excreted by the kidneys [2].

Additionally, to increase the performance of these carriers, it is necessary to guarantee a small particle size and high load capacities. In this sense, they need the property of circulating through the bloodstream long enough for the drug to exert its therapeutic effect and, preferably, accumulate in the required pathological zones. Therefore, biodegradable polymers have an essential function in improving the drug release kinetics and avoiding the accumulation of carriers [3]. The fact that biodegradable polymers can be degraded "in vivo" by enzymatic action or by chemical reactions allows their release from the body as biocompatible by-products, which avoids the surgical removal necessary in the cases of therapies with sustained-release drug implants. In addition, their degradation properties and the absence of toxicity make them ideal carriers of biomolecules for controlled release systems [4].

The manufacture of drug delivery micro or nanodevices is dependent on several factors such as the nature of the active agents, the physicochemical properties of the polymer, the end-use, as well the duration of the therapeutic treatment. Figure 7.1 shows some of the main methods used by different authors [4, 5].

Most of these methods are limited by the use of organic solvents or surfactants. In many cases, they are used for dissolving or dispersing poorly soluble

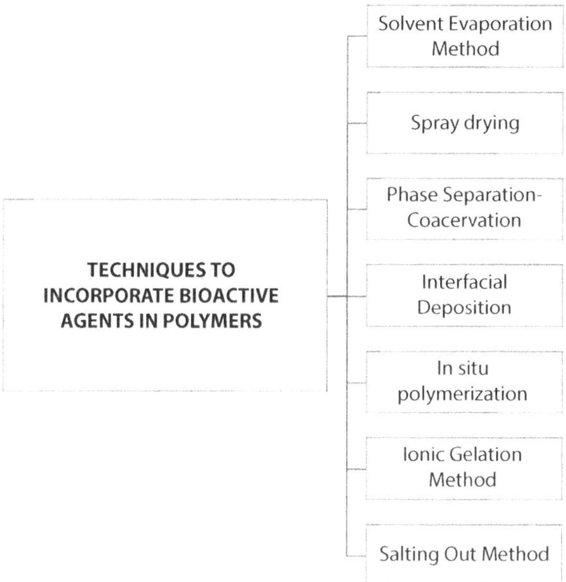

Figure 7.1 Main manufacturing methods for drug carrier systems (from the authors).

drugs that, by themselves, do not have good absorption and lead to poor bioavailability, producing serious side effects in the body. However, the residual solvent or surfactant often causes toxicity and other unwanted side effects. In addition, there is the possibility of drug precipitation after the preparation of aqueous solutions [1]. In this sense, the loading of drugs in biodegradable polymers through the use of supercritical fluids is presented as a "clean" alternative through the use of ecofriendly solvents. In this respect, a highly pure product can be achieved without solvent residues, which in turn, has a direct impact on the costs associated with solvent removal [6].

7.2 Supercritical Fluid Technology

Supercritical fluid technology (SCF) has had commercial relevance for more than 50 years, mainly due to its usefulness as an environmentally friendly technique replacing toxic solvents at the industrial and research level. In addition, SCF technology has potential use in liquid extraction and distillation operations, material processing, chemical reactions, purification, and drying, among other applications [7, 8].

Currently, the most favored industries from this technology are the pharmaceutical, textile [9], and food sectors. Specifically, the former has been able to substitute organic solvents for other more bening ones, such as water and carbon dioxide (CO_2), positioning SCF techniques as a great alternative to produce drug administration systems [10].

7.2.1 Supercritical Fluids

According to the phase rule, there is only one degree of freedom in the areas of two phases of a pure substance (PS), and the equilibrium pressure in each region is a function of temperature [7]. Figure 7.2 shows the equilibrium diagram of a PS, with the different phases as a function of temperature and pressure conditions.

The region of interest centered on the vapor-liquid curve or vapor pressure curve that begins at the triple point of the diagram (or the coexistence of the three states of matter) and ends at the critical point (CP) is shown in Figure 7.2. As the temperature grows, there is a decrease in the density of the liquid phase and a contrary tendency in the vapor density along the vapor pressure curve, until the convergence of these densities at the CP. Consequently, at the CP, there are no longer differences between the phases, and above it, there is no liquid or vapor state. In this sense, a fluid is in a supercritical state when its temperature and pressure values exceed the mentioned CP.

In the supercritical region, the pressure prevents the vaporization of the substance, and the temperature is high enough to avoid condensation. However, the increase in temperature promotes an increase in molecular mobility-limited in turn by pressure [11]. Under supercritical conditions,

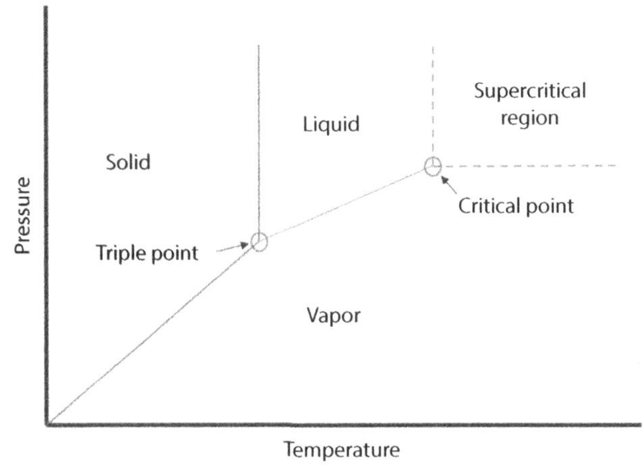

Figure 7.2 Model of an equilibrium diagram for a pure substance (from the authors).

it is impossible to liquefy a gas by increasing the pressure, thus supercritical fluids have unique properties between liquids and gases.

Operations with supercritical fluids depend on these properties, being able to vary them and the behavior of the system with an increase or decrease in temperature or pressure, as detailed in the physicochemical properties section.

Table 7.1 presents some supercritical fluids with their respective critical properties that can be selected as substitutes for organic solvents [7].

Within this group of fluids, one can differentiate those with a low critical temperature (LCT), such as CO_2, ethane, and propane, and those with a high critical temperature (HCT) such as water, methanol, and long-chain alkanes (greater than propane). These differences influence the power of the solvent and its selectivity. In general, those of low critical temperature show a low solvation capacity, with high selectivity for low molecular weight materials such as lipophilic low molecular weight, and low polarity organic compounds. However, its performance decreases in the presence of sugars, amino acids, and compounds that have polar functional groups, such as carboxyl or hydroxyl [7].

On one hand, the solvation capacity of fluids with HCT (between 200°C and 400°C) is higher than LCT fluids, and they are suitable for compounds with high molecular weights, although they present low selectivity. On the other hand, partial pyrolysis in high molecular weight or degradation of thermosensitive materials has been observed. Consequently, the

Table 7.1 Common fluids used for SCF technology (from the authors).

Supercritical fluid	Critical temperature, Tc (°C)	Critical pressure, Pc (MPa)	Critical density, ρc (kg/m³)
Carbon Dioxide	30.9	7.37	468
Ethane	32.2	4.88	203
Propane	96.6	4.25	217
Ammonia	132.3	11.35	235
Methanol	239.4	8.09	272
Ethanol	240.7	6.14	276
Toluene	318.5	318.5	292
Water	373.9	22.06	322

pharmaceutical and natural products industries have exhibited a trend for solvents with an LCT [7].

7.2.2 Physicochemical Properties

Supercritical technology has gain attention and use because of the particular physicochemical properties of chemicals under supercritical conditions. These fluids have intermediate characteristics between liquids and gases, easily adjustable through changes in pressure or temperature, according to the requirements of the process. Table 7.2 shows some of the typical physicochemical properties of SCF compared to the standard properties of gases and liquids.

One of the particular properties of SCFs is their density, which is usually similar to liquids but has better solvent capacity than gases. Therefore, under supercritical conditions, an increase of the pressure increases the density of SCF, the viscosity remains virtually unchanged, but the ability to dissolve substances and solvation capacity increases significantly. On the contrary, under ambient conditions, the capacity of gas to solubilize substances is almost negligible.

For its part, the diffusion coefficient of SCF is usually similar to that of gases, and the viscosity is significantly lower than liquids, which facilitates mass transfer or permeation of SCF in materials [11].

It should be noted that SCFs do not present appreciable surface tension, and this characteristic is relevant to develop processes that include interfacial phenomena [8].

7.2.3 Carbon Dioxide

All gases can reach a supercritical state, but high-temperature conditions are usually required to obtain them. This fact is particularly undesirable

Table 7.2 Physicochemical properties of SCF in comparison to liquids and gases (from the authors).

Property	Liquid	SCF	Gas
Density, kg/m^3	500-1500	200-500	0.5-2
Viscosity, mPa*s	0.2-3	0.01-0.03	0.01-0.3
Diffusion coefficient, m^2/s	10^{-9}	10^{-7}	10^{-5}
Heat conductivity, W/mK	0.1-0,2	0.05-1	0.01-0.02

when the samples contain thermolabile substances, such as a large proportion of pharmaceutical compounds. In this sense, supercritical CO_2 ($SCCO_2$) is considered the most viable alternative, because it has a low critical point at a critical temperature of 30.9°C (304.05 K) and 7.37 MPa (73.7 bar). Additionally, $SCCO_2$ is inert, and the residues that it can leave on the material are harmless. It is an inexpensive, nonflammable substance, easy to recycle or dispose of, and considered environmentally safe [9].

Furthermore, $SCCO_2$ is a nonpolar solvent, and it is ideal for solubilizing molecules with similar polarities. On the contrary, it is not a good option for solubilizing polar, hydrophilic molecules or compounds of very high molecular weight (proteins, fatty acids). Consequently, $SCCO_2$ is very favorable for processes of separation, extraction, drying, manufacture of particles, and impregnation of active agents [11].

7.3 Biodegradable Polymers

In recent decades, interest in biodegradable polymers as substitutes for conventional petroleum-derived polymers has increased, due to their "in vivo" degradation, and because of the high costs of extraction of conventional ones. Biopolymers can be obtained by enzymatic or nonenzymatic catalysis and generate biocompatible or harmless by-products that do not accumulate residues in the environment or organisms [12].

Two processes can be distinguished by which biopolymers can be integrated into the environment, usually called degradation and erosion. Degradation is associate with a rupture of polymeric chains of hydrolysis of links in shorter chains or oligomers, and erosion is related to the decrease in polymeric mass, due to the loss of water-soluble monomers, oligomers, and other products [13].

Depending on the specific type of biodegradation mechanism, polymers can be classified into those that degrade throughout their mass and those that degrade only on the surface. Mass degradation consists of a homogeneous transformation of the entire polymer matrix. Moreover, surface degradation is a phenomenon that occurs in a heterogeneous way on a thin surface layer of the polymer [13]. Figure 7.3 shows a representative scheme of these two types of degradation.

Biodegradable polymers can be classified into two broad categories according to their origin: biologically derived polymers, also known as natural polymers, and synthetic polymers (see Figure 7.4). Biological polymers are created from living organisms and obtained by direct biomass extraction in the form of proteins, polysaccharides, peptides, or

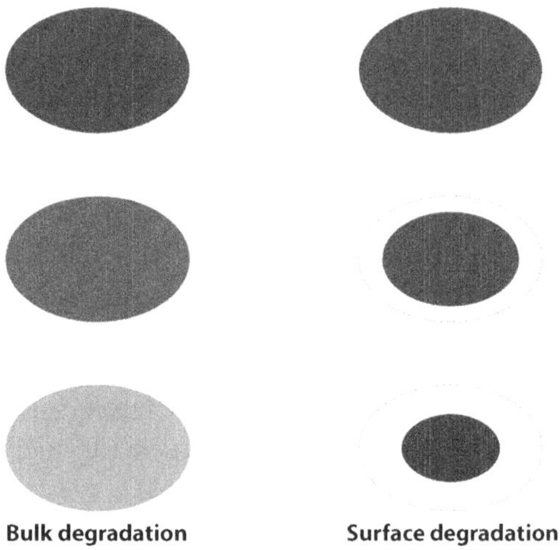

Figure 7.3 Biodegradation mechanisms (from the authors).

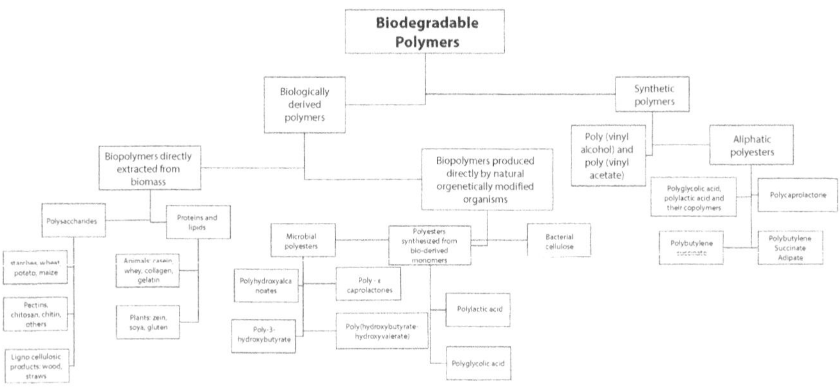

Figure 7.4 Classification of biodegradable polymers according to their origin and manufacturing method (from the authors).

produced directly from natural or genetically modified organisms, such as bacterial cellulose, polyesters synthesized from "bio-derived monomers" and microbial polyesters. These polymers have hydrophilic groups and possess a certain degree of crystallinity. However, despite of being appreciated for their high biocompatibility, they present certain drawbacks, such as antigenicity and the difficulty of carrying out a reproducible manufacturing process [14, 15].

On the other hand, synthetic polymers are those made in a laboratory. These polymers present the advantage of being easily modified for specific mechanical properties or a desired degradation rate by further chemical reactions, in comparison to natural polymers. Some examples of synthetic polymers are aliphatic polyesters, such as poly (lactic acid) and polycaprolactone, and the poly(vinyl alcohol), polyvinyl acetate [14, 15].

It should be noted that synthetic structures can usually be combined with natural ones, either as a copolymer or a blend, to achieve synergy of their properties of these two groups [16, 17].

Biodegradable polymers have advantages as drug carriers since their impregnation of active agents is straightforward, they have a high load-carrying capacity, and can be designed to have a sustained release from the polymeric matrix. Likewise, their nature usually gives them a biocompatible character [10].

Considering studies carried out since 2016, the use of biodegradable polymers for the impregnation of drugs with $SCCO_2$ predominates in a proportion of 1.7 times compared to nonbiodegradable polymers, as shown in Figure 7.5. Within the group of biodegradable polymers, natural materials include collagens, alginates, celluloses [18–20] and materials of synthetic origins such as polylactic acid, poly (lactic-co-glycolic acid), and poly (2-hydroxyethyl methacrylate) [21–23].

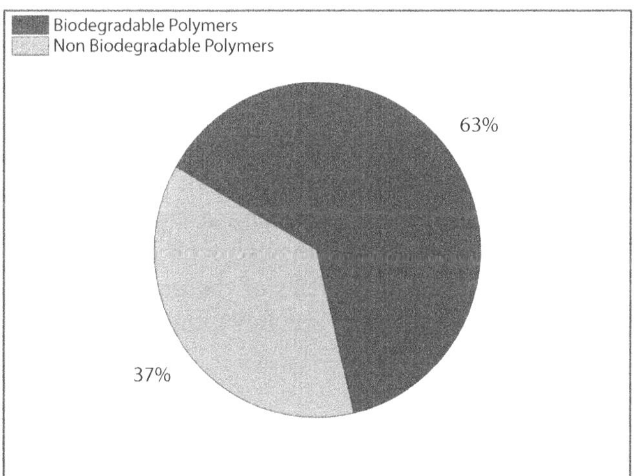

Figure 7.5 Uses of biodegradable polymers for drug loading using SCF technology based on bibliography of last 5 years (from the authors).

7.3.1 Main Biologically-Derived Polymers Used With SCF Technologies

7.3.1.1 *Cellulose*

Cellulose is a long-chain polysaccharide composed of a single repeating unit, cellobiose (see Figure 7.6a). It is characterized by elevated crystallinity, high molecular weight, infusible and insoluble in all organic solvents. For these reasons, it must be modified into derived substances (ethers, esters, and acetals) to facilitate its processing. At an industrial level, it is extracted mainly from wood and, to a lesser extent, from sugarcane bagasse stalks. Its main applications are in the manufacture of paper, explosives, textiles, dietary fibers, and membranes [24, 25].

7.3.1.2 *Chitosan*

Chitosan is a polysaccharide produced by the partial alkaline deacetylation of chitin (Figure 7.6b), which is the main component of crab shells. Chitosan, unlike chitin, is soluble in water, has biocompatible properties, antimicrobial activity, the moisturizing capacity, and can retain large amounts of water. These properties have allowed its use in broad applications, such as cosmetics, packaging, the synthesis of water-soluble prodrugs, the manufacture of absorbable sutures, and artificial skin [24, 25].

7.3.1.3 *Alginate*

Alginate is a polysaccharide extracted from brown algae using alkaline solutions. It is a biocompatible copolymer with different ratios between the monomers β-D-mannuronic acid and α-L-guluronic acid (Figure 7.6c). This relationship depends on the extraction source and influences the structural and chemical properties of the polymer. In the presence of divalent counterions (Ca^{2+}, Zn^{2+}, or Ba^{2+}), this biopolymer acquires a

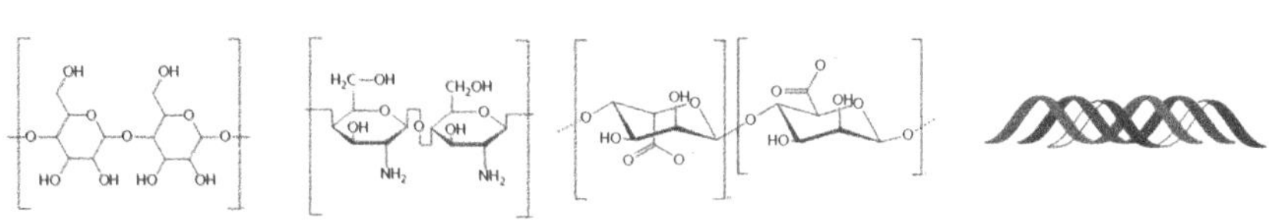

(**a**) Cellulose (**b**) Chitosan (**c**) Alginate (**d**) Collagen

Figure 7.6 Main biologically derived polymers used with SCF technologies (from the authors).

gelling character allowing the encapsulation of active agents. In addition, it is resistant to acids and is not toxic. Therefore, its use is appreciated for drug delivery with controlled release, bioengineering, and the food industry [25, 26].

7.3.1.4 Collagen

Collagen is the main protein of the connective tissues of animals, constituted by a variety of polypeptides conformed in a trimeric structure and with a primary structure dominated by lysine, glycine, hydroxyproline, and proline (Figure 7.6d). The glycine content in the sequence of this biodegradable polymer determines a good stiffness and low elongation, and a higher content of this amino acid gives it flexibility. From the denaturation or degradation of collagen, the gellatin, another biopolymer, is obtained. Most collagen applications have been focused in biomedicine and biomedical sciences [25, 27].

7.3.2 Main Synthetic Polymers Used With SCF Technologies

7.3.2.1 Polylactic Acid (PLA)

Polylactic acid, better known as PLA, is a thermoplastic polyester (Figure 7.7a) produced from a lactic acid monomer, by polycondensation or ring-opening polymerization of lactide. Lactic acid is a molecule that contains a chiral carbon and consequently has two optical isomers. This fact is responsible for the different PLA molecules that can be obtained, which have a broad range of properties that go from the amorphous state to the crystalline state. Some of the most relevant PLA properties are biodegradability, biocompatibility, and bioresorbability. These properties makes PLA suitable for various uses in the pharmacological industry, as a means of drug transport, and in the scaffolding of material as a mean for tissue regeneration. In addition, it has been used as absorbable suture material, absorbable implants, devices for internal fixation of bones, and in medical equipment [25].

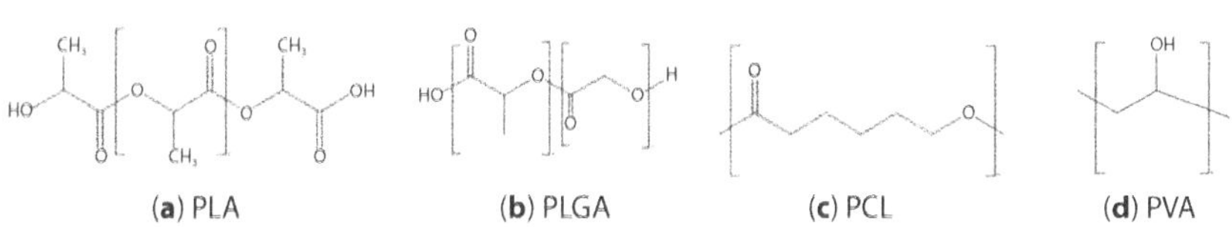

Figure 7.7 Main synthetic polymers used with SCF technologies (from the authors).

7.3.2.2 Poly (Lactic-co-Glycolic Acid) (PLGA)

Poly (lactic-co-glycolic acid) (PLGA) is synthesized from the copolymerization of L-lactide and DL-lactide (L) with glycolic acid (G). From the variation in the proportion of these monomers, different products such as amorphous polymers (25L: 75G) or semi-crystalline polymers (80L: 20G) can be obtained. One factor to keep in mind is that as the L/G monomer ratio increases, the degradability rate of the copolymer decreases. This biopolymer is often used as a nanoparticulate polymer layer in drug delivery systems. In addition, it has shown good cell adhesion for tissue engineering applications. The repetitive structure of this polymer is shown in Figure 7.7b [25].

7.3.2.3 Polycaprolactone (PCL)

Polycaprolactone or PCL is a biopolymer that is obtained from the ring-opening polymerization of the monomer ε-caprolactone. PCL is characterized by having a semi-crystalline linear structure with a broad solubility in different solvents and being quite resistant and semi-rigid when it has a high molecular weight (see Figure 7.7c). Its biodegradable nature makes it attractive as controlled drug release systems. Additionally, the low glass transition temperature of PLC allows its use as a compatibility agent or as a soft block in polyurethane formulations [25]. While PCL is degradable in various biotic environments, it degrades more slowly compared to biopolyesters and starch in most environments [27].

7.3.2.4 Poly (Vinyl Alcohol) (PVA)

Poly (vinyl alcohol) (PVA) is a linear synthetic biopolymer obtained by partial or total hydrolysis of polyvinyl acetate (Figure 7.7d). Its physicochemical and mechanical properties are dependent on the degree of hydroxylation although, its main characteristics are its high solubility in water and its resistance to organic solvents. This solubility requires crosslinking of the polymer to generate structural stability after swelling with water or biological fluids. Therefore, PVA is adaptable for the textile industry, paper industry, food packaging, and for the manufacture of medical devices [28].

7.4 Drug Delivery

Drug administration aims to transport active agents with therapeutic effects, preferably under controlled conditions that allow the molecule of interest to be delivered in the optimal amount, in the precise place and during the most suitable period. In this way, the frequency of administration is reduced, improving efficiency and reducing toxicity. On the other hand, drug delivery faces several challenges, such as the solubilization and diffusion of the active agent.

In order to overcome these limitations, in many formulations biodegradable polymers are used to encapsulate the drug, forming matrix structures that can be supplied as micro or nanoparticles [10]. Since the last decade, the hydrogels have been used as drug carriers because of their high swelling capacity. Also, microparticles are very popular for their simple manufacture and administration. These type of structure can be formed by solvent evaporation, spray drying, among other techniques. Nanometric systems have also had a great development, distinguishing between liposomes, nanoparticles, dendrimers, polymeric micelles and nanocrystals [29].

In this way, from the combination of materials science and drug administration, the particle synthesis process and its morphology can be controlled. However, conventional techniques for the manufacture of drug carriers have some limitations, such as chemical and thermal degradation of the active agent, the use of large volumes of organic solvents, a wide particle size distribution, and the presence of solvent residues in the final products [10].

In this sense, SCF technology is presented as an advantageous alternative, whose first report of this method based on the solubilization of active agents dates back to 1980, based on the work carried out by Krukonis *et al.* [11]. Since that time, the development of this technology has significantly improved, and supercritical CO_2 as been mostly used as in impregnation solvent due to it low critical point, which is ideal for impregnating thermosensitive therapeutic agents. Figure 7.8 shows the main supercritical fluid techniques currently used for impregnation and micronization of active compounds or polymer/drug composite particles.

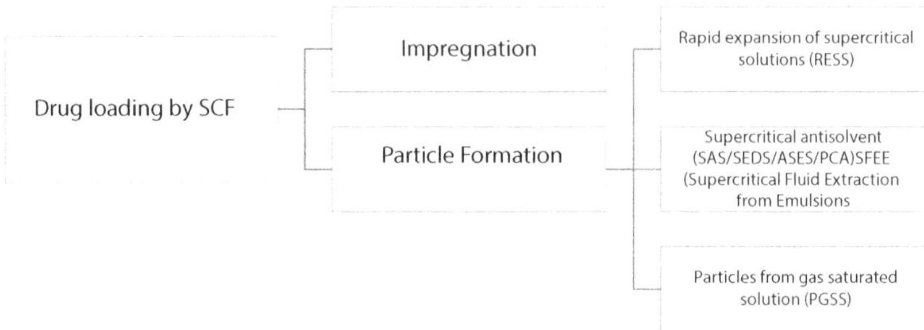

Figure 7.8 Main techniques with supercritical fluids used for drug loading (from the authors).

Supercritical impregnation process with CO_2

To carry out the supercritical impregnation process of drugs in a biodegradable polymeric matrix, the active agent must be totally or partially soluble in the supercritical fluid. However, when it is not possible to solubilize this molecule, solubilization can be increased using a low proportion of cosolvent (<10%), which is subsequently extracted from the polymeric matrix [30]. The supercritical impregnation process has been reported as a batch procedure, in which the polymer and the active substance are placed in a reactor physically separated, to avoid the deposition of the solute on the polymer as shown in Figure 7.9; which represents a typical configuration that consists of three phases.

In the first phase, the drug dissolves in $SCCO_2$ at set supercritical temperatures and pressures. Once the drug is solubilized, the charged $SCCO_2$ diffuses into the polymer matrix, resulting in the impregnation of the solute. During this process, depending on the temperature and pressure

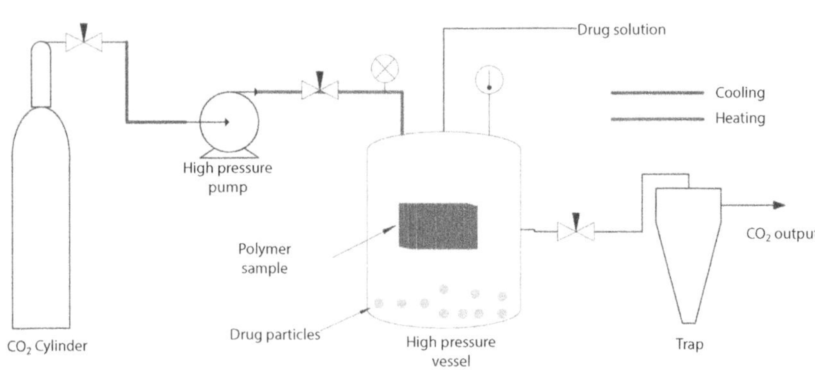

Figure 7.9 General process of supercritical impregnation with CO_2 (from the authors).

conditions, the swelling of the polymer may occur, and consequently, the dissolution is further facilitated. This impregnation process can be carried out in the presence or absence of agitation. In a third step, the system is depressurized, the drug precipitates leaving a part impregnated in the matrix, and the rest of it at the bottom of the reactor together with CO_2. In this stage, the $SCCO_2$ becomes gaseous CO_2 during venting, leaving the matrix completely. The recycling stages for CO_2 and nonimpregnated drugs are economical and environmentally friendly operations [31].

Therefore, to achieve good results by supercritical impregnation, the drug must be soluble in the fluid phase, and its partition coefficient must be highly favorable towards the impregnation support to allow significant impregnation amounts. Therefore, the efficiency of the impregnation process will be subject to the partition coefficient, which establishes the relative affinity of the drug for the supercritical fluid and the polymeric matrix under specific conditions of temperature and pressure. This coefficient varies depending on the experimental conditions, between 10^{-2} and 10^{4}, and it is expressed as:

$$K = \frac{C_{polymer}}{C_{CO_2}} \tag{7.1}$$

where

$C_{polymer}$: Drug concentration in the polymer matrix

C_{CO_2} : Drug concentration in CO_2

To determine the amount of drug impregnated in the polymeric matrix, "drug loading" is calculated through the following equation:

$$\%\,Drug\ loading = \frac{mass\ of\ drug}{mass\ of\ raw\ polymer} * 100 \tag{7.2}$$

The mass of drug in the crude polymer, or the mass percent of drug in the impregnated sample, should be used.

In general, the impregnation of drugs from $SCCO_2$ is widely extended in different industrial sectors, becoming a useful tool for loading drugs in polymeric matrices.

Microparticle formation

The rapid expansion of supercritical solutions (RESS) is a technique that allows the micronization of small and uniform particles. In addition, it is ideal for treating thermally labile compounds since it operates at moderate temperatures. The use of RESS for the micronization of drugs [32–34], of polymers [35–37], in the formation of polymer and drug administration systems [38, 39], among other uses.

Thus, to carry out the RESS process, the solute must have adequate solubility in the supercritical fluid. Therefore, it is limited to those polymers with high solubility in CO_2. In this process, the $SCCO_2$ is generated to flow together with the solute (i.e., a polymer) through a capillary nozzle towards an expansion chamber, generating a rapid depressurization under atmospheric conditions (see Figure 7.10); the expansion period is less than 10^{-5} s. This rapid decrease in operating conditions causes a diminution in the power of the solvent giving high supersaturation of the solute in the depressurized fluid, which leads to the precipitation of the solute [40]. This process is based on the phase separation induced by the difference in solute solubilities in the supercritical fluid at high and low pressures, respectively [35].

The supercritical antisolvent (SAS) technique is one of the most used to micronize solvent-free materials, either for the micronization of active compounds or their co-precipitation in polymeric vehicles. In this technique, the solute to be micronized is dissolved in an organic solvent and sprayed into a chamber containing $SCCO_2$; $SCCO_2$ dissolves in the liquid solvent, causing supersaturation of the solution, for this reason, it acts as an antisolvent agent, creating an unfavorable environment for the solute, for which the solute precipitates in the form of micro or nanoparticles. The principle of this technique is solvent-promoted phase separation [35, 41].

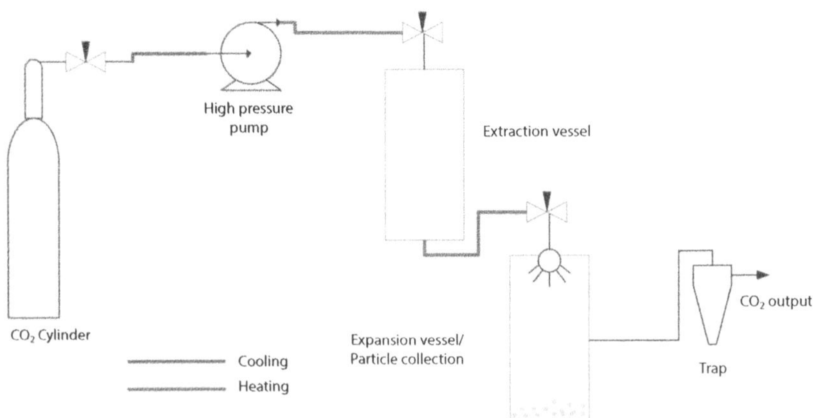

Figure 7.10 General scheme of RESS process (from the authors).

The SAS technique for particles micronization in oral, parenteral, transdermal, and topical drugs administration, as well as for aerosol preparation, medicinal patches, and active topical gels have been reported in the literature [42–48].

Figure 7.11 shows a typical scheme of the SAS process, which starts with the pumping of CO_2 at the pressure set in the precipitator, which is at a specific temperature, to establish supercritical conditions. The pure solvent is then introduced into the precipitator through a nozzle. Subsequently, more solvent solute solution is injected. At that time, rapid diffusion of $SCCO_2$ in the liquid solvent generates solute supersaturation, causing it to precipitate on a filter. The $SCCO_2$ stream is kept flowing for enough time to ensure complete solvent removal, then the system is depressurized, and precipitated dust is collected. Then, solvent/antisolvent mixtures are finally recovered downstream.

There are many modified versions of this process that differ in how the solvent containing the solute and the supercritical antisolvent come into contact, mainly due to the type of spray or injector used. In the supercritical fluid enhanced dispersion solution (SEDS) the solvents are mixed in a tube-in-tube injector or a coaxial nozzle, on the other hand, in the aerosol solvent extraction system (ASES), and the precipitation by compressed antisolvent (PCA) solution is sprayed from an injector [37, 41]. Moreover, in SFEE the solvent is replaced with O/W emulsion that provides an additional control over the particle size [49, 50]

The particle technique of gas saturated solutions, PGSS, is based on the interactions of $SCCO_2$ with polymers and low melting point fats. These compounds, in general, can dissolve large volumes of CO_2, even at intermediate pressures; CO_2 within these components causes a decrease in melting and glass transition temperatures and can cause a diminution

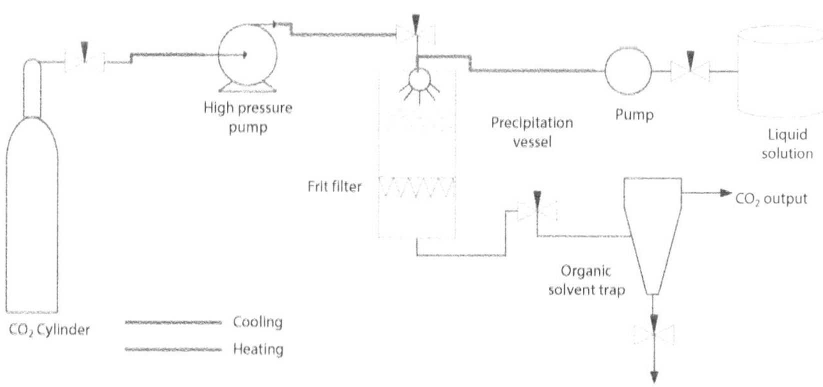

Figure 7.11 General scheme of SAS process (from the authors).

in viscosity. When these molten substances become saturated with CO_2, the gas expands at atmospheric pressure. This change in condition generates a rapid decrease in temperature due to the Joule-Thomson effect. In addition, an increase in the melting temperature to the original value at ambient pressure causes the rapid solidification of the polymer or fat. This technique is governed by "the pressure and temperature- and solvent-induced phase separation".

Then, to form composite microparticles, a microparticle suspension of the active agent is first created in the polymer matrix, which upon melting, is atomized to form composite microparticles containing the active substance suspended at random. It has been observed that directly melting the drug in PGSS causes its decomposition, even when the experimental studies were carried out, below its melting temperature. A general PGSS process is shown in Figure 7.12.

The PGSS technique has been used in the pharmaceutical and food sectors for the processing of a variety of products [51, 52]. Particularly, this process has been very successful for the creation of polymeric micro composites such as active agent carrier materials [53].

SCF technology uses biodegradable polymeric materials for the impregnation of drugs with different applications, which is not only restricted to the area of biomedicine. Most of the studies of supercritical impregnation with CO_2 are usually concentrated in applications related to the transdermal delivery of drugs through patches, dressings, or similar methodologies [18, 54–57], followed by the oral delivery of drugs [22, 58], and for use in active food packaging [16, 21, 57, 59, 60]. In turn, the aforementioned areas and others whose participation is less crucial, such as drug-eluting

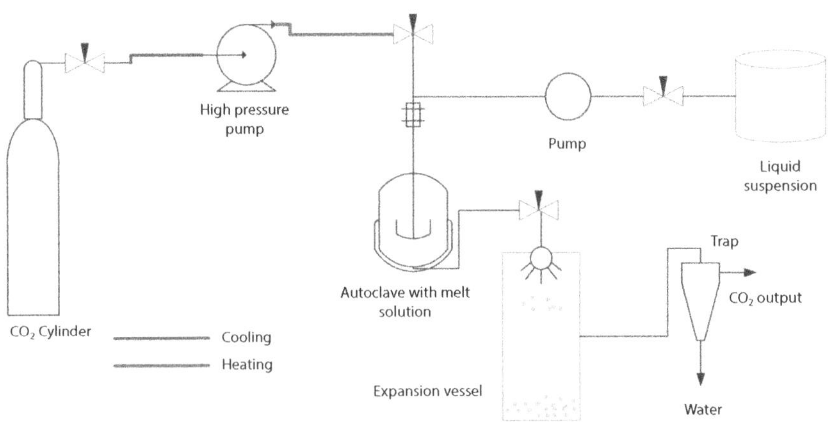

Figure 7.12 General scheme of PGSS process (from the authors).

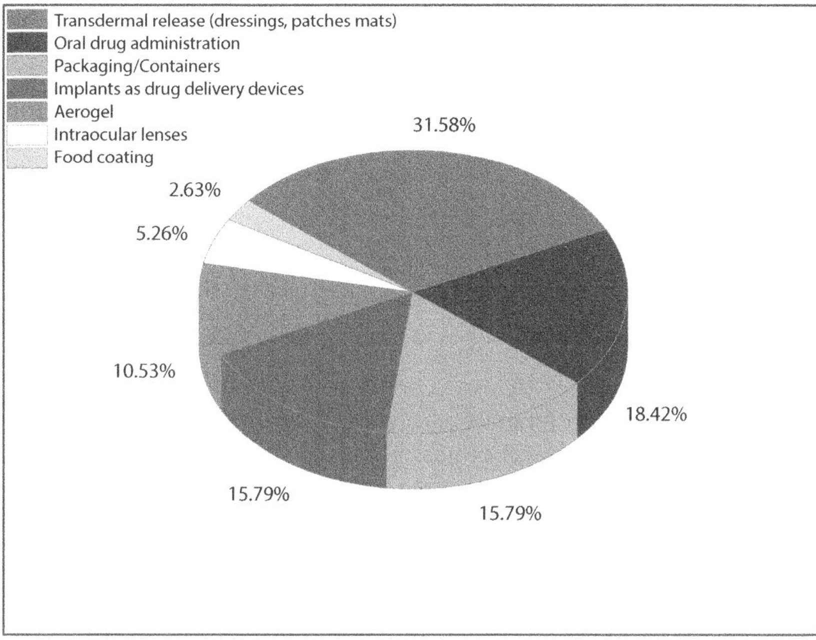

Figure 7.13 Applications of supercritical impregnation in biodegradable polymers (from the authors).

implants and aerogels, cover 82% of the applications currently being investigated (see Figure 7.13).

7.4.1 Types of Drugs

A wide variety of drugs are used in $SCCO_2$ impregnation studies, among which drugs synthesized for anti-inflammatory purposes stand out, such as nimesulide, ketoprofen, and acetylsalicylic acid [55, 61, 62], drugs with antibiotic properties, such as ciprofloxacin [23], and another group of substances with antimicrobial and bactericidal effects, studied mainly for use in active food packaging, among which are thymol [21], eugenol [58], and cinnamaldehyde [59]. Also, more specific drugs have been used, such as lansoprazole [63], which acts as an inhibitor of stomach acid secretion, and some antibiotics, such as ciprofloxacin [23], whose molecular structures are shown in Figure 7.14.

$SCCO_2$ impregnation has also been used to impregnate complex substances from natural extracts. Milovanovic *et al.* selected thyme extract to impregnate polylactic acid/poly (ε-caprolactone) films in order to create

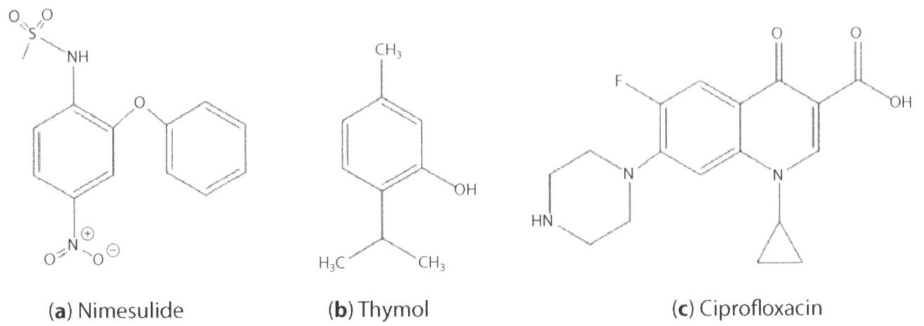

Figure 7.14 Examples of drugs used in $SCCO_2$ impregnation (from the authors).

food packaging with moderate antibacterial properties, since the load obtained was low and it was not possible to stop bacterial growth [16].

In the last 5 years of research, it has been observed that more than 85% of the studies of impregnation with SCF are based on anti-inflammatory and bactericidal or pesticide drugs, their predominant participation being around 85% (see Figure 7.15). Anti-inflammatory drugs are used mainly in the controlled administration of drugs [19, 22, 23, 55, 56, 62]. On the

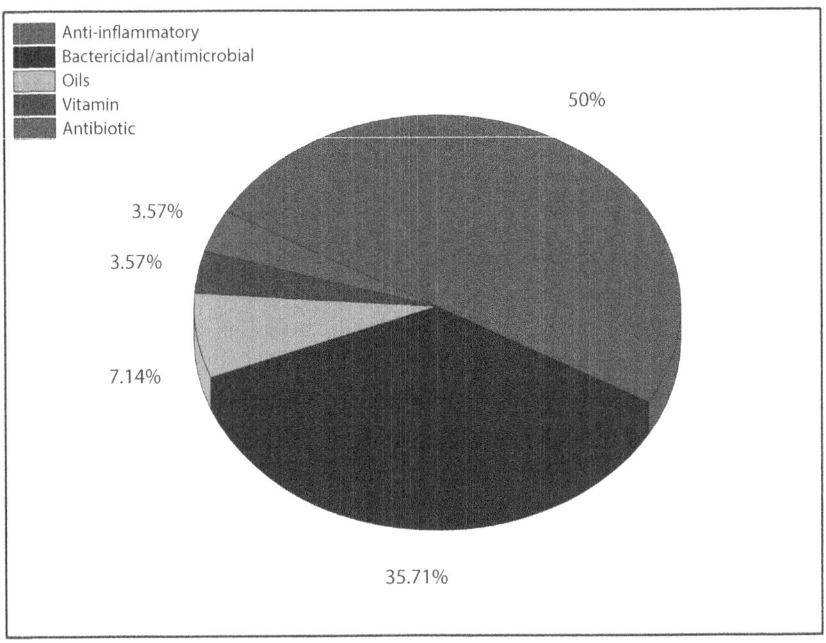

Figure 7.15 Different types of drugs used in supercritical impregnation with CO_2 (from the authors).

other hand, most bactericidal substances have been used for the creation of antioxidant, antimicrobial films, and packaging with food preservation capabilities [16, 21, 57, 59, 60], but also in the manufacture of functional textiles with pharmaceutical applications [17] and oral hygiene [58].

Effect of molecular size on the percentage of impregnation with $SCCO_2$

The type of drug and the impregnation loading are both influenced by the molecular size. In general, substances of low molecular sizes are selected for impregnation, although several ranges of interest can be differentiated: (a) Small range from 120 to 200 Da [20, 21, 58, 59], (b) Medium range between 200 and 380 Da [19, 55, 63], and (c) The upper range comprises molecules such as the dexamethasone salt (516.4 Da). Some researchers have carried out experiments with this substance with a higher molecular mass, such as that used in the impregnation of intraocular lenses, where high yields have been reported despite the low solubility of this compound in $SCCO_2$ [23].

Figure 7.16 shows a summary of the distribution of the impregnation percentage with the molecular weight of biodegradable and nonbiodegradable polymers. A trend towards the use of low molecular weights, between

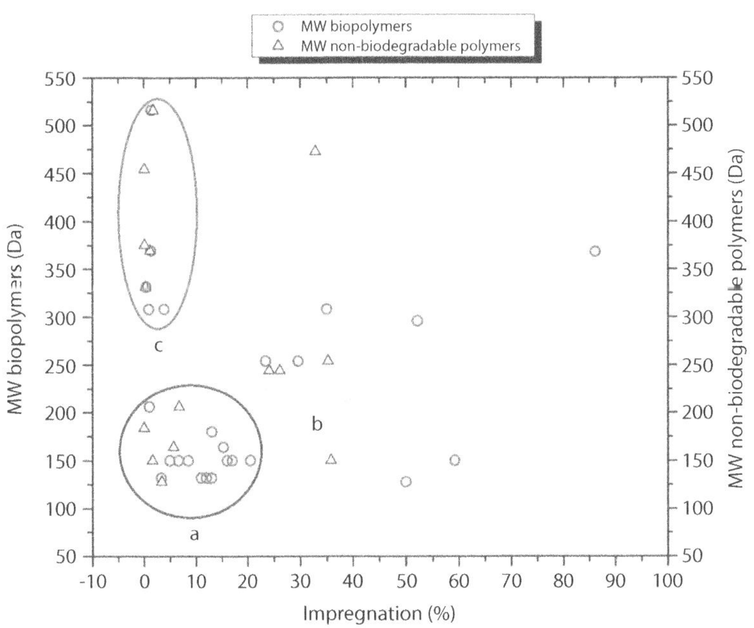

Figure 7.16 Molecular weight vs. impregnation rate (from the authors).

120 and 200 Da, can be observed, with a predominance in biodegradable polymers, observing an impregnation rate, with a maximum around 20% (Figure 7.16a). However, in other studies, it has been possible to achieve loads between 50% and 60% using biodegradable polymers under intermediate conditions of pressure and temperature [17, 20].

Additionally, in a small number of experiments it has been observed that the achieved impregnations show higher yields than the average (between 23% and 35%). In these cases, molecular weights belonging to the medium range (b) of 240 to 300 Da (Figure 7.16b) were used. Likewise, it is important to note that as the molecular weight increases, the probability of impregnation is lower, as observed in the region highlighted with a red circle (Figure 17.16c).

7.4.2 Influence of Experimental Conditions on the Drug Loading

Influence of Temperature on Impregnation with SCF

The influence of temperature on the impregnation of drugs with $SCCO_2$ is presented in Figure 7.17. It is important to note that this graph excludes other aspects of equal relevance, such as the nature of the polymer and the structure of the impregnated molecule.

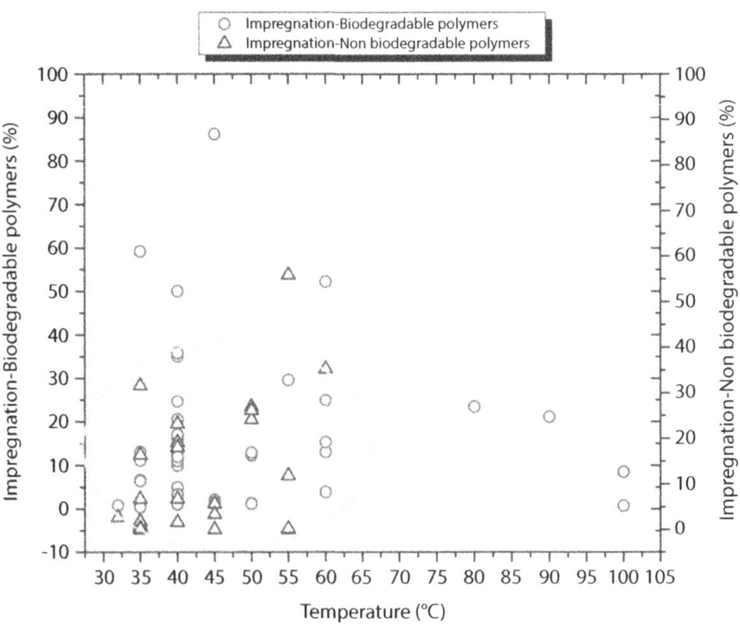

Figure 7.17 Temperature versus impregnation graph (from the authors).

Figure 7.17 shows that the tested temperature ranges from 32°C to 100°C for biopolymers, with a more limited range of temperatures for nonbiodegradable polymers. However, it is observed that more than 90% of the studies are carried out within the interval of 35°C to 60°C (circle area). Additionally, it has been observed that some authors have achieved impregnation percentages of up to 60% and with few exceptions reached 80% [64]. Better results and high yields of fillers have been achieved mainly using biodegradable polymers. Based on the mentioned trend, it is possible to adjust the test variables, and in optimal conditions reach impregnation percentages of up to 35%.

It should be borne in mind that the influence of temperature on the percentage of the impregnated drug, under isobaric conditions, varies according to the experimental study. Thus, taking some published research as examples, it is observed that by modifying the temperature the drug load can increase [17, 61, 63, 65] and, in some cases, decrease and then increase [62]. This impregnation behavior as a function of temperature can vary for the same drug and material depending on the pressure observed. Despite this disparity, in most studies, an increase in temperature favors drug impregnation.

Influence of pressure on impregnation with SCF

Like temperature, the influence of pressure on impregnation rates varies significantly between different studies. Figure 17.18 shows the effect of pressure on the load introduced to the polymeric material. The figure shows that a wide range of pressures from 75 bar to 500 bar has been tested. However, those studies at the upper-pressure level do not ensure a higher percentage of impregnation. In general, the highest proportion of studies (80%) is between pressures of 80 bar and 200 bar (circle area). Within this pressure range, it is observed that the impregnations are equivalent to those carried out at higher pressure. In addition, studies in which the operating conditions have favored higher impregnations [17, 19, 20, 64], especially in the studies carried out by Gracia and collaborators, where they obtained impregnations between 50% and 86% of curcumin in solids PLGA supports [64].

In summary, the most frequent pressure values (21% of cases) used for $SCCO_2$ impregnation in biodegradable polymers is 120 bar, followed by 100 bar and 200 bar representing 12.5% each, and in total around 50% of the conditions, either as a fixed parameter or as part of a range of evaluated pressures.

Conditions in which pressure increases provide some advantages over milder conditions and are generally selected. For example, in the study by Gañan *et al.* [66] the microencapsulation of chia oil is carried out in a soy protein matrix, through an experimental design at 100 bar and 160 bar, with temperature variations of 40°C and 60°C; whose results show an impregnation at 100 bar and 40°C of 22.1%, five times higher than when impregnating at 60°C. On the other hand, when the pressure increases, the impregnation increases of Δ2.5% is exclusively observed at 40°C. On the contrary, the impregnation of fibrous materials based on polyamide 6 with thymol increases the load by 11.6%, when the pressure rises from 100 to 200 bar, and at a constant temperature of 35°C. It should be noted that in the aforementioned research, Marković *et al.* make a comparison of the impregnation method with liquid CO_2, corroborating that the SCF techniques were better and produced a 25% loading improvement [17].

While another polyamide 6 impregnation studies have shown lower impregnation rates. In this sense, Mosquera *et al.* impregnated with eugenol at 60°C, showing a load of 13.62% at 100 bar and a progressive increase until 120 bar, with a maximum load of 15.27%. However, despite being a load lower than the average concerning the global statistical values (Figure 7.18), the mass of eugenol released showed antibacterial activity by inhibiting almost 100% of the bacteria tested [58].

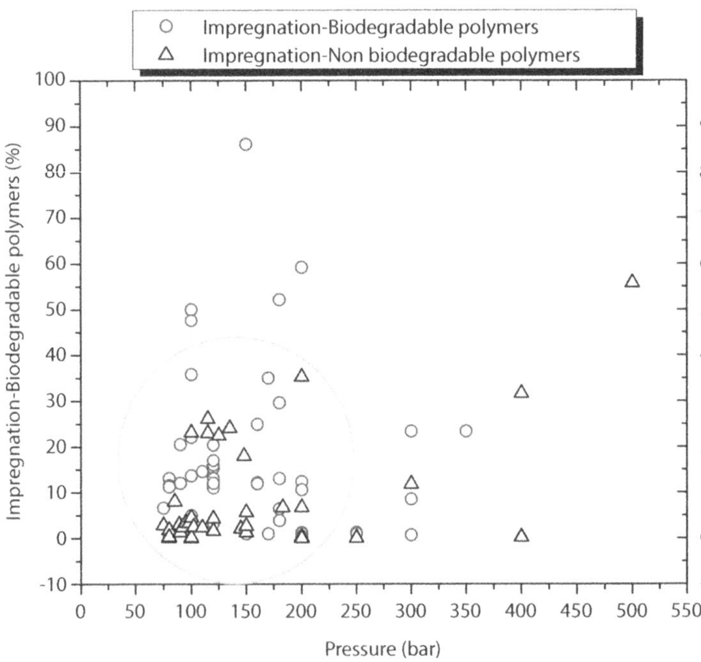

Figure 7.18 Effect of pressure on the percentage of impregnation with SCF (from the authors).

In general, the impregnation rates show a slight tendency of an increase in the load with increasing pressure [67–71]. This phenomenon could be a consequence of the improvement of the solubility of drugs in the fluid phase of $SCCO_2$ with pressure. This phenomenon produces an increase in the density of CO_2, together with the solvating power and plasticizing character, facilitating the swelling of the polymer and the absorption of CO_2 [21, 23, 58, 63]. It is also important to note that the solubility of the drug depends on CO_2 density and the intermolecular interactions in the fluid phase. For this reason, low pressures can produce a decrease in the density of CO_2 and, consequently, weak intermolecular forces that promote a low dissolution of the drug in the fluid phase [62].

7.5 Conclusion

In recent years, commercial and social interest in biopolymers, particularly biodegradable biopolymers, has increased, because of their environmental and economic benefits. Also, a variety of drugs can be incorporated into them, which expands the field of application of these materials. However, the lability of many active agents, particularly those of natural origin, makes the use of supercritical methods for their incorporation into the polymeric network practically essential. This synergy between biopolymers and SCF will surely be enhanced by emerging technologies such as 3D printing, which allow obtaining very complex geometries such as those of biological tissues with faithful fidelity. The combination of 3D printing and SCF impregnation of polymers and biopolymers should be considered as a possible evolution of the design of drug delivery systems and plattforms.

Acknowledgments

The authors would like to thank Prof. Dr. Inamuddin for providing the necessary funds to conduct this study. S.P. Fernandez Bordín and J.A. Chinellato Díaz would like to thank CONICET–Argentina for their doctoral scholarship.

References

1. Torchilin, V.P., Micellar nanocarriers: Pharmaceutical perspectives. *Pharm. Res.*, 24, 1, 2006.

2. Vilar, G., Tulla-Puche, J., Albericio, F., Polymers and drug delivery systems. *Curr. Drug Deliv.*, 9, 367, 2012.
3. Liechty, W.B., Kryscio, D.R., Slaughter, B.V., Peppas, N.A., Polymers for drug delivery systems. *Annu. Rev. Chem. Biomol. Eng.*, 1, 149, 2010.
4. Jana, P., Shyam, M., Singh, S., Jayaprakash, V., Dev, A., Biodegradable polymers in drug delivery and oral vaccination. *Eur. Polym. J.*, 142, 110155, 2021.
5. Park, J.H., Ye, M., Park, K., Biodegradable polymers for microencapsulation of drugs. *Molecules*, 10, 146, 2005.
6. Nunes, A. V., Rodriguez-Rojo, S., Almeida, A. P., Matias, A. A., Rego, D., Simplicio, A. L., Bronze, M. R., Cocero, M. J., Duarte, C. M. M., Supercritical fluids strategies to produce hybrid structures for drug delivery. *JCR*, 148, 1, 2010.
7. Martínez, J.L., *Supercritical fluid extraction of nutraceuticals and bioactive compounds*, CRC Press, Boca Raton, 2007.
8. Marre, S., Roig, Y., Aymonier, C., Supercritical microfluidics: Opportunities in flow-through chemistry and materials science. *J. Supercrit. Fluids*, 66, 251, 2012.
9. Goñi, M.L. Gañán, N.A. Martini, R.E. Supercritical CO2-assisted dyeing and functionalization of polymeric materials: A review of recent advances (2015–2020). *J. CO2 Util.*, 54, 101760, 2021.
10. Kankala, R.K., Zhang, Y.S., Bin Wang, S., Lee, C.H., Chen, A.Z., Supercritical fluid technology: An emphasis on drug delivery and related biomedical applications. *Adv. Healthc. Mater.*, 6, 1700433, 2017.
11. Brunner, G. *Gas Extraction: An Introduction to Fundamentals of Supercritical Fluids and the Application to Separation Processes*, Steinkopff, 1994.
12. Prajapati, S.K., Jain, A., Jain, A., Jain, S., Biodegradable polymers and constructs: A novel approach in drug delivery. *Eur. Polym. J.*, 120, 109191, 2019.
13. Lao, L.L., Peppas, N.A., Boey, F.Y.C., Venkatraman, S.S., Modeling of drug release from bulk-degrading polymers. *Int. J. Pharm.*, 418, 28, 2011.
14. Ghanbarzadeh, B. and Almasi, H., Biodegradable polymers, in: *Biodegradation - Life of Science*, R. Chamy and F. Rosenkranz (Eds.), pp. 141–185, InTech, Rijeka, 2013.
15. Zhang, Z., Ortiz, O., Goyal, R., Kohn, J., Biodegradable Polymers, in: *Handbook of Polymer Applications in Medicine and Medical Devices*, pp. 303–335, Elsevier Inc, 2014, ISBN 9780323228053.
16. Milovanovic, S., Hollermann, G., Errenst, C., Pajnik, J., Frerich, S., Kroll, S., Rezwan, K., Ivanovic, J., Supercritical CO_2 impregnation of PLA/PCL films with natural substances for bacterial growth control in food packaging. *Food Res. Int.*, 107, 486, 2018.
17. Marković, D., Milovanović, S., De Clerck, K., Zizovic, I., Stojanović, D., Radetić, M., Development of material with strong antimicrobial activity by high pressure CO_2 impregnation of polyamide nanofibers with thymol. *J. CO2 Util.*, 26, 19, 2018.

18. Pascoal, D.R.C., Cabral-Albuquerque, E.C.M., Velozo, E.S., de Sousa, H.C., de Melo, S.A.B.V., Braga, M.E.M., Copaiba oil-loaded commercial wound dressings using supercritical CO_2: A potential alternative topical antileishmanial treatment. *J. Supercrit. Fluids*, 129, 106, 2017.
19. Franco, P. and De Marco, I., Supercritical CO_2 adsorption of non-steroidal anti-inflammatory drugs into biopolymer aerogels. *J. CO2 Util.*, 36, 40, 2020.
20. Lopes, J.M., Mustapa, A.N., Pantić, M., Bermejo, M.D., Martín, Á., Novak, Z., Knez, Z., Cocero, M.J., Preparation of cellulose aerogels from ionic liquid solutions for supercritical impregnation of phytol. *J. Supercrit. Fluids*, 130, 17, 2017.
21. Torres, A., Ilabaca, E., Rojas, A., Rodríguez, F., Galotto, M.J., Guarda, A., Villegas, C., Romero, J., Effect of processing conditions on the physical, chemical and transport properties of polylactic acid films containing thymol incorporated by supercritical impregnation. *Eur. Polym. J.*, 89, 195, 2017.
22. Milovanovic, S., Markovic, D., Mrakovic, A., Kuska, R., Zizovic, I., Frerich, S., Ivanovic, J., Supercritical CO_2 - assisted production of PLA and PLGA foams for controlled thymol release. *Mater. Sci. Eng. C*, 99, 394, 2019.
23. Bouledjouidja, A., Masmoudi, Y., Sergent, M., Trivedi, V., Meniai, A., Badens, E., Drug loading of foldable commercial intraocular lenses using supercritical impregnation. *Int. J. Pharm.*, 500, 85, 2016.
24. Mitrus, M., Wojtowicz, A., Moscicki, L., Janssen, L.P.B.M., Janssen, L.P.B.M., Moscicki, F., Biodegradable polymers and their practical utility, in: *Thermoplastic Starch: A Green Material for Various Industries*, pp. 1–33, Wiley-VCH Verlag, Weinheim, Germany, 2009.
25. Vroman, I. and Tighzert, L., Biodegradable Polymers. *Mater*, 2, 307, 2009.
26. George, A., Shah, P.A., Shrivastav, P.S., Natural biodegradable polymers based nano-formulations for drug delivery: A review. *Int. J. Pharm.*, 561, 244, 2019.
27. Smith, R., (Ed.), *Biodegradable polymers for industrial applications*, Woodhead Publishing Limited and CRC Press, 2005.
28. Baker, M.I., Walsh, S.P., Schwartz, Z., Boyan, B.D., A review of polyvinyl alcohol and its uses in cartilage and orthopedic applications. *J. Biomed. Mater. Res. Part B Appl. Biomater.*, 100, 1451, 2012.
29. Kim, S., Kim, J.H., Jeon, O., Kwon, I.C., Park, K., Engineered polymers for advanced drug delivery. *Eur. J. Pharm. Biopharm.*, 71, 420, 2009.
30. Braga, M.E.M., Pato, M.T.V., Silva, H.S.R.C., Ferreira, E.I., Gil, M.H., Duarte, C.M.M., de Sousa, H.C., Supercritical solvent impregnation of ophthalmic drugs on chitosan derivatives. *J. Supercrit. Fluids*, 44, 245, 2008.
31. Champeau, M., Thomassin, J.M., Tassaing, T., Jérôme, C., Drug loading of polymer implants by supercritical CO_2 assisted impregnation: A review. *J. Control. Release*, 209, 248, 2015.
32. Gosselin, P., Lacasse, F.-X., Preda, M., Thibert, R., Clas, S.-D., McMullen, J.N., Physicochemical evaluation of carbamazepine microparticles produced

by the rapid expansion of supercritical solutions and by spray-drying. *Pharm. Devel. Technol.*, 8, 11, 2003.
33. Bolten, D. and Türk, M., Micronisation of carbamazepine through rapid expansion of supercritical solution (RESS). *J. Supercrit. Fluids*, 66, 389, 2012.
34. Türk, M. and Bolten, D., Polymorphic properties of micronized mefenamic acid, nabumetone, paracetamol and tolbutamide produced by rapid expansion of supercritical solutions (RESS). *J. Supercrit. Fluids*, 116, 239, 2016.
35. Yeo, S.-D. and Kiran, E., Formation of polymer particles with supercritical fluids: A review. *J. Supercrit. Fluids*, 34, 287, 2005.
36. Kiran, E., Supercritical fluids and polymers – The year in review – 2014. *J. Supercrit. Fluids*, 110, 126, 2016.
37. Reverchon, E., Adami, R., Cardea, S., Della Porta, G., The Journal of Supercritical Fluids Supercritical fluids processing of polymers for pharmaceutical and medical applications. *J. Supercrit. Fluids*, 47, 484, 2009.
38. Türk, M., Upper, G., Hils, P., Formation of composite drug–polymer particles by co-precipitation during the rapid expansion of supercritical fluids. *J. Supercrit. Fluids*, 39, 253, 2006.
39. Songtipya, L., Thies, M.C., Sane, A., Effect of rapid expansion of subcritical solutions processing conditions on loading capacity of tetrahydrocurcumin encapsulated in poly(l-lactide) particles. *J. Supercrit. Fluids*, 113, 119, 2016.
40. Müllers, K.C., Paisana, M., Wahl, M.A., Simultaneous Formation and Micronization of Pharmaceutical Cocrystals by Rapid Expansion of Supercritical Solutions (RESS). *Pharm. Res.*, 32, 702, 2015.
41. Cocero, M. J., Martín, A., Mattea, F., Varona, S., Encapsulation and co-precipitation processes with supercritical fluids: Fundamentals and applications. *J. Supercrit. Fluids*, 47, 3, 2009.
42. Lee, S., Nam, K., Kim, M.S., Jun, S.W., Park, J.-S., Woo, J.S., Hwang, S.-J., Preparation and characterization of solid dispersions of itraconazole by using aerosol solvent extraction system for improvement in drug solubility and bioavailability. *Arch. Pharmacal Res.*, 28, 866, 2005.
43. Wang, Y., Wang, Y., Yang, J., Pfeffer, R., Dave, R., Michniak, B., The application of a supercritical antisolvent process for sustained drug delivery. *Powder Technol.*, 164, 94, 2006.
44. Lee, S., Kim, M.S., Kim, J.S., Park, H.J., Woo, J.S., Lee, B.C., Hwang, S.J., Controlled delivery of a hydrophilic drug from a biodegradable microsphere system by supercritical anti-solvent precipitation technique. *J. Microencapsulation*, 23, 741, 2008.
45. Jung, I.-I., Haam, S., Lim, G., Ryu, J.-H., Preparation of peptide-loaded polymer microparticles using supercritical carbon dioxide. *Biotechnol. Bioprocess Eng.*, 17, 185, 2012.
46. Ha, E.-S., Kim, J.-S., Baek, I., Yoo, J.-W., Jung, Y., Moon, H.R., Kim, M.-S., Development of megestrol acetate solid dispersion nanoparticles for enhanced oral delivery by using a supercritical antisolvent process. *Drug Des. Devel. Ther.*, 9, 4269, 2015.

47. Sacchetin, P.S.C., Setti, R.F., Rosa, P.D.T.V.F., Moraes, Â.M., Properties of PLA/PCL particles as vehicles for oral delivery of the androgen hormone 17α-methyltestosterone. *Mater. Sci. Eng. C*, 58, 870, 2016.
48. Liu, M., Liu, Y., Ge, Y., Zhong, Z., Wang, Z., Wu, T., Zhao, X., Zu, Y., Solubility, antioxidation, and oral bioavailability improvement of mangiferin microparticles prepared using the supercritical antisolvent method. *Pharm.*, 12, 90, 2020.
49. Mattea, F., Martín, A., Matías-Gago, A., Cocero, M. J., Supercritical antisolvent precipitation from an emulsion: β-Carotene nanoparticle formation. *J. Supercrit. Fluids*, 51, 2, 2009.
50. Lévai, G., Albarelli, J., Santos, D., Meireles, M.A.A, Martín, A., Rodríguez-Rojo, S., Cocero, M. J., Quercetin loaded particles production by means of supercritical fluid extraction of emulsions: Process scale-upstudy and thermo-economic evaluation. *Food Bioprod. Process.*, 103, 2017.
51. Weidner, E., High pressure micronization for food applications. *J. Supercrit. Fluids*, 47, 556, 2009.
52. Varona, S., Kareth, S., Martín, Á., Cocero, M.J., Formulation of lavandin essential oil with biopolymers by PGSS for application as biocide in ecological agriculture. *J. Supercrit. Fluids*, 54, 369, 2010.
53. Fraile, M., Martín, Y., Deodato, D., Rodriguez-Rojo, S., Nogueira, I.D., Simplício, A.L., Cocero, M.J., Duarte, C.M.M., The Journal of Supercritical Fluids Production of new hybrid systems for drug delivery by PGSS (Particles from Gas Saturated Solutions) process. *J. Supercrit. Fluids*, 81, 226, 2013.
54. da Silva, C.V., Pereira, V.J., Costa, G.M.N., Cabral-Albuquerque, E.C.M., Vieira de Melo, S.A.B., de Sousa, H.C., Dias, A.M.A., Braga, M.E.M., Supercritical solvent impregnation/deposition of spilanthol-enriched extracts into a commercial collagen/cellulose-based wound dressing. *J. Supercrit. Fluids*, 133, 503, 2018.
55. Campardelli, R., Franco, P., Reverchon, E., De Marco, I., Polycaprolactone/nimesulide patches obtained by a one-step supercritical foaming + impregnation process. *J. Supercrit. Fluids*, 146, 47, 2019.
56. Morgado, P.I., Miguel, S.P., Correia, I.J., Aguiar-Ricardo, A., Ibuprofen loaded PVA/chitosan membranes: A highly efficient strategy towards an improved skin wound healing. *Carbohydr. Polym.*, 159, 136, 2017.
57. López de Dicastillo, C., Villegas, C., Garrido, L., Roa, K., Torres, A., Galotto, M.J., Rojas, A.R., Romero, J., Modifying an active compound's release kinetic using a supercritical impregnation process to incorporate an active agent into PLA electrospun mats. *Polymers*, 10, 479, 2018.
58. Mosquera, J.E., Goñi, M.L., Martini, R.E., Gañán, N.A., Supercritical carbon dioxide assisted impregnation of eugenol into polyamide fibers for application as a dental floss. *J. CO2 Util.*, 32, 259, 2019.
59. Villegas, C., Torres, A., Rios, M., Rojas, A., Romero, J., de Dicastillo, C.L., Valenzuela, X., Galotto, M.J., Guarda, A., Supercritical impregnation of

cinnamaldehyde into polylactic acid as a route to develop antibacterial food packaging materials. *Food Res. Int.*, 99, 650, 2017.

60. Kuska, R., Milovanovic, S., Frerich, S., Ivanovic, J., Thermal analysis of polylactic acid under high CO_2 pressure applied in supercritical impregnation and foaming process design. *J. Supercrit. Fluids*, 144, 71, 2019.
61. Champeau, M., Coutinho, I.T., Thomassin, J.M., Tassaing, T., Jérôme, C., Tuning the release profile of ketoprofen from poly(l-lactic acid) suture using supercritical CO_2 impregnation process. *J. Drug Deliv. Sci. Technol.*, 55, 101468, 2020.
62. Salgado, M., Santos, F., Rodríguez-Rojo, S., Reis, R.L., Duarte, A.R.C., Cocero, M.J., Development of barley and yeast β-glucan aerogels for drug delivery by supercritical fluids. *J. CO2 Util.*, 22, 262, 2017.
63. Ameri, A., Sodeifian, G., Sajadian, S.A., Lansoprazole loading of polymers by supercritical carbon dioxide impregnation: Impacts of process parameters. *J. Supercrit. Fluids*, 164, 104892, 2020.
64. Gracia, E., García, M.T., Rodríguez, J.F., de Lucas, A., Gracia, I., Improvement of PLGA loading and release of curcumin by supercritical technology. *J. Supercrit. Fluids*, 141, 60, 2018.
65. Franco, P., Pessolano, E., Belvedere, R., Petrella, A., De Marco, I., Supercritical impregnation of mesoglycan into calcium alginate aerogel for wound healing. *J. Supercrit. Fluids*, 157, 104711, 2020.
66. Ganañ, N., Bordón, M.G., Ribotta, P.D., González, A., Study of chia oil microencapsulation in soy protein microparticles using supercritical CO_2-assisted impregnation. *J. CO2 Util.*, 40, 101221, 2020.
67. Alessi, P., Kikic, I., Cortesi, A., Fogar, A., Moneghini, M., Polydimethylsiloxanes in supercritical solvent impregnation (SSI) of polymers. *J. Supercrit. Fluids*, 27, 309, 2003.
68. Dias, A.M.A., Braga, M.E.M., Seabra, I.J., Ferreira, P., Gil, M.H., De Sousa, H.C., Development of natural-based wound dressings impregnated with bioactive compounds and using supercritical carbon dioxide. *Int. J. Pharm.*, 408, 9, 2011.
69. Milovanovic, S., Markovic, D., Aksentijevic, K., Stojanovic, D.B., Ivanovic, J., Zizovic, I., Application of cellulose acetate for controlled release of thymol. *Carbohydr. Polym.*, 147, 344, 2016.
70. Bouledjouidja, A., Masmoudi, Y., Sergent, M., Badens, E., Effect of operational conditions on the supercritical carbon dioxide impregnation of anti-inflammatory and antibiotic drugs in rigid commercial intraocular lenses. *J. Supercrit. Fluids*, 130, 63, 2017.
71. Villegas, C., Torres, A., Rios, M., Rojas, A., Romero, J., de Dicastillo, C.L., Valenzuela, X., Galotto, M.J., Guarda, A., Drug impregnation for laser sintered poly(methyl methacrylate) biocomposites using supercritical carbon dioxide. *J. Supercrit. Fluids*, 136, 29, 2018.

8

Neural Network for Screening Active Sites on Proteins

Johanna Bustamante-Torres[1]*, Samantha Pardo[2] and Moises Bustamante-Torres[3,4]

[1]*Faculty of Philosophy, Letters and Education Sciences, Universidad Central del Ecuador, Quito City, Ecuador*
[2]*Environmental Engineering Faculty, Universidad Politécnica Salesiana, Quito City, Ecuador*
[3]*Biomedical Engineering Department, School of Biological and Engineering, Yachay Tech University, Urcuqui City, Ecuador*
[4]*Department of Radiation Chemistry and Radiochemistry, Institute of Nuclear Sciences, National Autonomous University of Mexico, Mexico City, Mexico*

Abstract

The study and understanding of proteins fields are excellent in the biosciences field. The interactions of proteins provide essential information about life. Therefore, many techniques have been developed for this analysis, such as *in vitro*, *in vivo*, and *in silico*. Despite each technique having advantages, *in silico* methods are a terrific alternative for analyzing the proteins and their interactions using computer tools by its versatility through algorithms. The active sites are of great interest because of their significance in the structure of the protein to interact with another molecule. This chapter details some of the main techniques currently applied to study the active sites on proteins, the database where the information is available, such as Protein Data Bank (PDB), Dali server, structural alignment program (SSAP), structural alignment of multiple proteins (STAMP), catalytic site atlas (CSA), or protein families' database (Pfam). Besides, it describes relevant information about some algorithms that have been developed based on machine learning, such as PDBSiteScan program, patterns in nonhomologous tertiary structures (PINTS), genetic active site search (GASS), site map, computed atlas of surface topography of proteins (Castp), etc. These programs allow getting trustful information about the site actives and other interactions.

**Corresponding author*: jpbustamante@uce.edu.ec

Inamuddin, Tariq Altalhi, Jorddy N. Cruz and Moamen Salah El-Deen Refat (eds.) Drug Design Using Machine Learning, (225–246) © 2022 Scrivener Publishing LLC

Keywords: Active sites, proteins, machine learning, *in silico* techniques, *in vivo* techniques, *in vitro* techniques

8.1 Introduction

Biomolecules play an outstanding role in nature, such as protein and enzymes [1]. The gist term that encompasses the study of proteins is known as the proteome. The proteome is the entire complement or database or set of proteins produced by a living organism from the alterations or modifications produced in native protein when organisms are subjected to many changes [2]. Protein was first discovered and named in the 1800s, but it was noted for its central role in living organisms in the 1900s, meanwhile, it was identified (structure) in the 1950s [3]. Since then, proteins have been extensively studied due to the significant variety of proteins. Based on the binding approach, there is a term "protein-protein interaction" (PPI). PPI handles many biological processes, including cell-to-cell interactions and metabolic and developmental control [4]. The PPI presents an appealing actives site, the binding site of the proteins with other molecules that are often called the substrate.

PPI are critical for cellular processes, such as macromolecular structures, enzyme complexes, and the regulation and transduction of signals. Understanding interactions provide information about cell function and helps design targeted drugs and treat pathogens [5]. A wide range of techniques has characterized PPIs and its function. For example, chemical and biology techniques are also employed to determine the PPIs *in vitro* and *in vivo*. However, nowadays, because of the advance in technology, computerized techniques are performed on a computer or via simulation known as *in silico*. The PPI analysis through *in silico* techniques consisted of several methods that are described below in this chapter [6]. Currently, *in silico* methods, through machine learning, are a great alternative to study proteomics.

Machine learning (Ml) contains ideas inherited over time and adapted from several disciplines, rendering it a real multidisciplinary and interdisciplinary field [7]. The term prediction is a primary task in machine learning research, which has increasingly popular in biomedical, medical, clinical, and drug development fields after the Precision Medicine Initiative was established by the 44th US president, Obama Barack [8]. Practically, Ml tries to build algorithms that can receive input data and use statistical analysis to predict an output value within an acceptable range. Table 8.1 describes the common uses of the Ml.

Table 8.1 Summarize of MI uses.

Machine learning uses	Reference
Gather understanding of the cyber phenomenon that produce the data under study. Abstract the understanding of underlying phenomena in the form of a model Predict future values through a pre-stablished model Detect anomalous behavior	[9]

In recent years, there has been a notable advance in computational chemistry calculation methods oriented to the modeling and evaluating proteins. Ml has advantages over the non-learning-based method because the last one has been designed for specific applications. Nevertheless, Ml is adaptive to other scenarios, and it does not require a software adaptation [10]. The protein interactions can be analyzed *in silico* to become a viable alternative to save time in designing experiments with better expectations of success and reduce costs in materials and reagents. Currently, through these computational methods, some models and schemes can be generated and made available that can allow the discovery of potential therapeutic targets to treat specific pathologies with new clinical treatment options [11].

8.2 Structural Proteomics

Proteomics is a fast and powerful discipline to study the sum of all proteins from an organism under specific conditions [12]. Proteins perform a variety of functions, including enzymatic catalysis, transporting ions and molecules from one organ to another, nutrients, the contractile system of muscles, tendons, cartilage, antibodies, and regulating cellular and physiological activities [13, 14]. Proteomic technologies have advanced various drug discovery and development areas through the comparative assessment of normal and diseased-state tissues, transcription, and/or expression profiling, and the identification of biomarkers [15].

The analysis of the various properties of the proteome requires an equally diverse range of technologies and methods for data integration and mining [16]. As a discipline, proteomics has grown at the interface of physical and biochemistry, computer science, and bioinformatics, emphasizing high throughput and reduced user bias [17].

8.2.1 PPIs

PPIs are vital for researching biology systems approaches due to their particular physical contact established between two or more protein molecules. As a result, several biochemical events such as electrostatic forces, hydrogen bonds, and hydrophobic interactions are produced [4]. Besides, other biochemical events, such as the kinetic properties of enzymes, substrate channeling, inactivate or suppression proteins, or regulatory role are affected by PPIs [6, 18]. The biological (surface) recognition, like in the immune system, is also mediated by PPIs as in the case of binding of lymphocyte function-associated antigen (LFA)-1 presented on the surface of immune cells to intracellular adhesion molecule (ICAM)-1 found on the surface of endothelial cells [19]. Table 8.2 describes some of the main Ml program to study the PPIs.

In vitro methods, such as affinity chromatography, crystallography, NMR spectroscopy, coimmunoprecipitation, and protein arrays, are used to characterize PPI. Nowadays, because of the advance in technology *in-silico* approach has grown significantly to study the PPI. For instance, Zhang *et al.*, developed an exciting algorithm known as PrePPI to predict the three-dimensional structural information of PPI based on nonstructural evidence with high accuracy, combining the structural information with other functional clues [20]. Likewise, an algorithm called Coev2Net was developed to investigate the PPIs. This method involves predicting the binding interface, evaluating the interface's compatibility with an interface coevolution-based model [21].

8.2.2 Active Sites in Proteins

Active sites are binding sites present in the enzyme/protein surface capable of getting interactions with another molecule (also known as substrate).

Table 8.2 Summarize of the main Ml program to study the PPIs.

Gist Ml to study PPIs	Reference
Support Vector Machine k-Nearest Neighbour Principal Component Analysis Ensemble Learning Algorithm Artificial Neural Networks Random Forest Deep architectures	[22]

Structures of enzyme-substrate/product complexes have been studied for over four decades, but their knowledge during the chemical reaction is limited [23]. The active site is considered the enzyme's specific place where the substrate binds (E and S), forming a structural complementarity. Figure 8.1 illustrates the interaction between enzyme and substrate and the active site on the enzyme.

The enzyme/protein first binds to its substrate, and then it forms a complex known as enzyme-substrate complex (E+S =P), as shown in Figure 8.2. Subsequently, a chemical operation is produced in this complex by forming the final product [24], then the product leaves the active site.

The active site of amino acids that bind functional groups in the substrate ensures an adequate substrate location and formation of the transition intermediary, subjected to catalysis [25], where the reaction occurs. However, there are other important factors to consider, such as pH and temperature. For example, when the pH or solvent conditions are changed, a partial denaturation of the enzyme is possible [26], and the interaction with the substrate can be affected.

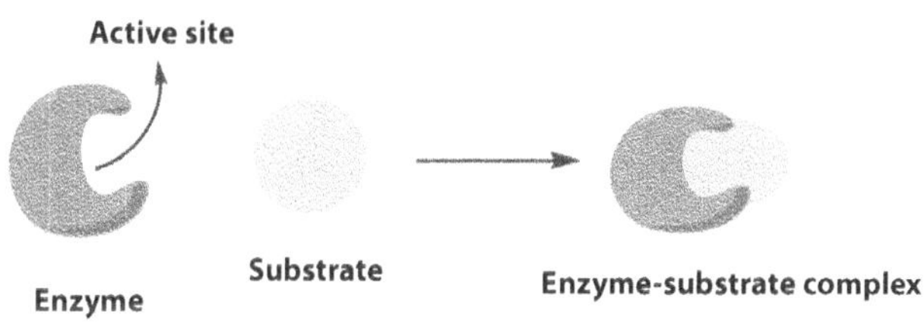

Figure 8.1 Scheme representation of the interaction of enzyme and substrate through the active site.

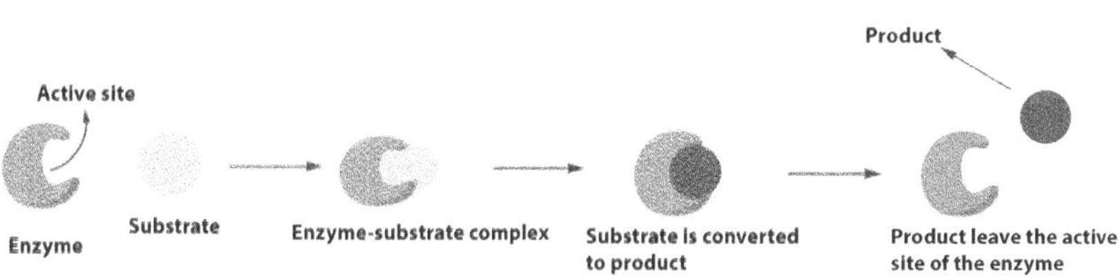

Figure 8.2 Scheme representation of the whole process from a substrate to becoming product.

8.3 Gist Techniques to Study the Active Sites on Proteins

Diverse techniques have been applied to determine the essential information of enzyme/substrate behavior. The active sites on proteins have been widely studied *in vitro*, *in vivo*, or the most studied lastly *in silico*. Even though each technique has thriving advantages, *in vitro* and *in vivo* are more expensive, high time consuming and less accurate than *in silico* techniques, which are based on computerized tools. Figure 8.3 illustrates the conventional and *in silico* approach to study the proteins and their interactions currently.

8.3.1 *In Vitro*

8.3.1.1 Affinity Purification

In vitro methodology refers to an experiment in a test tube, that is, a controlled environment. *In vitro* data are often used to fully or partially satisfy information requirements that would otherwise require data generation with tests on living organisms (*in-vivo* tests). Several methods use this type of experimental technique to determine active sites in proteins, such as

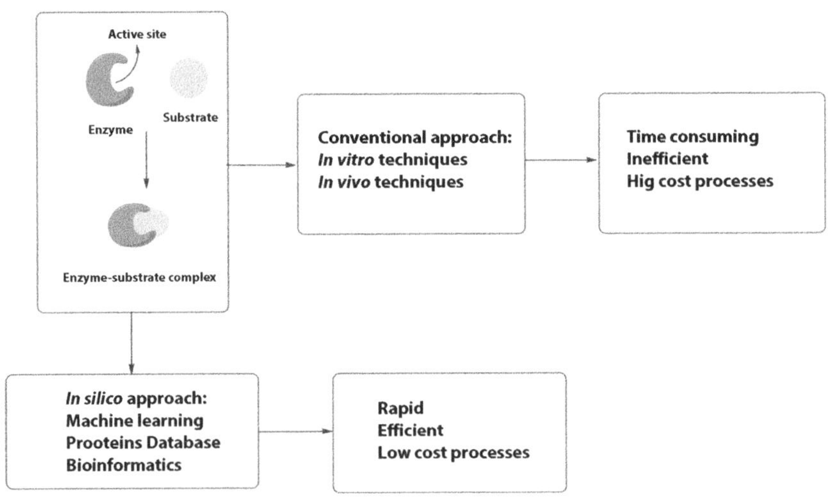

Figure 8.3 Conventional and *in silico* techniques employed to study active sites on proteins.

affinity purification, which consists of purification of the protein by specific binding to another molecule for which it has high affinity.

Researchers have studied the use of highly magnetic chitosan particle preparations with a coercive force of up to 3500 Oe, where the surface of the particles was joined with aldehyde groups to provide binding of affinity ligands, concluding that the proposed method is successful for affinity purification of aprotinin [27]. On the other hand, studies have shown that to purify the enzyme that activates ubiquitin, the affinity column requires ATP and Mg^{2+}, and a high pH to displace the protein, which is why it is suggested to increase the concentrations of a thiol compound or by joint supplementation of AMP and pyrophosphate [28].

8.3.1.2 Affinity Chromatography

Many proteins may be studied using affinity chromatography, which takes advantage of the binding properties of proteins and ligands as shown in Figure 8.4. A recombinant protein mixture is passed through a chromatography column with an immobilized ligand that binds to affinity-tagged proteins [29]. Contaminants and leftovers are then washed away, followed by a rinse of purified bound proteins. As a result, this method relies on ligands limited to beads that bind to the protein of interest and may subsequently be rinsed out with a solution of free ligands. This yields the purest protein samples with the highest specific activity of any technology now in use. Besides, this technique can be classified as structures of amino acid of

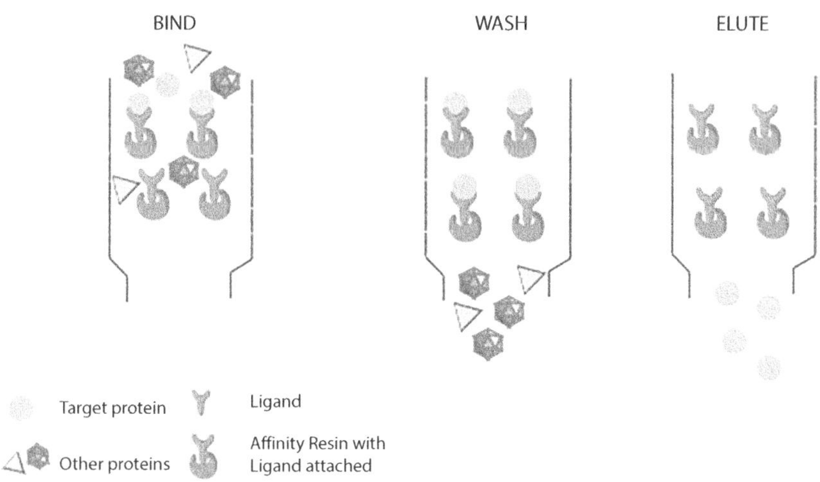

Figure 8.4 Scheme representation of the affinity chromatography.

only one use or series in the protein as the point of attachment for purification, and as targeted proteins involving an additional set amino acid set, the "tag."

8.3.1.3 Coimmunoprecipitation

PPIs are essential for biological processes. For example, the PPI of signaling molecules mediates the passage of signals from outside into the cell. Moreover, the protein can be transported to another place and/or interact with another protein, acquiring new modifications by itself. Therefore, this information aims to understand some diseases and develop new treatments to solve them [30]. Coimmunoprecipitation (CoIP) is considered the best assay to detect PPI, mainly when performed with endogenous proteins, as shown in Figure 8.5. CoIP is based on immunoprecipitation, a technique to pull apart an antibody-bound target protein from other proteins. CoIP involves the binding of an antibody protein to a protein that usually rejects it. This is followed by a separation process that preserves complex proteins [31].

8.3.1.4 Protein Arrays

Protein arrays have been considered a futuristic method for identifying PPI, protein phospholipid, and protein kinase substrates. They are also helpful for clinical diagnosis and disease monitoring. Protein arrays have emerged as a promising approach for a wide variety of applications, including identifying PPI, protein-phospholipid interactions, small molecule targets, and protein kinase substrates. They can also be used for clinical diagnosis

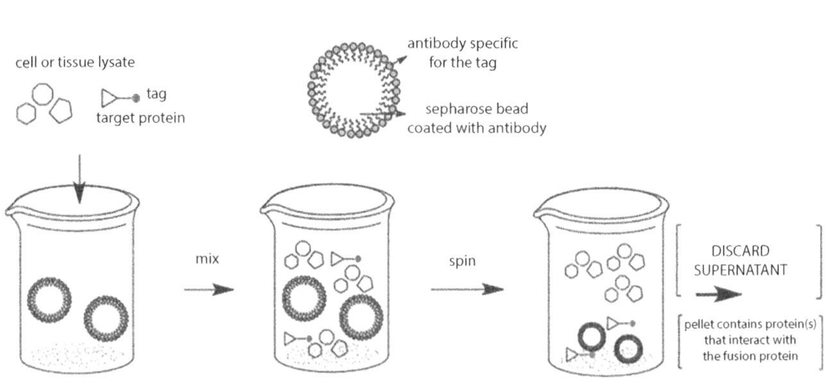

Figure 8.5 Scheme representation of the coimmunoprecipitations technique.

and monitoring of disease states. Understanding complex cell systems will necessitate identifying and analyzing each component and determining how they interact and are regulated. Determining the biochemical actions of proteins and how they are controlled and modified by other proteins is crucial in this process. Individual molecules have traditionally been studied one at a time to understand the biochemical functions of proteins. This method is inefficient since it is sluggish and labor-intensive [32].

Protein arrays are used to determine PPI, track protein expression levels, and count the number of target analytes in biological samples. The matrices are utilized in disease state research, diagnosis, quality control, and monitoring. Most antibodies, such as cancer, apoptosis, and cell cycle biomarker antibody arrays, are accessible in matrix format. Protein arrays can be bought in bulk or made in-house. There are equipments and chemicals available to create, run, and analyze matrices; there is also an extensive range of vendor software, scanners, and printed slides. Protein arrays must consider the protein of interest, the detection feature, and the ease of array manufacturing.

8.3.1.5 *Protein Fragment Complementation*

The PPI is linked to the refolding of enzymes from related fragments in this approach, where the restoration of enzymatic activity functions as a detector of protein interaction.

Protein Fragment Complementation Assays (PCA) is a class of assays for detecting PPI designed to give easy and uncomplicated methods for studying PPI in any live cell, multicellular organism, or *in vitro*. PPIs can be detected and expressed at endogenous levels via PCAs between proteins of any molecular size. Proteins are expressed in their proper cellular compartments and can go through any posttranslational modification or degradation that they would generally go through, except for the consequences of PCA fragment fusion.

8.3.1.6 *Phage Display*

Phage display is a molecular biology technique whereby phage genomes are modified so that the coat proteins of the assembled virions fuse with other proteins or peptides of interest (of any origin), thus showing them to the external environment. A gene fragment is introduced into a gene with a functional purpose on the protein, resulting in a new and advanced protein covered by the phage with potential activity. In recent years, proteins and protein domains have been exposed in the capsid of filamentous phages.

In current molecular biology, there are three fundamental applications of the methodology for exposing proteins in phages. The first achieves a direct evolution of the molecule to obtain mutants with a marked increase in biological activity; the second consists of selecting high-affinity antibodies, and the third corresponds to the expression and screening of cDNA libraries [33].

8.3.1.7 X-Ray Crystallography

Initially, X-ray crystallography could only examine solid crystals with a regular atomic arrangement. Crystallographers can examine biological materials, such as proteins or DNA by forming crystals out of them through this technique. The breakthrough occurred when the increasing capacity of computers enabled the modeling of the structure of these increasingly complicated crystals. As a result, this method is frequently utilized in medication development. When a pharmaceutical firm looks for a novel medicine to combat a specific bacteria or virus, it must first identify a tiny chemical capable of inhibiting active proteins (enzymes) that are implicated in attacking human cells. As the importance of proteins grows, researchers in many fields have found that a working knowledge of X-ray diffraction is an indispensable tool. Ilari, Carmelinda Savino (2008) studied the molecular replacement method using a downloaded search model of the PDB through computerized tools to obtain macromolecular structures of proteins. They were demonstrating the benefit of using increasingly sophisticated computer programs for the resolution of structures [34].

8.3.1.8 Nuclear Magnetic Resonance Spectroscopy (NMR)

Nuclear magnetic resonance (NMR) spectroscopy is the most potent structural determination tool in the structural determination of chemical compounds. It is based on the magnetic properties of atomic nuclei, based on the interaction of the nuclear magnetic moment with an external magnetic field, which leads to different energy levels. The response to the transition between these levels by the absorption of radiofrequency energy by the atomic nuclei can be detected, amplified, and recorded in what would be a spectral line or resonance signal. In this way, the NMR spectra are generated for compounds with nuclei of the nonzero magnetic moment.

In terms of its applications, NMR is very valuable in drug design since it is a method from which very diverse information can be obtained, such as knowing the structural information of a molecule, distinguishing between two conformations of the same compound, or detect interactions between different molecules, such as drug-receptor interactions. NMR applications in various classes of MPCs, including G-protein-coupled receptors, ion channels, and retinal proteins, extending the discussion to protein-protein complexes that span entire cellular compartments or orchestrate processes such as protein transport across or within membranes [35]. Table 8.3 describes some of the gist information from the proteins obtained from the NMR.

Mass spectrometry (MS) heightened the way to determine and analyze proteomes and is typically the method for identifying proteins present in biological systems. Several methodologies based on MS have been developed to analyze proteomes [36].

It can be understood to obtain more information of new ligands for a specific pharmacological target through chemical displacement and other parameters and the development of these new ligands. By knowing the interaction between ligand and the target protein is critical in drug design. This is where NMR plays a crucial role since it allows to correlate the changes in a target molecule when a ligand binds to it, with the chemical shifts observed when comparing the spectra before and after the union. The interaction that occurs can be studied by focusing on the ligand or the target, and although there are various techniques within each type, there are more than study the ligand. In contrast, the techniques that study the target are more specific and have higher performance.

8.3.2 *In Vivo*

8.3.2.1 In-Silico Two-Hybrid

The techniques employed *in vivo* methods are designed to detect the interactions with the yeast double hybrid system. So far, protein interaction prediction methods have been proposed based on sequence or structure

Table 8.3 Essential information obtained by the NMR.

NMR information from proteins	Reference
Provides information of functional groups such as ionization states, pKa, and hydrogen bonds Determine and identify contacts between individual atoms of proteins and its binding partners. Backbone and side-chain dynamics motions	[37]

information [38]. In response, many methods are developed to predict the PPIs structure, although many are still studied. One of the main disadvantages is the high false-positive and high false-negative results. Thus, *in silico-two hybrid* (Y2H) method arises as a promising technique to detect the physical interactions of pairs of proteins. Besides, this technique can determine the binding sites or active sites. According to Rao *et al.* (2014), two protein domains are required in the Y2H [6]:

(i) A DNA binding domain (DBD) that helps binding to DNA, and
(ii) An activation domain (AD) responsible for activating transcription of DNA.

The main advantage of *in-silico* two-hybrid is distinguishing the true or false interactions in even many cases [39]. Therefore, a unique algorithm was developed to analyze the PPIs among 16 Bd Mitogen-activated protein kinases (BdMAPKs) and 86 BdPP2Cs (which can recognize and docking the BdMAPKs) in B. distachyon using a novel docking approach (D-site). The results showed an optimistic prediction of PPIs and the visualization of a three-dimensional structure [40]. On the other hand, Jia et al. uses the gist component in the venom of snakes, phospholipase A2s (PLA2s), as a "bait" to identify the interactions between PLA2s and 14 of the most common proteins in Western diamondback rattlesnake (*Crotalus atrox*) venom by using Y2H analysis, a technique used to detect PPIs, and finally, the three-dimensional structure was determined using computerized program MODELLER [41].

8.3.3 *In-Silico* and Neural Network

Since the 1970s, protein structure comparison methods have become increasingly sophisticated [42]. There are many algorithms developed to analyze the active sites based on structural data. Besides, the protein structure and function can be found in those databases. Some *in-silico* techniques include docking, tree-based methods phylogenetic, chromosomal proximity, or gene fusion.

8.3.3.1 Data Base

8.3.3.1.1 Protein Data Bank

The Protein Data Bank (PDB) (http://www.rcsb.org/pdb/) is a single worldwide server of structural data of biological macromolecules established at

Brookhaven National Laboratories (BNL) [43, 44]. Currently, PDB is under the control of the Worldwide Protein Data Bank (wwPDB), whose mission is to "maintain a single PDB archive of macromolecular structural data that is freely and publicly available to the global community" [45]. This server can manage the PDB archive's data processing and distribution center and offers various tools and resources for data analysis [46].

PDB records contain secondary structures, helix, strand, coil, and turn, but it does not have secondary structure information [47]. PDB contains approximately 83900 biological structures [45]. For example, the Research Collaboratory for Structural Bioinformatics (RCSB) PDB Web site provides tools for searching, visualizing, and analyzing PDB data, including easy exploration of chemical interactions that stabilize macromolecules [48].

8.3.3.1.2 DALI

DALI server provides information about the structure found in PDB. This database measures structural relatedness in terms of similarities of intramolecular distance matrices. The alignments are determined only by comparing the three-dimensional coordinates [49].

8.3.3.1.3 Structural Alignment Program (SSAP)

This algorithm gets to obtain information related to the motifs among proteins through a multiple comparison method. This algorithm has evolved into several versions that allow identifying proteins. All versions of structural alignment program (SSAP) require an input WOLF file (which is PDB) that generates information about hydrogen bonding patterns and secondary structure assignments [42].

8.3.3.1.4 Structural Alignment of Multiple Proteins (STAMP)

In order to reduce the need for visual verification of dehydrogenase fold domains, globins, and serine proteinases, two similarity indices are introduced to determine the quality of each generated structural alignment through structural alignment of multiple proteins (STAMP) method. STAMP technique contains information related to groups of proteins and the alignment of each residue. Moreover, it provides information about the structural motifs through Sc and Pij's values [50].

8.3.3.1.5 Catalytic Site Atlas

Catalytic site atlas (CSA) method provides information concerning residue annotation for enzymes in the PDB. This dataset works in two ways:

(1) an original hand-annotated set containing information extracted from the primary literature and (2) a homologous addition set containing annotation inferred by PSI-BLAST and sequence alignment to one of the original sets [51].

8.3.3.1.6 Protein Families' Database (Pfam)

Fin *et al.* (2013) developed a database containing protein families known as Pfam (http://pfam.sanger.ac.uk/, for the UK) and (http://pfam.janelia.org/, for the USA), which employ the Hidden Markov Model and two alignments. This database shows relevant information through representative graphs or interactive access to the data [52] of active sites on proteins.

8.3.3.2 Sequence-Based Approaches

Sequences for a wide variety of genomes are now available, including, of course, the human. The order of the bases A, T, G, and C of a genome says little if there are no ways to decode the information it contains. Thus, one of the outstanding achievements related to genome sequencing is developing various computational algorithms designed to translate biological meaning. Bioinformatics is a science that arises from the need to interpret the information contained in DNA, RNA, and protein sequences. Since DNA and protein sequencing techniques spread and the volume of sequences in data banks increased, the need arose to develop algorithms to catalog sequences, analyze their similarity, and discover their structural and functional properties. *In silico* studies have been carried out from the analysis of primary sequences through pre-established models based on algorithms, which should present an adequate biological reproducibility employing molecular coupling [11].

8.3.3.3 Structure-Based Approaches

Years ago, the only procedures that allowed determining the structure and function of a protein were sequencing, X-ray crystallography, and nuclear magnetic resonance. However, thanks to advances in bioinformatics during the 1960s, different types of software were developed that allow comparisons between amino acid sequences found in databases such as genebank (gene bank) and National Center for Biotechnology Information (NCBI) to provide essential information about the proteins, avoiding the use of the laboratory [53, 54]. The development of these new prediction mechanisms has made it possible to mitigate the tremendous theoretical problem that constitutes the ignorance of the function and structure of thousands of hypothetical proteins [53]. When comparisons of a hypothetical protein sequence with other proteins are made with the help of these bioinformatics programs, it is possible to infer a function if the results show significant similarities in specific highly conserved regions of the proteins, since it is possible that a sequence with function unknown is similar to another sequence whose function has already been determined [54, 55]. It is essential to know that through the analysis of amino acid sequences, it is possible to detect two types of fundamental structures to determine the function of a protein; motives and domains. Motifs are conserved amino acid sequences (that is, they are very similar in related proteins) that fold in specific ways and give proteins stability and functionality. The domains are also conserved sequences that fold independently of the rest of the protein and constitute distinct regions within its structure; in fact, the association of the different domains originates the tertiary structure [56]. The detection of similarities in the motifs and domains of proteins can indicate the presence of homologies, that is, of a common evolutionary origin. Thus, the study of the protein composition of the organism is essential to understand its infective and pathogenic mechanisms since many of them involve the interaction of various proteins and enzymes.

8.3.3.4 Phylogenetic Tree

The use of protein-protein coupling methods to predict protein complexes' interaction regions and structure is still a challenge. Several researchers have used the information contained in genomes (domain fusion, conservation of order gene, phylogenetic distribution) to predict interactions between proteins. If two polypeptide chains are subunits of the same protein or complex, their genes are frequently adjacent in the genome and are jointly expressed and regulated at the DNA level [57, 58], by applying this criterion to loosely related genomes. Pellegrini *et al.*, elaborated an exciting method called phylogenetic profiles, which determines the coevolution of interacting proteins, in other words, the presence-absence of orthologous genes in different genomes [59]. If the pattern of orthologous proteins (presence-absence) is conserved in organisms of the same species, it is probably because one of the proteins cannot exert its function without the other. Huynen *et al.*, applied this method to the genome of Mycoplasma genitalium, predicting 34% of the pairs as interacting and an additional 29% belonging to the same metabolic pathway or functional process [60].

8.3.3.5 Gene Fusion

Gene fusion is based on the fusion between two separate proteins in another species [61]. It is a traditional genetic tool for studying the regulation and constructing a hybrid gene [62]. The functional consequences and biological significance of either or both the fusion genes are determined by constitutive activation of the gene with intact functional domains, irrespective of the expression level [63].

Marcotte *et al.* and Enright *et al.* created a novel technique employing domain fusion. These methods use the principle that when two proteins A and B contain domains homologous to different domains of the third protein in another organism, but A and B are not homologous, they can interact between them [64, 65]. The method developed by Marcotte *et al.* is known as the "Rosetta stone method" because it uses the information recorded from inaccessible databases [64]. Enright and colleagues used BLAST method to determine protein orthology and find 64 fused genes in four prokaryotic genomes [65].

The limitation of the methods described is that they are only applicable to completely sequenced genomes to ensure the absence of specific genes; on the other hand, they are applicable only in bacteria, where the order of the genes is a relevant characteristic; and finally, dependence on the quality of the multiple alignments of the proteins under study.

8.4 Neural Networking Algorithms to Study Active Sites on Proteins

8.4.1 PDBSiteScan Program

Ivanisenko *et al.*, develop the PDBSiteScan program (at http://wwwmgs.bionet.nsc.ru/mgs/systems/fastprot/pdbsitescan.html) to determine the active sites and posttranslational modification sites in 3D protein structure. This algorithm has outstanding advantages due to its versatility to recognizes active sites [66].

8.4.2 Patterns in Nonhomologous Tertiary Structures (PINTS)

The method patterns in nonhomologous tertiary structures (PINTS), available on http://pints.embl.de, can determine the whole residue pattern on a target protein through database comparison. This PINTS algorithm compares the predefined patterns against databases (DALI, VAST, SSAP, STAMP) of complete structures and entire structures to databases of particular residues likely to be functionally important [67].

8.4.3 Genetic Active Site Search (GASS)

Genetic active site search (GASS) is an accessible and user-friendly web server (http://gass.unifei.edu.br/) that uses protein servers such as PDB [43] or 1691 catalytic site templates found on CSA [68] to determine similar active sites. GASS-WEB works in two scenarios: searching and matching [69], where it employs the information into the database to determine the active sites on the proteins. The main advantage of this technique is the active site template to search similar active sites in a protein database, which can generate an average accuracy of approximately 99% [70].

8.4.4 Site Map

SiteMap determines potential binding sites by linking together "site points" most likely to contribute to tight protein-ligand or protein-protein binding [71]. SiteMap correctly identifies the known binding site as the top-ranked site in 86% of the cases, with the best results (>98%) [72]. This method provides an algorithm for binding site identification that can help researchers locate binding sites (active sites). SiteMap analyzes the specific regions within the binding site that are suitable for occupancy by hydrophobic groups, ligand hydrogen-bond donors, acceptors, or metal-binding functionality [73].

8.4.5 Computed Atlas of Surface Topography of Proteins (CASTp)

The computed atlas of surface topography of proteins (CASTp) method generates a comprehensive and detailed quantitative characterization of interior voids and surface pockets of proteins' characteristics in active sites [74]. CASTp determines the delineation of all atoms participating in their formation. Besides, CASTp measures the volume and area of each pocket and voids analytically, using the solvent accessible surface and molecular surface models, which helps assess the accessibility of binding sites to various ligands and substrates [75].

8.5 Conclusion

The continuous technology advantage has facilitated the investigation of biosciences. This arises as an ease manipulation through the computerized method. PDB, DALI, SSAP, STAMP, CSA, Pfam are databases containing information related to protein families, bondings, coil, secondary and tertiary structure, and sometimes these programs are freely available. For example, the PDBSiteScan program determines the active sites and binding sites in a protein structure, while PINTS allows determining and comparing information based on trustful databases. GASS is highly used because it is based on PDB and CSA, generating an average accuracy of almost 99%. On the other hand, the Site Map algorithm determines the active sites (protein-protein binding), while CASTp measures the accessibility of active sites to ligands and substrate.

References

1. Bustamante-Torres, M., Romero-Fierro, D., Estrella-Nuñez, J., Bucio, E., Microbial degradation of lipids, in: *Recent Adv. In Microbial Degradation*, pp. 251–272, Springer Link, Springer, Singapore, 2021.
2. Shah, T. and Misra, A., Proteomics, in: *Challenges In Delivery Of Therapeutic Genomics And Proteomics*, pp. 387–427, 2011.
3. Marcus, J., Protein Basics: Animal and vegetable proteins in food and health. *Culinary Nutr.*, 189–230, 2013.
4. Braun, P. and Gingras, A., History of protein-protein interactions: From egg-white to complex networks. *Proteomics, 12*, 1478–1498, 2012.
5. De La, V., Russis, T., Valles, A., Gómez, R., Chinea, G., Pons, T., Interacciones proteína-proteína: Bases de datos y métodos teóricos de predicción. *Biotecnol. Apl.*, 20, 201, 2003.
6. Rao, V., Srinivas, K., Sujini, G., Kumar, G., Protein-protein interaction detection: Methods and analysis. *Int. J. Proteomics*, 2014, 147648, 12, 2014.
7. Subasi, A., Machine learning techniques, in: *Practical Machine Learning For Data Analysis Using Python*, pp. 91–202, 2020.
8. Zou, Q. and Ma, Q., The application of machine learning to disease diagnosis and treatment. *Math. Biosci.*, *320*, 108305, 2020.
9. Edgar, T. and Manz, D., Research methods for cyber security, in: *Machine Learning*, pp. 53–173, 2017.
10. Sommer, C. and Gerlich, D., Machine learning in cell biology—Teaching computers to recognize phenotypes. *J. Cell Sci.*, 216, 5529, 2013.
11. Caballero, D., Serrano E, M., Reyes, V., Llerena, P., Cuadro, M., Salgado, C., Rodríguez, P., Modelación por homología de la proteína Luxs de

Porphyromonas gingivalis cepa W83, Modelling by homology of Luxs protein in Porphyromonas gingivalis strain W83. *Rev. Clin. Periodoncia Implantol. Rehabil. Oral.*, 105, 105–103, 2012.
12. Husi, H. and Albalat, A., Proteomics, in: *Handbook of Pharmacogenomics and Stratified Medicine*, pp. 147–179, 2014.
13. Gromiha, M., Proteins. *Protein Bioinf.*, 1–27, 2009.
14. Bustamante-Torres, M., Romero-Fierro, D., Estrella-Nuñez, J., Bucio, E., Microbial degradation of proteins, in: *Recent Advances in Microbial Degradation*, pp. 351–371, Springer Link, 2021.
15. Joshi, K. and Patil, D., Proteomics, in: *Innovative Approaches in Drug Discovery*, pp. 273–294, 2017.
16. Twyman, R., Proteomics, in: *Encyclopedia of Applied Ethics*, pp. 642–649, 2012.
17. Coorssen, J., Proteomics, in: *Brenner's Encyclopedia of Genetics*, pp. 508–510, 2013.
18. Phizicky, E. and Fields, S., Protein-protein interactions: Methods for detection and analysis. *Microbiol. Rev.*, *59*, 94, 1995.
19. Lawson, C. and Wolf, S., ICAM-1 signaling in endothelial cells. *Pharmacol. Rep.*, 61, 22, 2009.
20. Zhang, Q., Petrey, D., Deng, L., Qiang, L., Shi, Y., Aye Jue, C., Bisikirka, B., Lefebvre, C., Accili, D., Hunter, T., Maniatis, T., Califano, A., Honig, B., Structure-based prediction of protein–protein interactions on a genome-wide scale. *Nature*, 490, 556, 2012.
21. Hosur, R., Xu, J., Bienkowska, J., Berger, B., iWRAP: An interface threading approach with application to prediction of cancer-related protein– protein interactions. *J. Mol. Biol.*, *405*, 1295, 2011.
22. Zhang, M., Su, Q., Lu, Y., Zhao, M., Niu, B., Application of machine learning approaches for protein-protein interactions prediction. *Med. Chem.*, 13, 506–514, 2017.
23. Samara, N., Gao, Y., Wu, J., Yang, W., Detection of reaction intermediates in Mg 2+ -dependent DNA synthesis and RNA degradation by time-resolved X-ray crystallography. *Meth. Enzymol.*, 283–327, 2017.
24. Robeva, R. and Yildirim, N., Bistability in the lactose operon of escherichia coli: A comparison of differential equation and boolean network models, in: *Mathematical Concepts And Methods In Modern Biology*, pp. 37–74, 2013.
25. Blanco, A. and Blanco, G., Enzymes. *Med. Biochem.*, 153, 153–175, 2017.
26. Purich, D., Covalent enzyme-substrate compounds: Detection and catalytic competence, in: *Enzyme Kinetics and Mechanism—Part F: Detection and Characterization of Enzyme Reaction Intermediates*, 2002.
27. An, X., Su, Z., Zeng, H., Preparation of highly magnetic chitosan particles and their use for affinity purification of enzymes. *J. Chem. Technol. Biotechnol.*, 78, 596, 2003.
28. Ciechanover, A., Elias, S., Heller, H., Hershko, A., Covalent affinity" purification of ubiquitin-activating enzyme. *J. Biol. Chem.*, 257, 2537, 1982.

29. Cossío, F., Disparidades econômicas inter-regionais, capacidade de obtenção de recursos tributários, esforço fiscal e gasto público no federalismo brasileiro, in: *Encyclopedia of Immunology*, vol. 1, p. 131, 1998.
30. Hemmings, H.C. and Girault, J.A., Cell signaling, in: *Foundations of Anesthesia*, pp. 31–50, 2006.
31. Iqbal, H., Akins, D.R., Kenedy, M.R., Co-immunoprecipitation for identifying protein-protein interactions in Borrelia burgdorferi, in: *Methods in Molecular Biology*, vol. 1690, Clifton, N.J. (Ed.), p. 47, 2018.
32. Hall, D.A., Ptacek, J., Snyder, M., Protein microarray technology. *Mech. Ageing Dev.*, 128, 161, 2007.
33. Santiago Vispo, N., García Ojalvo, A., Cesareni, G., Exposición de proteínas foráneas en plll, Combinatoria, Molecular, pp. 133–159 , Elfos Scientiae, 2004.
34. Ilari, A. and Savino, C., Protein structure determination by X-ray crystallography. *Methods Mol. Biol.*, 452, 63, 2008.
35. Kaplan, M., Pinto, C., Houben, K., Baldus, M., Nuclear magnetic resonance (NMR) applied to membrane–protein complexes. *Q. Rev. Biophys.*, 49, 2016.
36. Hixson, K., Lopez-Ferrer, D., Robinson, E., Paša-Tolić, L., Proteomics, in: *Encyclopedia Of Spectroscopy And Spectrometry*, vol. 766, 2017.
37. Gao, G., Williams, J., Campbell, S., Protein–protein interaction analysis by nuclear magnetic resonance spectroscopy. *Methods Mol. Biol.,* 261, 79–92, 2014 vol. 79, 2004.
38. Kamal, H., Minhas, F., Farooq, M., Tripathi, D., Hamza, M., Mustafa, R., Tripathi, D., Hamza, M., Mustafa, R., Zuhaib Khan, M., Manssor, S., Pappu, H., Amin, I., *In silico* prediction and validations of domains involved in gossypium hirsutum SnRK1 protein interaction with cotton leaf curl multan betasatellite encoded βC1. *Front. Plant Sci.*, 10, 1–14, 2019.
39. Pazos, F. and Valencia, A., *In silico* two-hybrid system for the selection of physically interacting protein pairs. *Proteins: Struct. Funct. Genet.*, 47, 219, 2002.
40. Jiang, M., Niu, C., Cao, J., Ni, D., Chu, Z., *In silico*-prediction of protein–protein interactions network about MAPKs and PP2Cs reveals a novel docking site variants in Brachypodium distachyon. *Sci. Rep.*, 8, 1–11, 2018.
41. Jia, Y. and Lopez, I., Kowalski. Toxin transcripts in Crotalus atrox venom and *in silico* structures of toxins. *J. Venom Res.*, 10, 18–22, 2020.
42. Orengo, C. and Taylor, W., SSAP: Sequential structure alignment program for protein structure comparison. *Meth. Enzymol.*, 266, 617–635, 1996.
43. Bernstein, F., Koetzle, T., Williams, G., Meyer, E., Brice, M., Rodgers, J., Kennard, O., Shimanouchi, T., Tasumi, M., The protein data bank: A computer-based archival file for macromolecular structures. *J. Mol. Biol.*, *112*, 535, 1977.
44. Berman, H., The Protein Data Bank. *Nucleic Acids Res.*, *28*, 235, 2000.
45. Tong, J. and Ranganathan, S., Scientific publications and databases, in: *Computer-Aided Vaccine Design*, vol. 21, 2013.

46. Dutta, S., Zardecki, C., Goodsell, D., Berman, H., Promoting a structural view of biology for varied audiences: An overview of RCSB PDB resources and experiences. *J. Appl. Crystallogr.*, 1224, 2010.
47. Gromiha, M., Protein Structure Analysis. *Protein Bioinf.*, 63–105, 2010.
48. Zardecki, C., Dutta, S., Goodsell, D., Voigt, M., Burley, S., RCSB Protein data bank: A resource for chemical, biochemical, and structural explorations of large and small biomolecules. *J. Chem. Educ.*, 2016.
49. Holm, L. and Sander, C., Dali: A network tool for protein structure comparison. *Trends Biochem. Sci.*, *20*, 478, 1995.
50. Russell, R. and Barton, G., Multiple protein sequence alignment from tertiary structure comparison: Assignment of global and residue confidence levels. *Proteins: Struct. Funct. Genet.*, *14*, 309, 1992.
51. Porter, C., The Catalytic Site Atlas: A resource of catalytic sites and residues identified in enzymes using structural data. *Nucleic Acids Res.*, 32, 129, 2004.
52. Finn, R., Bateman, A., Clements, J., Coggill, P., Eberhardt, R., Eddy, S., Heger, A., Hetherigton, K., Holm, L., Mistry, J., Sonnhammer, E., Tate, J., Punta, M., Pfam: The protein families database. *Nucleic Acids Res.*, *42*, 222, 2013.
53. Barreto, H., Bioinformática: Una oportunidad y un desafío. *Bioinf. presents both an opportunity challenge, Rev. Colomb. Biotecnol.*, 1, 132, 2008.
54. Ellis, J. and Morrison, D.A., Application of bioinformatics to parasitology. *Int. J. Parasitol.*, 35, 463, 2005.
55. Brock, O. and Brunette, T.J., *Predicting Protein Structure with Guided Conformation Space Search*, 2015.
56. Cozzone, A.J., *Proteins: Fundamental Chemical Properties*, Wiley Online Library, 2021, www.els.net.
57. Overbeek, R., Fonstein, M., D'Souza, M., Pusch, G., Maltsev, N., The use of gene clusters to infer functional coupling. *Proceedings of the National Academy of Sciences of the United States of America*, vol. 96, p. 2896, 1999.
58. Torno, W., Snel, B., Bork, P., Gene context conservation of a higher order than operons. *Trends Biochem. Sci.*, 25, 474, 2000.
59. Pellegrini, M., Marcotte, E., Thompson, M., Eisenberg, D., Ye, T., Assigning protein functions by comparative genome analysis: Protein phylogenetic profiles. *Proceedings of the National Academy of Sciences of the United States of America*, vol. 96, p. 4285, 1999.
60. Huynen, M., Snel, B., Lathe, W.,., IIIII, Bork, P., Predicting Protein Function by Genomic Context: Quantitative Evaluation and Qualitative Inferences. *Genome Res.*, 10, 1204, 2000.
61. Tripathi, L., Chen, Y., Mizuguchi, K., Murakami, Y., Network-based analysis for biological discovery, in: *Encyclopedia of Bioinformatics and Computational Biology*, vol. 283, 2019.
62. Weinstock, G., Microbial Genetics, in: *Brenner's Encyclopedia of Genetics*, p. 392, 2013.
63. Chinnaiyan, A. and Palanisamy, N., Chromosomal aberrations in solid tumors. *Prog. Mol. Biol. Transl. Sci.*, 95, 55–94, 2010.

64. Marcotte, E.M., Pellegrini, M., Ng, H.L., Rice, D.W., Yeates, T.O., Eisenberg, D., Detecting protein function and protein-protein interactions from genome sequences. *Science*, *285*, 751, 1999.
65. Enright, A., Iliopoulos, I., Kyrpides, N., Ouzounis, C., Protein interaction maps for complete genomes based on gene fusion events. *Nature*, 402, 86, 1999.
66. Ivanisenko, V., Pintus, S., Grigorovich, D., Kolchanov, N., PDBSiteScan: A program for searching for active, binding and posttranslational modification sites in the 3D structures of proteins. *Nucleic Acids Res.*, 32, 549, 2004.
67. Stark, A. and Russell, R., Annotation in three dimensions. PINTS: Patterns in Non-homologous Tertiary Structures. *Nucleic Acids Res.*, 31, 3341, 2003.
68. Furnham, N., Holliday, G., de Beer, T., Jacobsen, J., Pearson, W., Thornton, J., The catalytic site atlas 2.0: Cataloging catalytic sites and residues identified in enzymes. *Nucleic Acids Res.*, *42*, 485, 2013.
69. OpenEBechn, 2017. https://openebench.bsc.es/tool/gass-web.
70. Moraes, J., Pappa, G., Pires, D., Izidoro, S., GASS-WEB: A web server for identifying enzyme active sites based on genetic algorithms. *Nucleic Acids Res.*, 45, 315, 2017.
71. Halgren, T., New method for fast and accurate binding-site identification and analysis, in: *Chemical Biology & Drug Design*, vol. *69*, p. 146, 2007.
72. Halgren, T., Identifying and characterizing binding sites and assessing druggability. *J. Chem. Inf. Model.*, *49*, 377, 2009.
73. SiteMap | Schrödinger, 2021. https://www.schrodinger.com/products/sitemap.
74. Laskowski, R.A., Luscombe, N.M., Swindells, M.B., Thornton, J.M., Protein clefts in molecular recognition and function, in: *Protein Science: A Publication of the Protein Society*, vol. 5, p. 2438, 1996.
75. Binkowski, T., CASTp: Computed atlas of surface topography of proteins. *Nucleic Acids Res.*, *31*, 3352, 2003.

9

Protein Redesign and Engineering Using Machine Learning

Zhuha Basit[1], Hira Akram[2], Muhammad Mudassir Iqbal[2*], Gulzar Muhammad[3†], Muhammad Shahbaz Aslam[2], Iram Gul[2], Muhammad Jamil[4] and Mudassir Hussain Tahir[5]

[1]*School of Biological Sciences, University of the Punjab, Lahore, Lahore, Pakistan*
[2]*School of Biochemistry and Biotechnology, University of the Punjab, Lahore, Lahore, Pakistan*
[3]*Department of Chemistry, GC University Lahore, Lahore, Pakistan*
[4]*Institute of Chemistry, University of Sargodha, Sargodha, Pakistan*
[5]*Department of Chemistry, Division of Science and Technology, University of Education, Lahore, Lahore, Pakistan*

Abstract

Several proteins are employed in the diagnosis, prevention, cure, or treatment of the disease. Mutations in the pathogenic organisms at a faster rate, the emergence of zoonotic diseases, and complications in malignancies demand the enhanced specificity, affinity, activity, and efficacy of protein drugs. A particular function of a protein molecule depends mainly upon the structural characteristics of the protein molecule. The sequence of amino acids in a polypeptide chain determines the secondary and tertiary structure of the protein molecule and hence its function. Protein redesign improves the structural and functional capability of therapeutic proteins significantly. The application of various machine learning techniques enables us to redesign novel protein drugs by predicting secondary and tertiary structural features, solubility, stability, and specificity. In redesigning protein structure, different mutations are investigated for beneficial, harmful, or neutral effects on characteristics and the functions of the therapeutic protein. Introduction of beneficial mutations in the primary sequence of proteins and structural modifications augment protein's function. Machine learning methods use principles of computation and algorithms and constitute models from data

**Corresponding author*: mudassiribb@gmail.com
†*Corresponding author*: mgulzar@gcu.edu.pk

Inamuddin, Tariq Altalhi, Jorddy N. Cruz and Moamen Salah El-Deen Refat (eds.) Drug Design Using Machine Learning, (247–282) © 2022 Scrivener Publishing LLC

collected. This chapter discusses recent advancements in various machine learning methods employed for redesigning protein drugs in detail.

Keywords: Protein, drug, machine learning, neural network, ensemble, deep learning

9.1 Introduction

Proteins are polymers of mere 20 amino acids, but how amino acids can interact and fold is the reason behind the sophisticated functions of the proteins in living organisms. Proteins mediate all fundamental processes of life, diversity of folding, and variation in functions of proteins have intrigued biologists for the past 50 years, and the study of protein function became the core of biomedical research. It is quite surprising that for protein comprised of 200 residues, 20^{200} sequences are possible and an infinitesimal number of subsets has been sampled through natural evolution. The full sequence space can be explored through de novo design of proteins that follow physical protein folding principles. Computational technology has unfolded an entirely new era in protein design and engineering. Now it is possible to design and synthesize any protein from scratch with atomic-level accuracy. No doubt, by far, most of the proteins which have been engineered are actual modifications of naturally occurring proteins but through advanced knowledge, it should be possible to design and synthesize proteins with entirely new functions to tackle up various challenges in fields of drug design, nanotechnology, and biomedicine [1]. EvoDesign server designs protein sequences with desired features from the sequences in a database. Figure 9.1 illustrates steps in de novo design of protein with the help of EvoDesign server [2].

Structures of proteins have been usually determined primarily through different sophisticated and complex techniques, such as NMR spectroscopy [3], cryoelectron microscopy [4], and X-ray crystallography [5]. The expansion of crystallographic data of proteins helps to construct various protein sequences by using short fragments which frequently reappear. In de novo designing of proteins, another milestone is the development and synthesis of proteins with quite complex functions. Proteins are designed in a way that they can bind with various porphyrins, metals, and other co-factors [6]. Methods based on computational approaches are widely employed in predicting secondary and tertiary structural features of proteins and depict their biological functions when experimental approaches are limited [7]. The scientific revolution is being driven by deep

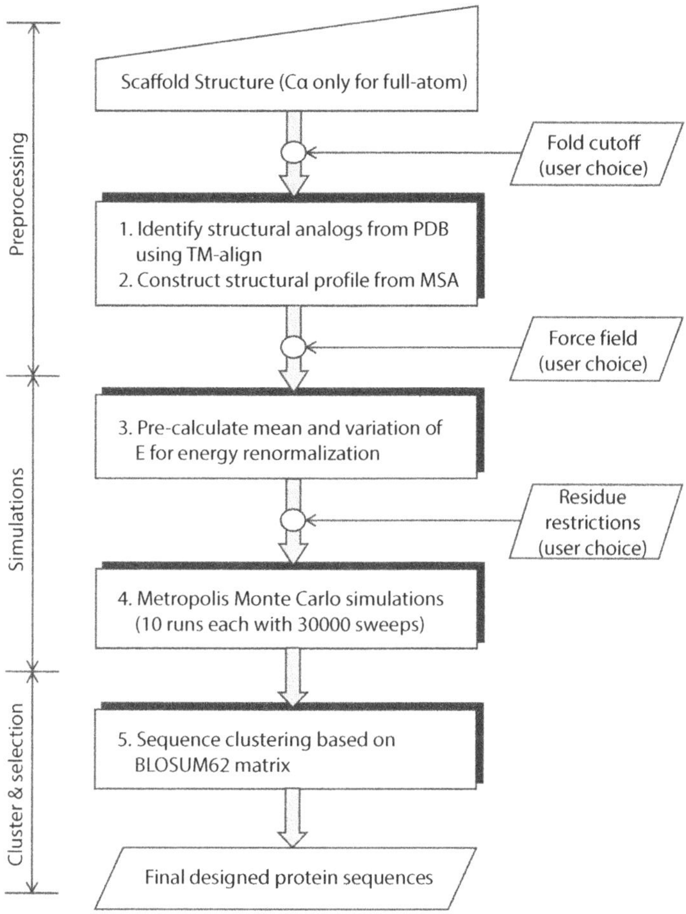

Figure 9.1 A simple illustration of EvoDesign server showing the steps in de novo protein designing (reprinted with permission under creative commons license from [2]).

learning through the availability of more significant data, toolkits that can be accessed easily, and influential computational resources, which have opened avenues in many fields including structural modelling of proteins. The structural modeling of proteins, such as prediction of their structure from evolutionary information and sequence of amino acids, engineering them to achieve anticipated functionality or to predict the behavior and properties of proteins, is crucial to comprehend and modify various biological systems even at a molecular level [8].

Deep learning methods have opened new arenas in the engineering of proteins. Based on the stacked neural network layers, deep learning can be categorized as various machine learning techniques in which functions are parameterized based on non-linear activation functions and the configuration of an affine transformation. Their main superiority over traditional methods lies in their ability to extract domains that possess specific features. Deep learning has revolutionized various digital applications such as speech recognition [9], classification of images [10], and game-playing [11]. Inspired by these features, attention turned towards deep learning applications in more complex and sophisticated things, such as the structure and design of proteins [12]. Figure 9.2 illustrates major steps in modelling of proteins.

This chapter describes the use of various machine learning methods to formulate various protein drugs. Initially, steps in the design of sequence-function models for proteins are introduced to the reader. This section provides information about the evaluation and training of

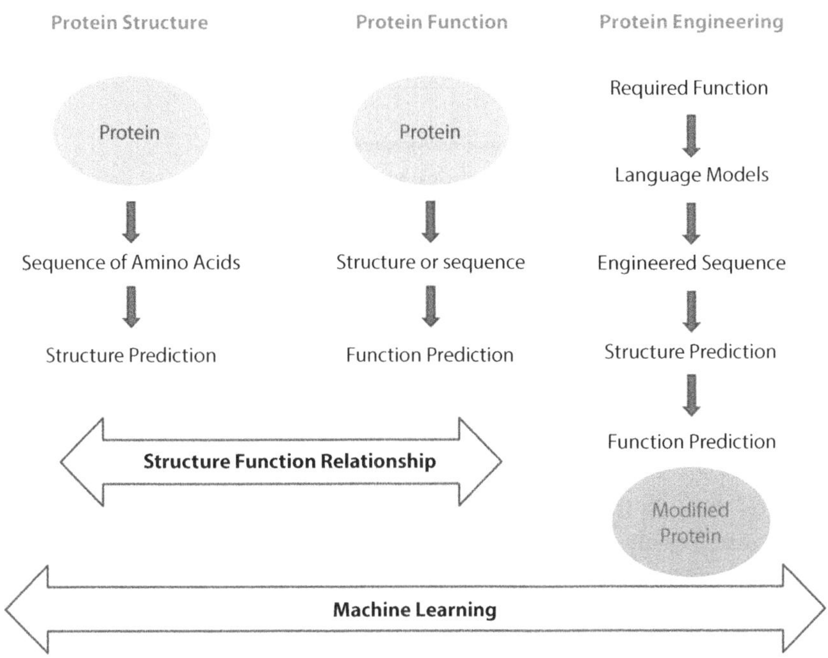

Figure 9.2 Comparison of the major tasks in modelling proteins: Structure Prediction: In this case, input sequence and structure of the protein are computationally predicted. Function Prediction: In this case, structure/sequence is known and the neural network predicts function as output. The most advanced case starts with the desired function and output gives a sequence that can fold three-dimensionally to provide the desired function.

models, representation of proteins by vectors, and guidance in predicting the sequence and function of proteins. In the following part of the chapter, types of features and prediction of thermo-stability of protein with single point mutations are explained. Afterward, different machine learning methods like support vector machine, neural network, Bayesian network, ensemble learning, and deep learning are discussed. In the last, the application of machine learning in enzyme engineering is enlightened.

9.2 Designing Sequence-Function Model Through Machine Learning

The models of machine learning acquire information from examples of sequences of proteins and then measurement of respective functions of proteins. The learning of a model depends on the criteria chosen. The library can be screened randomly to select variants [13] or enhance information for various mutations [14–19]. Undoubtedly, the easiest method is a random selection of variants, but it sometimes becomes crucial to exploit information gathered from experiments of higher cost to improve the model's accuracy. The process to obtain maximum information about mutations in the rest of the library is a challenge and almost the same as obtaining maximum diversity in the training sequences. Once the training data are collected, the next step is to decide which machine learning model can be employed and then the information is represented in an amenable form to the model and the model is trained [20]. In a novel strategy, the amino acids are represented audibly through the sonification method that converts amino acid signals into vibrations. Artificial intelligence generates this de novo musical data and then translates it into a specific protein sequence, hence obtaining a de novo design of protein with specific characteristics. It provides a way to understand specific patterns, mutations, variations, and channels to explain the importance of the protein sequence [21].

Many algorithms exist for machine learning, however not a single is optimized to perform all tasks [22]. For directed evolution guided by machine learning, we want methods that can take various sequences and output values associated with them and then take unseen sequences and predict output in the same vein. A linear transformation is applied to the input features in the simplest machine learning models like absence or presence of mutation [13], location of amino acid at each position or sequence block in a library composed of chimeric proteins [23]. Before shifting to the most potent models, linear models are usually employed in the prediction of baseline. Regression and classification trees are employed to move from input characteristics such as from branches to the labels. In ensemble methods, decision tree models, such as boosted trees [24] and random forests, are used to merge various models into the most precise meta predictor. Random forests act as a computationally efficient and robust baseline in small data sets, such as those we encounter during protein engineering experiments. They have been employed to predict the thermostability of enzymes [25–27].

To calculate similarities between input pairs, kernel methods, such as kernel ridge regression [28], support vector machines [29], and kernel function are employed. They project the features of input to form a space that is characterized by high dimensions. In this approach, coordinates are not computed into a new space. However, on protein inputs general-purpose kernels can be used, other kernels have been designed to be employed on proteins, such as mismatch string and spectrum kernels [30, 31] and they count the subsequences shared among proteins and the three-dimensional structure of a protein is accounted by weighted decomposition kernels [32]. Support vector machines predict the expression and localization of membrane proteins, thermostability of proteins [33–35], and enantioselectivity of enzymes [36].

Probabilistic predictions have been made by employing Gaussian process (GP) which merges Bayesian learning with kernel methods [37]. These models provide guidelines about experimental design by capturing uncertainty. One problem associated with Gaussian process is its run time. A greater number of training models demand significantly increased run time to complete the job. Hence, it is inappropriate for larger data sets. However, now most accurate and fast approximations are available [38, 39]. Protein sequences are represented in embedded form and the predictive ability of Gaussian process model is trained on embeddings. Accurate predictions are made by using embeddings. The explanation of embeddings is quite easy as there is no need for structural data, alignment or selection of properties [40]. Photoproperties of channel rhodopsin, fluorescence [41], thermostability [42], and membrane localization have been predicted through Gaussian process.

Neural networks, which are deep learning models, extract features of high level from inputs that are structured. For tasks that have large labelled data sets, the neural networks are most feasible. They have been successfully employed for prediction of the binding site [43], nucleic acid-protein binding [44], secondary structure [45], thermostability [46], functional class, and solubility [47]. Now they have been exploited for three-dimensional

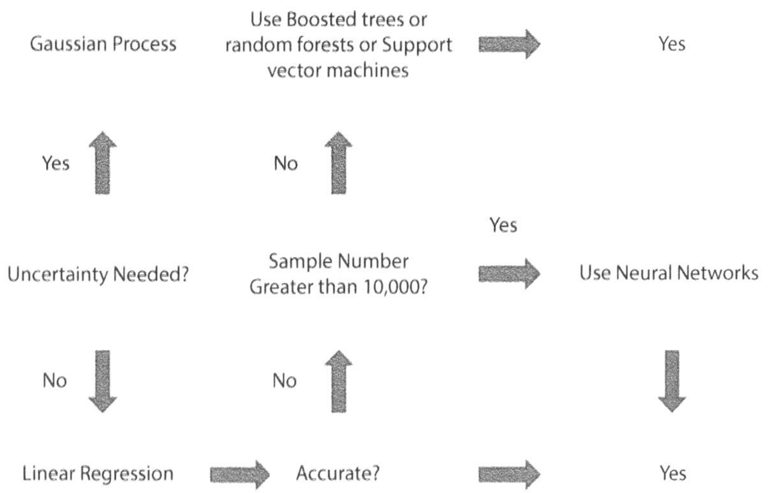

Figure 9.3 The most general illustration to choose sequence function model for machine learning.

structure as well. Figure 9.3 illustrates the choice of the sequence-function model for machine learning.

9.2.1 Training of Model and Evaluation

The process in which various parameters are tuned to enhance the productive accuracy is known as tuning of model bases on machine learning. Accurate prediction of the input labels that were not seen during the training is a prime goal of training. So, in the model training process, efficiency must be forecasted for the date that is not in the training set. Therefore, withholding about 20% of data, also called a test set, is essential for evaluating the model. Besides parameters, the form of a model is estimated by various hyper-parameters, and model families can also be categorized as hyper-parameter. The parameter is directly extracted from the data. They are set manually or estimated by various random searches, grid search, or Bayesian optimization [48]. In the case of a neural network, the various parameters are the size, number, and connectivity of each layer. The accuracy may be affected significantly through minor changes in values of hyper-parameters and the assortment of optimum values is much laborious computationally as for every set of parameters, the training of a new model is required.

Once the test is removed, data that remains should be bifurcated into a validation set and training set for selecting hyper-parameters and comparing the model. Parameters are learned from the training set whereas hyper-parameters are chosen from the validation set by estimating test error. Cross-validation is done when there is small training. When there is n-fold cross-validation, there is a splitting of the training set into complementary subsets. Then prediction of each subset is made by employing a model which is manipulated on other subsets. The estimation of the correctness of the model with the subsets gives an approximation of the correctness of the tests. More time for training is required in case of cross-validation but it provides better estimation than constant validation. To get a better estimation of the performance of a model under given conditions, it is recommended to split data sets into validation, training, and test sets. When data sets are of mutagenic studies, the best way is to train on those variants characterized during the former round of mutagenesis and evaluate the model's performance on advanced rounds [20].

9.2.2 Representation of Proteins by Vector

The models of machine learning cannot be applied directly on sequences of proteins rather their enforcement is on vectors of numbers. What can be estimated depends now on how the protein sequence is vectorized [49, 50]. A protein sequence can be considered a string having a definite length, and each amino acid can be regarded as a sample from a set of alphabets. The easiest means to code such a cord is to denote amino acids by number but this method requires some order. In the case of amino acids, there exists no biological or physical basis. Each length position is represented by one-hot encoding in signifying every location by a single number. When structural information is present, it is possible to one-hot encode the individuality of couples of amino acids that are present at a certain distance [14, 15].

It is possible to utilize physical properties of protein for encoding such as the representation of amino acids can be made based on volume, charge or hydrophobic nature and then whole protein may be denoted by merging properties of individual amino acids. Protein Feature Engineering Toolkit [51] and amino acid index [52] contain large libraries of physical features describing sequences of proteins. Efforts are made to bifurcate amino acids into two dimensions concerning hydrophobicity and volume [53] or by merging structural information with physical properties [54]. This merging occurs when each position is encoded as an amalgamation of the amino acids in its arithmetical vicinity. Molecular characteristics usually govern functional features and they are not known. No doubt, in databases, many sequences have been deposited but their majority is unlabelled.

These unlabelled sequences of amino acids encompass data that describes the dispersal of those amino acids nominated through evolutionary processes and constitute protein molecules, so they help predict nature. AAIndex2-style and BLOSUM can be categorized as the most straightforward encodings integrating evolutionary information, and these substitution matrices are based on relative frequencies of amino acids [55].

Learned encoding is usually low dimensional, and they improve their performance through a transfer of information present in the unlabelled sequences to more specific tasks of prediction; however, specification of learned encodings for the particular task of prediction is a laborious task. No vectorization method can be considered universally optimum as no model can be regarded as optimum for the performance of all the tasks [22]. There is a need to employ a combination of heuristics and domain expertise to select encodings for the comparison. One-hot encoding is preferred in small data sets, whereas domain knowledge can make accurate predictions. Learned encodings can help to improve performance when there is insufficient accuracy [56].

9.2.3 Guiding Exploration by Employing Sequence-Function Prediction

Once the model for a sequence of amino acids and protein function is achieved, the choice of other sequences that need to be scrutinized may be made either based on direct optimization over different sequences or by employing a library of beneficial mutations. In the latter case, linear models can be learned for mutational effects, and they can be investigated to find out whether mutations are deleterious, neutral or beneficial. Then, these mutations may be eliminated, corrected, or reevaluated in further optimal series [13]. Sequences can then be further optimized. When there is a need for multiple rounds for optimization and probabilistic predictions are provided through the sequence function model, learned information and investigation of unseen regions could balance through Bayesian optimization [48]. Uncertainty can be estimated through probabilistic predictions; the model knows well about things it does not know. These approaches have been amalgamated with recombination guided by structure for optimization of thermostability of cytochrome and conductance of light-activated channel rhodopsin [16]. In the absence of high throughput screening for properties of channel rhodopsin, conductance cannot be optimized with traditional methods of directed evolution.

9.3 Features Based on Energy

Recently, hot spots are predicted from the features based on energy. The energetically important residues have been predicted by Kortemme and his colleagues through a linear combination of Lennard Jones potential, hydrogen bonding potential dependent on orientation, implicit solvation model, and by taking into account approximation of reference state, which is unfolded [57]. Tuncbag and his colleagues improved the accuracy for predicting hot spots by applying statistical pair potentials of inter residues [58, 59]. For predicting hot spot residues, Lise and his co-workers made calculations of intermolecular energies of side chains, Van der Waal potential, intramolecular energies of side chains, and solvation energies [60, 61]. Residual energy, combined score of energy calculated through ENDES [62, 63], the energy of side chain, and interface propensity were incorporated by Deng and his colleagues [64].

9.4 Features Based on Structure

The amino acid chain with its secondary structural features folds in a three-dimensional structure known as the tertiary structure of a protein. The tertiary structure facilitates us to understand the functions of a protein. Modifications in the structure of proteins improve functions compared to modifications in the sequences [65, 66]. Definition of the secondary structure of proteins (DSSP) is used to calculate the surface areas accessible to solvent [67]. Features related to accessible surface areas have been widely employed for predicting hot spots and protein-protein interactions on the interface [58, 64, 68, 69]. Various biochemical contacts such as salt bridges, atom contacts, hydrogen bonding, and residue contacts are vital structural characteristics helpful to predict hot spots [70–72]. The calculations are performed for fold recognition of protein molecules [62, 73] and further employed in PredHS [64].

9.5 Prediction of Thermostability of Protein with Single Point Mutations

One of the main issues in the engineering of proteins is their thermostability. If the thermostability of mutant variants could be predicted, it would help make decisions about engineering proteins through mutagenesis. To do the most specific mutation and find out hot spots in-silico scanning method of point mutations is used. Thousands of mutant proteins whose thermostability is measured experimentally are available on the publically available database ProTherm. Two different data sets based on two other properties of proteins that depend upon their thermostability, named change in melting temperature and change in free energy of unfolding, were extracted from the mentioned database. Information about the physical properties of amino acids, structural information about the point mutations, and calculations of free energy change of folding were derived from building up models of thermostability prediction by utilizing tools of informatics modelling. To build up prediction models, partial least square regression and five primary machine learning methods named naive Bayes classifier, support vector machine, K nearest neighbour, artificial neural network, and random forest are mainly used to build up prediction models. Apart from this, binary and ternary classification and the regression models were built up, and later on, they were evaluated. Among various prediction models, the Rosetta calculation for free energy change ranked at the top [27].

9.6 Selection of Features

Performance of prediction can be enhanced to a significant level by employing feature selection and it also helps to escape overfitting. Moreover, it provides pretty deep insight into the means used to generate data [74]. Algorithms that are used generally for the selection of features are maximum relevance maximum distance [75], support vector machines [76], random forest, and F-score [77]. Hot spots have been predicted through various feature selection approaches such as Decision tree is used by MINERVA [70] and F-score is used by APIS [69]. Random forest was used by Moreira and his colleagues [78] and Wang and his colleagues [79] in predicting hot spots. The algorithm of sequential backward elimination and random forest were combined through PredHS [68] for the selection of optimum features in predicting hot spots. Qiao and his co-workers [80] developed the hybrid feature strategy to predict hot spots and combine mRMR, F-score, and decision tree.

9.6.1 Extraction of Features

Another dimensional reduction approach employed to apply machine learning is the extraction of features. The two most commonly used techniques for the extraction of features are linear discriminant analysis (LDA) and principal component analysis (PCA) [81–83]. Principal component analysis transforms data orthogonally to convert correlated variables to set variables that are not linearly correlated, the principle components. Melo and his colleagues employed principal component analysis to improve the prediction of hot spots and narrow down the data set's dimensionality [84]. Moreira and his co-workers used principal component analysis to produce a variety of data sets, such as PCAUp, PCA, PCADown, and their performance was assessed in predicting hot spots [78].

9.7 Force Field and Score Function

In structural modelling of proteins, one of the significant requirements is score function or force field for ranking models and/or samples [85]. A force field describes the surface potential energy of protein. Some knowledge-based terms may also be present in the score function, but sometimes, they do not have any physical meaning and have been designed to distinguish non-native conformations from near-native ones [86]. The appropriate statistical behaviors of various biomolecules can be reproduced through Monte Carlo simulation or by molecular dynamics [87–89]. Currently, efforts based on deep learning to comprehend the force field are categorized into two main types: graph-derived and fingerprint-derived. Some rotational and translational constant characteristics, such as Behler Parrinello fingerprint, were developed by Parrinello and Behler [90] to code the atoms in surrounding to construct neural networks. They did so to study possible surfaces through calculations involving computations based on quantum mechanical models. Smith and his colleagues extended this framework and the accuracy of the system was tested through simulation of systems up to 312 atoms conditional language models are used for the sequences of proteins that condition directly on graph specification of a certain target structure. Various complex dependencies in protein structure are captured by focusing on those residues which are local in three-dimensional space but long-range in the sequence. This approach offers comparative advantages over a neural network and conventional approaches with generative models for designing the targeted biomolecules [91, 92]. Graph convolutions are employed by SchNet and deep tensor neural networks to get information about representative of every atom within the vicinity of its chemical environment [93, 94]. No doubt, within a chemical environment, the ability to learn about representative atoms and quality of prediction has made approaches based on graphs quite popular but their applications usually give rough results when applied to larger systems and therefore, their main focus has been remained on small molecules [95].

The paradigm is shifting toward deep learning methods based on score function due to massive gains in speed and efficiency. Forces, energies, and time-averaged properties can be reproduced through molecular dynamic simulation on neural networks [96]. Though these score functions are generalizable to a more extensive system, there is a dearth to apply such potential directly to construct a model of the complete protein molecule. On Chignolin composed of 10 residues and Trp cage consisting of 20 residues, ANI-x and AIMNet have been trained with ANI-MD data set [92, 97]. Molecular mechanics/quantum mechanics strategy [98] have been merged with neural potential by Wang and his colleagues [99] and Lahey and Rowley [100] to model docking with larger proteins and small-sized ligands.

9.8 Machine Learning for Prediction of Hot Spots

Besides selecting appropriate features or combinations, employing a practical machine learning approach also helps predict hot spots significantly. Various approaches of machine learning such as support vector machines, nearest neighbor [101], neural networks [102], decision trees, ensemble learning [103] and Bayesian networks [104] have been employed in predicting hot spots in protein-protein interaction.

9.8.1 Support Vector Machines

One of the most widely employed techniques of machine learning is the support vector machine. Support vector machines are binary classifiers and extend the principle of the optimal hyperplane. Support vector machines minimize the structural risk. The main pros of support vector machines are accuracy and efficiency, whereas it also has some cons, such as labels are required for input data, and it is found appropriate only for classification problems of two types. Through support vector machines, several models of hot spot prediction have been built [64, 69, 80, 105, 106]. MINERVA was proposed by Cho and his co-workers, which considers 54 features of molecular, sequence, and structural interactions. Then, the selection of the top three features is made using a decision tree. Then support vector machine was used for the creation of a model which could predict hot spots of protein-protein interaction [70]. Xia and his colleagues studied sixty-two structural and sequential features and removed redundant features through F score. Then, for identifying hot spots by support vector machines, APIS predictor was developed. It came out that more hot spots can be predicted through support vector machines than predicted by employing traditional methods [69]. Two models, namely KFC2a and KFC2b, were developed by Zhu and his colleagues in predicting hot spots using support vector machines [107]. Thirty-eight features were selected and then used in PredHS [64] to the training of models by support vector machines and remarkable improvement in performance was observed. A subset of 58 features was selected by Ye and his co-workers, which contained features of microenvironment and 10 networks through random forest algorithm [106] and then the prediction model was built using support vector machines. HEP [105] utilized 108 various structural, sequential, and domain features, and then selection of top 2 was made by two-step selection methods and a support vector machine was employed for the construction of a final model.

9.8.2 Nearest Neighbor

One of the simplest methods of machine learning is the nearest neighbor algorithm [101]. Hu and his colleagues proposed a model based on the sequence of a protein. The classifier's implementation was done through the IBK algorithm, which helped address the issues associated with the recent neighbor algorithm as it was much sensitive to data [108]. Jiang and his co-workers also used IBK algorithm to propose a model-based on sequence to get better projections using the training set [109].

9.8.3 Decision Trees

One of the supervised learning methods is the decision tree, as it depicts the relationship map among tags and features the predictive model. Every branch in the tree represents forecast output and each leaf node describes some category. Decision-making methods prune the branches which help in achieving some balance tree. Simplicity in preparation of data and easy comprehension are the main pros of decision trees whereas the main shortcomings associated with decision trees are increased rate of error associated with each category and prediction of continuous fields is also a gruesome task. Two models of decision trees, K-FADE and K-CON have been combined on the classical KFC model [71].

9.8.4 Neural Networks

Simulation of human intuitive thinking is done by artificial neural networks [102], which makes distributed patterns of data storage and can process them in a parallel manner. Each node represents the output of the function. In this approach, the linking between nodes signifies the signal quantitatively. Artificial neural networks have demonstrated outstanding and remarkable characteristics in recognizing patterns, and immense applications have been described in medicine and biology. Amino acid is a hot spot that interacts with the sequence constituting the single protein. In this case, there is no need to get knowledge about a partner of interaction [110].

9.8.5 Bayesian Networks

Bayesian network [111] established as an extended branch of Bayesian method in contrast with Bayesian foundation [112], in which each variable is assumed as discrete, magnifies independent hypothesis of variables. The foundation of this mathematical model lies upon probabilistic reasoning, which combines features of graph theory and Bayesian principle and showed impressive results in addressing the issues of strong correlation. The main problem lies with its inability to sort out variables. Three fundamental information sources named structure, energy, and evolutionary determinants of Bayesian network were combined with the PCRPi method [113]. For the implementation of Bayesian Network, BNT was used, and to get into the structural insight of BNs, R package deal was employed. Through experiments, it has been proven that accurate and consistent predictions about the hot spots can be made through PCRPi. One of the main advantages of PCRPi is its ability to handle missing data of protein.

9.8.6 Ensemble Learning

Methods based on ensemble involve algorithms of machine learning that syndicate various classifier algorithms in a single model that can give predictions to get better performance. Many algorithms such as AdaBoost, Random Forest, xgboost, and gradient tree boosting exist for ensemble [114–117]. Wang and his colleagues proposed a novel model of Random Forest that combines various features, such as huge information on account of target residue and neighboring ones to predict various hotspots involved in the interaction of proteins [118]. Unbalanced data were processed by Huang and his co-workers [119] through SMOTE [120] and hot spots were predicted through the application of AdaBoost. PredHS-Ensemble was proposed by Deng and his colleagues [64], which employs decision fusion technique and ensemble composed of n classifiers on the training data. Subsets were generated through the adoption of an approach of asymmetric bootstrap resampling. In this case, random sampling is done by replacing the class which is present in greater number so that the number of classes equals the number of several samples belonging to the class less in number and there is an arrangement of minority samples in appropriate subsets. Bagging predictor is a way of generating the various versions of predictor and subsequently achieve aggregated predictor, which averages over those versions when the numerical outcome is predicted. Bootstrap generates these multiple versions used in new learning sets [121].

Integrated bagging is much powerful with undersampling rather than with over-sampling. The most precise extension of bagging is roughly balanced bagging. Two versions are considered for neighborhood balanced bagging. In the first version, the bootstrap samples are larger whereas in the second the size is kept small. The first version works far better than the over-sampling bagging extension [122]. Random forests are the combination of various tree predictors and there is a dependence of each tree on the random vector value which is sampled independently. The distribution is the same for all the trees. The value of generalization error is linked with the strength of trees and the association among trees [123]. The generalization error rate is minimized by using stacked generalization as it deduces the biases of various generalizers to the learning set. It is a much sophisticated and advanced version of cross-validation [124]. In negative correlation learning the individual networks are trained through the ensemble method and they are combined in the same learning process. Individual networks in negative correlation are simultaneously and interactively trained in ensemble with penalty term of correlation in error functions. Cooperation and specialization are created among individual networks through the negatively correlated network [125]. Deep neural networks with a wide range of parameters are much strong machine learning systems but the main problem associated with these networks is overfitting. It is difficult to use such networks as they are quite slow. This is addressed through the random dropout of samples during training from neural networks [126].

The ensemble learning model is designed based on heterogeneous ensemble frameworks for the prediction of default risk. XGBoost is used initially for ensemble learning and deep neural network, XGBoost and logistic regression are considered as individual learners that undergo linear weighted fusion [127]. A new prediction method is proposed for the creation of a weighted combination of various candidate learners to build the super learner. V-fold cross-validation is used to construct super learner during the prediction by a fast algorithm. Weights are selected by v-fold cross-validation and candidate learners are combined [128]. Ensemble methods are impressive in supervised learning as they train various learners and combine their predictions. The ensemble comprises multiple clusters trained with a k-mean algorithm.

Table 9.1 Various techniques of ensemble learning.

Ensemble technique	Application	Reference
PredHS-Ensemble	Increases efficiency for predicting hot spot	[64]
AdaBoost	Statistical classification tool	[114]
Xgboost	Adds information to weak predictions	[116]
Gradient Boosting	Function approximation	[117]
SMOTE	Adjusts class distribution	[120]
Bagging	Reduces variation in imbalanced data	[121, 122]
Random Forest	Prediction of hot spots in protein	[118, 123]
Stacked Regression	Improves prediction accuracy	[124]
Negative correlation learning	Controls diversity in ensemble	[125]
Explicit/Implicit ensembles	Prevents neural networks from overfitting	[126]
Heterogeneous ensemble	Classifies different types from the same data	[127]
Supper learner	Cross-validates efficiency of multiple models	[128]
Unsupervised	Clusters unlabeled data	[129]
Semisupervised	Able to predict from labeled and unlabeled data	[130]

Ensemble aligns clusters and improves clustering to a significant extent [129]. The supervised learning learns mapping and trains set made of pairs. The focus of most of the tasks is on classification. The oldest semi-supervised method of learning is generative models. If large data is unlabeled, it is possible to identify components of a mixture [130]. Different techniques of ensemble learning are depicted in Table 9.1.

9.9 Deep Learning—Neural Network in Computational Protein Designing

Nevertheless, a diverse range of applications is associated with the computational designing of proteins. Still, protein engineering for a given function

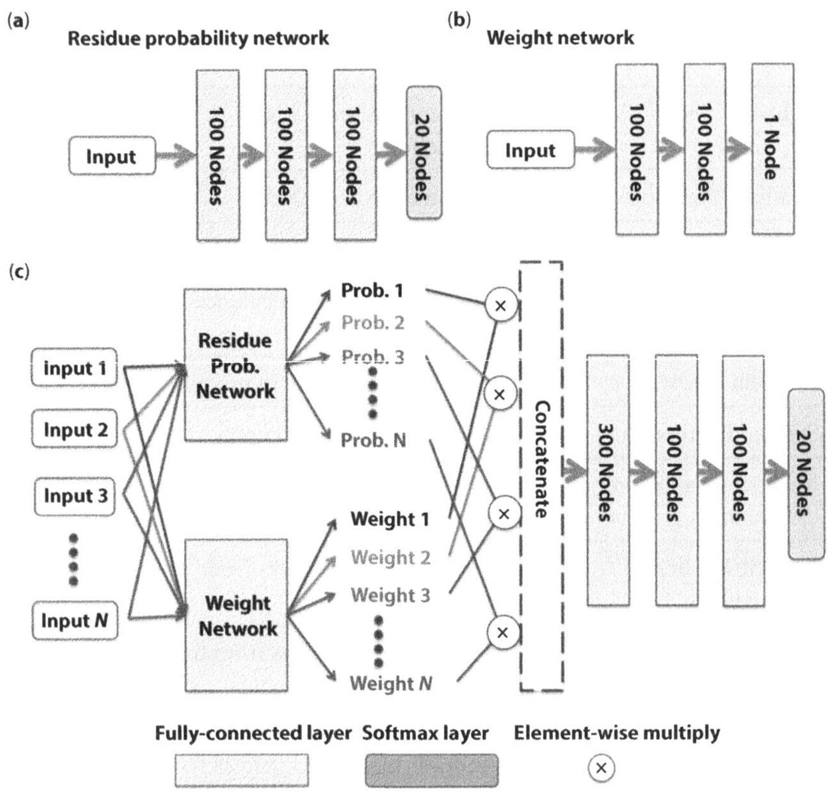

Figure 9.4 A framework of three neural networks. A represents the network to estimate the probability of residue, B represents the network to estimate weight assigned to ties among nodes, and C represents a fully connected network (reprinted with permission under creative commons license from [131]).

presents a daunting task. Whereas at one side, the number of solved structures of proteins is growing day by day. On the other hand, the number of unique protein folds has attained a steady number which depicts that on each fold, there is an accumulation of more structural information. Deep learning neural network is a much superior approach to machine learning and it offers great opportunities to handle robust and wide data. Wang and his co-worker used neural networks for computational designing of proteins as the probability of naturally occurring amino acids was predicted by them on every amino acid of the protein. Collection of a larger number of structures of a protein was initially made, then there was the construction of a multi-layer neural network. Several characteristics defining structure were dug out as input properties. Employment of network output using a residue type restraint approach significantly increases the sequence identity. The strategy has been used to engineer three different proteins through an online server, Rosetta. The sequence identity was 3% higher than achieved through already existing methods which may help in further improving the methods of computational designing of proteins. A framework of three neural networks is illustrated in Figure 9.4 [131].

9.10 Machine Learning in Engineering of Proteins

Although machine learning is quite a new approach, it has been applied successfully in challenging predictions faced during the engineering of enzymes. One of the toughest challenges in biochemistry has remained as the prediction of protein structure as the number of structures that have been resolved are dramatically less than the number of known sequences. About 215 million sequences of proteins are available publically but only 145,000 structures are available in the repository of the most famous database, the Protein Data Bank (PDB) [132].

The training of AlphaFold network was done by the entries of PDB to predict the distance present between the C-beta atoms of residues employing multiple sequence alignments [133] and the highest scores were received at the competition. About one-third of the total 124 targets predicted by AlphaFold had GDT_TS score greater than 50, which showed that the structure is correct topologically [134]. Recently, a novel machine learning technique, element-specific persistent homology has been employed to investigate Protein-ligand binding affinity [135]. Mutant serotonin designed through machine learning shows an ability to give fluorescence [136].

No doubt, the results of CASP12 observed significant improvements but still, there is much room for further betterment of protein structure predictors [137]. Using techniques of machine learning antibodies, are engineered to neutralize the SARS-CoV-2, a virus that provoked from a zoonotic source into the human in 2019. The process to design antibodies against the corona virus comprises several steps involving data mining, model training, feature extraction, use of modern techniques of ensemble, and selection of sequence with most specificity to virus illustrated in Figure 9.5 [138].

In biological processes, the most critical role is played by various posttranslational modifications. The forthcoming posttranslational modification comprises a central position with amino acid residues in the vicinity as they are basic residues of a protein sequence. Understanding these sequences is crucial as it will help explore their purposed biological functions and contribute significantly to understanding various molecular mechanisms that act as the base of protein and drug design. Various shortcomings such as lower accuracy and stability, are associated with present algorithms. Support vector machines and multilayer neural networks have been invoked to predict such potential sites by exploiting features such as E-H description of segments of proteins, the composition of residues of amino acids, and some properties of amino acids obtained from the amino acid index database. When redundant information is available, it is easy to select various features in the pro-processing step. In this way, the issue of accuracy in the classification can be addressed [139].

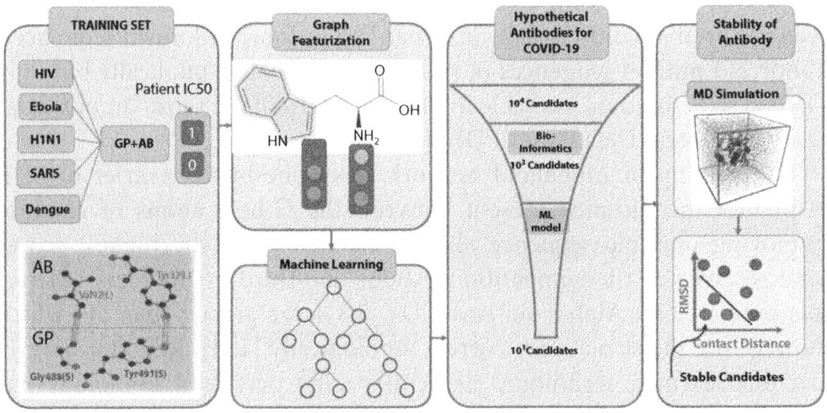

Figure 9.5 The process to design antibodies against SARS-CoV-2 using advanced techniques of machine learning (reprinted with permission under creative commons license from [138]).

Machine learning methods predict the interactions among amino acids, their characteristics, and beneficial mutants. A prognostic model of the protein built from the sequence and effectiveness of the mutants describes the characters of proteins after different mutations. The use of this technique improves the enantioselectivity of the epoxide hydrolase [140]. Due to immune responses, therapeutic proteins become unproductive. Without changing the structure and function of proteins, epitopes of T-cells are removed to reduce immunogenicity by different computational protein design processes [141]. Protein engineering optimizes protein functions. In a novel strategy, the functions of the protein are analyzed through sequence maps. These methods of machine learning significantly enhance mutations through directed evolution by knowledge of the characteristics of thus produced variants and their improved properties. Unknown functions of different proteins are also discovered [20].

"Loop walking method" is used to enhance protein thermostability. Different mutations are induced in 12 loops of *Burkholderia cepacia* lipase and on analysis it is discovered that loop 7 has a great effect on the thermostability of the protein. A model is built using data of different thermostable variants to check thermostability potentials. 20 combinations are studied out of 7786 combinations and just three mutants (P233D/L234P/V235S) have 66% action after heat processing for 30 min at 60°C which is greater than wild type variants [142]. Different factors like obesity, psychosocial stress, sleep habits, malnutrition, environmental toxins affect the host's susceptibility and immune responses on exposure to a viral pathogen (COVID-19). The machine learning methods help in predicting the person's risk of getting an infection and then advise to treat or prevent it [143]. Protein-protein interactions play an important role in cell functioning and also identify targets for drug discoveries. From experimentally obtained PPI data, PPI networks are built for new drug discoveries or PPIN-based biological research [144]. Bone morphogenetic protein-2 possesses two types of epitopes, conformational wrist epitopes, and linear knuckle epitopes. These epitopes interact with Type-I and Type-II receptors respectively. Through machine learning methods, knuckles peptides are redesigned to interact with receptor Type-II. 32 different knuckles derived peptides are formed that interact with type-II recombinant receptors with different affinities. Eight different peptides showing a high affinity for receptors are selected and their activity is analyzed by alkaline phosphatase assay for further working [145]. By using biological information and computing powers, scientists are continuously working to discover new non-natural allosteric drugs and cope with different challenges like the selection of ligands. For information recovery, different computational approaches like molecular docking and molecular dynamics work together [146]. During protein therapeutics development, protein aggregation is the most common challenge at all stages. Aggregation is predicted by different approaches or algorithms like SAP, CamSol, Solubis, Aggrescan3D, etc. Such studies help to enhance the solubility of proteins. These methods enable a researcher in the selection of proteins, save time and cost [147].

Besides making predictions about the structure of proteins, another area of active research is making predictions about catalytic sites. Computational methods for making predictions about the function of proteins range from gene to genome and from sequence to structure and those based on interactions [148]. To overcome the challenges associated with the functional annotation of enzymes, various initiatives, such as CAFA, COMBREX, and EFI, have been proposed. Machine learning has also been exploited for assigning EC numbers to enzymes based on purposed 3D structure [149]. Deep learning has also been used in predicting enzymes EC number based on the sequence of a protein by employing both features which depend upon the length of the sequences of proteins such as one-hot encoding and which do not depend on the length of the sequence of proteins such as encoding of the functional domain. Nonuniformity was introduced in the dimensions of features through the employment of features that rely upon sequence length. To address this issue, a framework was presented that can simultaneously select features, uniformization of dimensions, and classification of model training. To ensure the performance of this newly introduced framework, the activity of five isoforms of Aurora kinase B and three isoforms of glutamine was predicted. There was excellent correspondence with experimental data. Deep learning has been utilized for the engineering of enzymes and their catalytic site [137]. However, the main issue lies with enzyme activity profiles as the nomenclature is much complex and a large number of mechanisms are possible [3].

If machine learning is restricted to a specific enzyme family, then it is possible to predict the function of enzymes and for this training, available smaller data sets are used. However, this issue can be addressed through high throughput methods of data collection. Glycosyltransferase superfamily 1 was selected by authors [150] for analysis as this group of enzymes has a wide range of substrates. When this diversity was joined with scaffold conservations, the significance of background mutations increased many folds. Data of 54 enzymes and 91 substrates were derived from *Arabidopsis thaliana* from assay based on mass spectroscopy, and these data were utilized in functional prediction. Later on, various physiochemical properties such as molecular area, log P and type or number of various nucleophilic groups, decision trees based on sequence, and structural information like functional group and type of scaffold were trained. Then the predictor was tested on two enzyme families and four individual sequences of genes. It demonstrated the enormous potential associated with Machine Learning predictors on data acquired. However, prediction for other families by predictor from one family will also achieve the target needs to be demonstrated. eSol database has been exploited to ensemble all proteins of *E. coli* in predicting protein solubility [151]. Seven different continuous and binary algorithms which include Naive Bayes, decision tree, XGboost, logistic regression, conditional random forests, support vector machines, and artificial neural networks have been combined by Han and his colleagues [152] with the highest accuracy was represented by Support Vector Machines.

Attempts were made to generate a generative adversarial network, which was directed toward synthesizing more data. In this network, two neural networks work opposite to each other. One network generates artificial examples, and the second distinguishes them from real examples. But, the data of protein solubility was scarce, so the predictor could not be evaluated by designing some independent test and there is much need for more data. R^2 value was obtained around 0.4 which demonstrated much room in this area to design some reliable predictor. The prediction about protein solubility can also be made by seeing the effect of individual mutations. It is anticipated that the most complex predictors based on machine learning would be available to predict their solubility in the near future as remarkable work has been done and success achieved in collecting data about changes in solubility of proteins upon mutations through the exploitation of deep mutational scanning [153]. The substituting amino acid affects solubility, catalytic efficiency, stability, enantio-selectivity, and specificity of the substrate.

The issues, which were associated with ProTherm database, are addressed through the recent PON-tstab [154] database. Random forest classifier was presented by which undertook 1106 features for training from various groups such as coevolution and conservation scored for substituted or mutated positions, experimental conditions, the substitution of amino acids, and their physiochemical properties and thermodynamic features based on sequence and extracted through ProtDCal [155]. PON-tstab predictor is a good predictor of stability of proteins as it attained an accurate prediction ratio of about 0.5 compared to 0.33 which was achieved through some random predictor. So, it implies that predicting the stability of proteins is still a gruesome and challenging task [156]. Designing combinatorial libraries through machine learning for the directed evolution of proteins is another exciting application in protein engineering [157].

This is somewhat revolution as it has reduced the efforts significantly and in this case, multiple positions can be mutated simultaneously through which improvements were made in exploring sequence space. It can also help in further screening rounds through suggestions and the selection of a set of refined variants.

Table 9.2 Applications of machine learning in protein redesign.

Application of machine learning	Reference
Channel rhodopsin for efficient eukaryotic expression and plasma membrane localization	[15]
Channel rhodopsin for minimum invasive optogenetics	[16]
Directed evolution for protein engineering	[20]
Thermostability prediction for protein	[27]
Mutant fluorescent proteins	[41]
Neutralizing antibodies discovery for novel coronavirus	[138]
Mutant proteins from combinatorial libraries	[158]
Prediction of Protein Translational Modification Sites	[139]
Glycosyltransferase activity prediction	[150]
Protein solubility distribution of *Escherichia coli* proteins	[151]
Directed evolution of enantioselective enzymes	[140]
Protein-ligand binding affinity prediction	[135]
Removal of T-cell epitopes	[141]
Enhanced protein thermostability	[142]
Mutant serotonin sensor	[136]
Therapeutics for COVID-19 care	[143]
Prediction and redesign of protein-protein interactions	[144]
Mutant BMP-2 knuckle Epitope-Derived osteogenic peptides	[145]
Predicting activity of drugs	[146]
Improved solubility of proteins	[147]

Wu and his co-workers used direct evolution assisted by machine learning to engineer enzymes in forming a new carbon-silicon bond that was stereo-divergent [158]. For this reaction of ethyl 2-diazopropanote with phenyl-dimethyl silane was chosen with nitric oxide dioxygenase was used as a catalyst, and it was obtained from *Rhodothermus marinus.* A range of machine learning algorithms such as kernel and linear models, ensemble methods, and neural networks were tested. The starting S enantiomer was improved to a great degree. After a few rounds of evolution experiments guided by machine learning, a novel variant of the enzyme was discovered with high enzyme efficiency for R enantiomer. Two standard approaches for directed evolution were also compared and one was supported with shallow neural networks. A total of 149361 measurements which were published from a total of 160,000 variants by doing saturation mutagenesis at four positions of domain B1 of protein G were employed. Optimization was enhanced to two folds through machine learning methods as variant numbers were reduced by 30% through approaches guided by machine learning methods. Various applications of machine learning in protein redesign are depicted in Table 9.2.

9.11 Conclusion

Structure redesign is essential to augment the function of protein drugs. Several pharmaceutically significant proteins have been redesigned with improved functional activity. The primary sequence determines the structure and function of proteins. Techniques of machine learning enable us to predict the structures of novel proteins and assign functions to the protein through the prediction of interaction with other molecules. Methods of machine learning also allow us to redesign protein molecules with improved structure and functional performance by incorporating changes in the primary sequence and predicting sequence gaps and physical or chemical changes during the induction of mutations in proteins. Protein drug redesign through machine learning algorithms involves data mining, data labeling, classification of data into clusters extraction of features, and identification of hot spots, etc. The machine learning algorithms utilize principles of statistics to solve problems in multiple steps. Recently developed techniques in machine learning include neural networks, kernel method, Gaussian process, ensemble, deep learning, unsupervised, and supervised learning, etc. Current and future research canvas of protein drug redesign using machine learning is not only vast but versatile too and includes upgradation of grand processing units and servers, development of novel and efficient algorithms, and application of algorithms to improve the efficiency of pharmaceutically important proteins.

References

1. Huang, P.S., Boyken, S.E., Baker, D., The coming of age of *de novo* protein design. *Nature*, 537, 320, 2016.
2. Mitra, P., Shultis, D., Zhang, Y., EvoDesign: *De novo* protein design based on structural and evolutionary profiles. *Nucleic Acids Res.*, 41, W273, 2013.
3. Markwick, P.R.L., Malliavin, T., Nilges, M., Structural Biology by NMR: Structure, dynamics, and interactions. *PLoS Comput. Biol.*, 4, e1000168, 2008.
4. Jonic, S. and Vénien-Bryan, C., Protein structure determination by electron cryo-microscopy. *Curr. Opin. Pharmacol.*, 9, 636, 2009.
5. Slabinski, L., Jaroszewski, L., Rodrigues, A.P.C., Rychlewski, L., Wilson, I.A., Lesley, S.A., Godzik, A., The challenge of protein structure determination-lessons from structural genomics. *Protein Sci.*, 16, 2472, 2007.
6. Korendovych, I.V. and DeGrado, W.F., *De novo* protein design, a retrospective. *Q. Rev. Biophys.*, 53, e3, 2020.
7. Hollingsworth, S.A. and Dror, R.O., Molecular dynamics simulation for all. *Neuron*, 99, 1129, 2018.
8. Gao, W., Mahajan, S.P., Sulam, J., Gray, J.J., Deep learning in protein structural modeling and design. *Patterns*, 1, 100142, 2020.
9. Young, T., Hazarika, D., Poria, S., Cambria, E., Recent trends in deep learning based natural language processing. *IEEE Comput. Intell. Mag.*, 13, 55, 2018.
10. Guo, Y., Liu, Y., Oerlemans, A., Lao, S., Wu, S., Lew, M.S., Deep learning for visual understanding: A review. *Neurocomputing*, 187, 27, 2016.
11. Silver, D., Schrittwieser, J., Simonyan, K., Antonoglou, I., Huang, A., Guez, A., Hubert, T., Baker, L., Lai, M., Bolton, A., Chen, Y., Lillicrap, T., Hui, F., Sifre, L., van den Driessche, G., Graepel, T., Hassabis, D., Mastering the game of Go without human knowledge. *Nature*, 550, 354, 2017.
12. Senior, A.W., Evans, R., Jumper, J., Kirkpatrick, J., Sifre, L., Green, T., Qin, C., Žídek, A., Nelson, A.W.R., Bridgland, A., Penedones, H., Petersen, S., Simonyan, K., Crossan, S., Kohli, P., Jones, D.T., Silver, D., Kavukcuoglu, K., Hassabis, D., Protein structure prediction using multiple deep neural networks in the 13th Critical Assessment of Protein Structure Prediction (CASP13). *Proteins: Struct. Funct. Bioinform.*, 87, 1141, 2019.
13. Fox, R.J., Davis, S.C., Mundorff, E.C., Newman, L.M., Gavrilovic, V., Ma, S.K., Chung, L.M., Ching, C., Tam, S., Muley, S., Grate, J., Gruber, J., Whitman, J.C., Sheldon, R.A., Huisman, G.W., Improving catalytic function by ProSAR-driven enzyme evolution. *Nat. Biotechnol.*, 25, 338, 2007.

14. Romero, P.A., Krause, A., Arnold, F.H., Navigating the protein fitness landscape with Gaussian processes. *Proc. Natl. Acad. Sci.*, 110, E193, 2012.
15. Bedbrook, C.N., Yang, K.K., Rice, A.J., Gradinaru, V., Arnold, F.H., Machine learning to design integral membrane channelrhodopsins for efficient eukaryotic expression and plasma membrane localization. *PLoS Comput. Biol.*, 13, e1005786, 2017.
16. Bedbrook, C.N., Yang, K.K., Robinson, J.E., Mackey, E.D., Gradinaru, V., Arnold, F.H., Machine learning-guided channelrhodopsin engineering enables minimally invasive optogenetics. *Nat. Methods*, 16, 1176, 2019.
17. Liao, J., Warmuth, M.K., Govindarajan, S., Ness, J.E., Wang, R.P., Gustafsson, C., Minshull, J., Engineering proteinase K using machine learning and synthetic genes. *BMC Biotechnol.*, 7, 6750, 2007.
18. Govindarajan, S., Mannervik, B., Silverman, J.A., Wright, K., Regitsky, D., Hegazy, U., Purcell, T.J., Welch, M., Minshull, J., Gustafsson, C., Mapping of amino acid substitutions conferring herbicide resistance in wheat glutathione transferase. *ACS Synth. Biol.*, 4, 221, 2014.
19. Musdal, Y., Govindarajan, S., Mannervik, B., Exploring sequence-function space of a poplar glutathione transferase using designed information-rich gene variants. *Protein Eng. Des. Sel.*, 30, 543, 2017.
20. Yang, K.K., Wu, Z., Arnold, F.H., Machine-learning-guided directed evolution for protein engineering. *Nat. Methods*, 16, 687, 2019.
21. Yu, C.H., Qin, Z., Martin-Martinez, F.J., Buehler, M.J., A Self-consistent sonification method to translate amino acid sequences into musical compositions and application in protein design using artificial intelligence. *ACS Nano*, 13, 7471, 2019.
22. Wolpert, D.H., The lack of a priori distinctions between learning algorithms. *Neural Comput.*, 8, 1341, 1996.
23. Li, Y., Drummond, D.A., Sawayama, A.M., Snow, C.D., Bloom, J.D., Arnold, F.H., A diverse family of thermostable cytochrome P450s created by recombination of stabilizing fragments. *Nat. Biotechnol.*, 25, 1051, 2007.
24. Friedman, J.H., Stochastic gradient boosting. *Comput. Stat. Data Anal.*, 38, 367, 2002.
25. Tian, J., Wu, N., Chu, X., Fan, Y., Predicting changes in protein thermostability brought about by single- or multi-site mutations. *BMC Bioinf.*, 11, 370, 2010.
26. Li, Y. and Fang, J., PROTS-RF: A robust model for predicting mutation-induced protein stability changes. *PLoS One*, 7, e47247, 2012.
27. Jia, L., Yarlagadda, R., Reed, C.C., Structure based thermostability prediction models for protein single point mutations with machine learning tools. *PLoS One*, 10, e0138022, 2015.
28. Nadaraya, E.A., On estimating regression. *Theory Probab. Its Appl.*, 9, 141, 1964.
29. Dietrich, R., Opper, M., Sompolinsky, H., Statistical mechanics of support vector networks. *Phys. Rev. Lett.*, 82, 2975, 1999.

30. Leslie, C., Eskin, E., Noble, W.S., The spectrum kernel: A string kernel for svm protein classification, in: *Pacific Symposium on Biocomputing 2002*, Hawaii, World scientific, pp. 564–575, 2001.
31. Leslie, C.S., Eskin, E., Cohen, A., Weston, J., Noble, W.S., Mismatch string kernels for discriminative protein classification. *Bioinformatics*, 20, 467, 2004.
32. Jokinen, E., Heinonen, M., Lähdesmäki, H., mGPfusion: Predicting protein stability changes with Gaussian process kernel learning and data fusion. *Bioinformatics*, 34, i274, 2018.
33. Capriotti, E., Fariselli, P., Casadio, R., I-Mutant2.0: Predicting stability changes upon mutation from the protein sequence or structure. *Nucleic Acids Res.*, 33, W306, 2005.
34. Cheng, J., Randall, A., Baldi, P., Prediction of protein stability changes for single-site mutations using support vector machines. *Proteins: Struct. Funct. Bioinf.*, 62, 1125, 2005.
35. Buske, F.A., Their, R., Gillam, E.M.J., Bodén, M., *In silico* characterization of protein chimeras: Relating sequence and function within the same fold. *Proteins: Struct. Funct. Bioinf.*, 77, 111, 2009.
36. Liu, J. and Kang, X., Grading amino acid properties increased accuracies of single point mutation on protein stability prediction. *BMC Bioinf.*, 13, 44, 2012.
37. Quinonero-Candela, J., Rasmussen, C.E., Williams, C.K., Approximation methods for gaussian process regression, in: *Large-Scale Kernel Machines*, L. Bottou, *et al.* (Eds.), pp. 203–223, The MIT Press, US, 2007.
38. Wilson, A. and Nickisch, H., Kernel interpolation for scalable structured Gaussian processes (KISS-GP). *PMLR*, pp. 1775–1784, 2015.
39. Wang, K., Pleiss, G., Gardner, J., Tyree, S., Weinberger, K.Q., Wilson, A.G., Exact Gaussian processes on a million data points. *Adv. Neural Inf. Process. Syst.*, 32, 14648, 2019.
40. Yang, K.K., Wu, Z., Bedbrook, C.N., Arnold, F.H., Learned protein embeddings for machine learning. *Bioinformatics*, 34, 2642, 2018.
41. Saito, Y., Oikawa, M., Nakazawa, H., Niide, T., Kameda, T., Tsuda, K., Umetsu, M., Machine-learning-guided mutagenesis for directed evolution of fluorescent proteins. *ACS Synth. Biol.*, 7, 2014, 2018.
42. Pires, D.E.V., Ascher, D.B., Blundell, T.L., mCSM: Predicting the effects of mutations in proteins using graph-based signatures. *Bioinformatics*, 30, 335, 2013.
43. Jiménez, J., Doerr, S., Martínez-Rosell, G., Rose, A.S., De Fabritiis, G., DeepSite: Protein-binding site predictor using 3D-convolutional neural networks. *Bioinformatics*, 33, 3036, 2017.
44. Alipanahi, B., Delong, A., Weirauch, M.T., Frey, B.J., Predicting the sequence specificities of DNA- and RNA-binding proteins by deep learning. *Nat. Biotechnol.*, 33, 831, 2015.

45. Panda, B., Majhi, B., A novel improved prediction of protein structural class using deep recurrent neural network. Evol. Intel., 14, 253, 2021.
46. Giollo, M., Martin, A.J.M., Walsh, I., Ferrari, C., Tosatto, S.C.E., NeEMO: A method using residue interaction networks to improve prediction of protein stability upon mutation. *BMC Genomics*, 15, s7, 2014.
47. Khurana, S., Rawi, R., Kunji, K., Chuang, G.-Y., Bensmail, H., Mall, R., DeepSol: A deep learning framework for sequence-based protein solubility prediction. *Bioinformatics*, 34, 2605, 2018.
48. Snoek, J., Larochelle, H., Adams, R.P., Practical bayesian optimization of machine learning algorithms. *Adv. Neural Inf. Process. Syst.*, 25, 12062944, 2012.
49. Bengio, Y., Courville, A., Vincent, P., Representation learning: A review and new perspectives. *IEEE Trans. Pattern Anal. Mach. Intell.*, 35, 1798, 2013.
50. Domingos, P., A few useful things to know about machine learning. *Commun. ACM*, 55, 78, 2012.
51. Ofer, D. and Linial, M., ProFET: Feature engineering captures high-level protein functions. *Bioinformatics*, 31, 3429, 2015.
52. Kawashima, S., Pokarowski, P., Pokarowska, M., Kolinski, A., Katayama, T., Kanehisa, M., AAindex: Amino acid index database, progress report 2008. *Nucleic Acids Res.*, 36, D202, 2007.
53. Barley, M.H., Turner, N.J., Goodacre, R., Improved descriptors for the quantitative structure–activity relationship modeling of peptides and proteins. *J. Chem. Inf. Model.*, 58, 234, 2018.
54. Qiu, J., Hue, M., Ben-Hur, A., Vert, J.P., Noble, W.S., A structural alignment kernel for protein structures. *Bioinformatics*, 23, 1090, 2007.
55. Henikoff, S. and Henikoff, J.G., Amino acid substitution matrices from protein blocks. *Proc. Natl. Acad. Sci.*, 89, 10915, 1992.
56. Alley, E.C., Khimulya, G., Biswas, S., AlQuraishi, M., Church, G.M., Unified rational protein engineering with sequence-based deep representation learning. *Nat. Methods*, 16, 1315, 2019.
57. Kortemme, T., Kim, D.E., Baker, D., Computational alanine scanning of protein-protein interfaces. *Sci. Signaling*, 2004, pl2, 2004.
58. Tuncbag, N., Gursoy, A., Keskin, O., Identification of computational hot spots in protein interfaces: Combining solvent accessibility and inter-residue potentials improves the accuracy. *Bioinformatics*, 25, 1513, 2009.
59. Tuncbag, N., Keskin, O., Gursoy, A., HotPoint: Hot spot prediction server for protein interfaces. *Nucleic Acids Res.*, 38, W402, 2010.
60. Lise, S., Archambeau, C., Pontil, M., Jones, D.T., Prediction of hot spot residues at protein-protein interfaces by combining machine learning and energy-based methods. *BMC Bioinf.*, 10, 365, 2009.
61. Lise, S., Buchan, D., Pontil, M., Jones, D.T., Predictions of hot spot residues at protein-protein interfaces using support vector machines. *PLoS One*, 6, e16774, 2011.

62. Liang, S. and Grishin, N.V., Effective scoring function for protein sequence design. *Proteins: Struct. Funct. Bioinf.*, 54, 271, 2003.
63. Liang, S., Meroueh, S.O., Wang, G., Qiu, C., Zhou, Y., Consensus scoring for enriching near-native structures from protein-protein docking decoys. *Proteins: Struct. Funct. Bioinf.*, 75, 397, 2009.
64. Deng, L., Guan, J., Wei, X., Yi, Y., Zhang, Q.C., Zhou, S., Boosting prediction performance of protein–protein interaction hot spots by using structural neighborhood properties. *J. Comput. Biol.*, 20, 878, 2013.
65. Liu, S., Liu, C., Deng, L., Machine learning approaches for protein–protein interaction hot spot prediction: Progress and comparative assessment. *Molecules*, 23, 2535, 2018.
66. Lee, B. and Richards, F.M., The interpretation of protein structures: Estimation of static accessibility. *J. Mol. Biol.*, 55, 379, 1971.
67. Joosten, R.P., te Beek, T.A.H., Krieger, E., Hekkelman, M.L., Hooft, R.W.W., Schneider, R., Sander, C., Vriend, G., A series of PDB related databases for everyday needs. *Nucleic Acids Res.*, 39, D411, 2010.
68. Deng, L., Guan, J., Dong, Q., Zhou, S., Prediction of protein-protein interaction sites using an ensemble method. *BMC Bioinf.*, 10, 426, 2009.
69. Xia, J.-F., Zhao, X.-M., Song, J., Huang, D.-S., APIS: Accurate prediction of hot spots in protein interfaces by combining protrusion index with solvent accessibility. *BMC Bioinf.*, 11, 174, 2010.
70. Cho, K.-i., Kim, D., Lee, D., A feature-based approach to modeling protein–protein interaction hot spots. *Nucleic Acids Res.*, 37, 2672, 2009.
71. Darnell, S.J., Page, D., Mitchell, J.C., An automated decision-tree approach to predicting protein interaction hot spots. *Proteins: Struct. Funct. Bioinf.*, 68, 813, 2007.
72. Keskin, O., Ma, B., Nussinov, R., Hot regions in protein–protein interactions: The organization and contribution of structurally conserved hot spot residues. *J. Mol. Biol.*, 345, 1281, 2005.
73. Lee, D.T. and Schachter, B.J., Two algorithms for constructing a Delaunay triangulation. *Int. J. Comput. Inf. Sci.*, 9, 219, 1980.
74. Saeys, Y., Inza, I., Larranaga, P., A review of feature selection techniques in bioinformatics. *Bioinformatics*, 23, 2507, 2007.
75. Zou, Q., Zeng, J., Cao, L., Ji, R., A novel features ranking metric with application to scalable visual and bioinformatics data classification. *Neurocomputing*, 173, 346, 2016.
76. Guyon, I., Weston, J., Barnhill, S., Vapnik, V., Gene selection for cancer classification using support vector machines. *Mach. Learn.*, 46, 389, 2002.
77. Chen, Y.-W. and Lin, C.-J., Combining SVMs with various feature selection strategies, in: *Feature Extraction*, I. Guyon, *et al.* (Eds.), pp. 315–324, Springer, Berlin Heidelberg, 2006.

78. Moreira, I.S., Koukos, P.I., Melo, R., Almeida, J.G., Preto, A.J., Schaarschmidt, J., Trellet, M., Gümüş, Z.H., Costa, J., Bonvin, A.M.J.J., SpotOn: High accuracy identification of protein-protein interface hot-spots. *Sci. Rep.*, 7, 8007, 2017.
79. Wang, L., Zhang, W., Gao, Q., Xiong, C., Prediction of hot spots in protein interfaces using extreme learning machines with the information of spatial neighbour residues. *IET Syst. Biol.*, 8, 184, 2014.
80. Qiao, Y., Xiong, Y., Gao, H., Zhu, X., Chen, P., Protein-protein interface hot spots prediction based on a hybrid feature selection strategy. *BMC Bioinf.*, 19, 14, 2018.
81. Jia, C., Zuo, Y., Zou, Q., O-GlcNAcPRED-II: An integrated classification algorithm for identifying O-GlcNAcylation sites based on fuzzy undersampling and a K-means PCA oversampling technique. *Bioinformatics*, 34, 2029, 2018.
82. Liang, Y.Z., Kvalheim, O.M., Keller, H.R., Massart, D.L., Kiechle, P., Erni, F., Heuristic evolving latent projections: Resolving two-way multicomponent data. 2. Detection and resolution of minor constituents. *Anal. Chem.*, 64, 946, 1992.
83. Du, L., Meng, Q., Jiang, H., Li, Y., Using evolutionary information and multi-label linear discriminant analysis to predict the subcellular location of multi-site bacterial proteins via Chou's 5-steps rule. *IEEE Access*, 8, 56452, 2020.
84. Melo, R., Fieldhouse, R., Melo, A., Correia, J., Cordeiro, M., Gümüş, Z., Costa, J., Bonvin, A., Moreira, I., A Machine learning approach for hot-spot detection at protein-protein interfaces. *Int. J. Mol. Sci.*, 17, 1215, 2016.
85. Nerenberg, P.S. and Head-Gordon, T., New developments in force fields for biomolecular simulations. *Curr. Opin. Struct. Biol.*, 49, 129, 2018.
86. Derevyanko, G., Grudinin, S., Bengio, Y., Lamoureux, G., Deep convolutional networks for quality assessment of protein folds. *Bioinformatics*, 34, 4046, 2018.
87. Alford, R.F., Leaver-Fay, A., Jeliazkov, J.R., O'Meara, M.J., DiMaio, F.P., Park, H., Shapovalov, M.V., Renfrew, P.D., Mulligan, V.K., Kappel, K., Labonte, J.W., Pacella, M.S., Bonneau, R., Bradley, P., Dunbrack, R.L., Das, R., Baker, D., Kuhlman, B., Kortemme, T., Gray, J.J., The rosetta all-atom energy function for macromolecular modeling and design. *J. Chem. Theory Comput.*, 13, 3031, 2017.
88. Best, R.B., Zhu, X., Shim, J., Lopes, P.E.M., Mittal, J., Feig, M., MacKerell, A.D., Optimization of the additive CHARMM all-atom protein force field targeting improved sampling of the backbone ϕ, ψ and side-chain $\chi1$ and $\chi2$ dihedral angles. *J. Chem. Theory Comput.*, 8, 3257, 2012.
89. Weiner, S.J., Kollman, P.A., Case, D.A., Singh, U.C., Ghio, C., Alagona, G., Profeta, S., Weiner, P., A new force field for molecular mechanical simulation of nucleic acids and proteins. *J. Am. Chem. Soc.*, 106, 765, 1984.

90. Behler, J. and Parrinello, M., Generalized neural-network representation of high-dimensional potential-energy surfaces. *Phys. Rev. Lett.*, 98, 146401, 2007.
91. Smith, J.S., Isayev, O., Roitberg, A.E., ANI-1: An extensible neural network potential with DFT accuracy at force field computational cost. *Chem. Sci.*, 8, 3192, 2017.
92. Smith, J.S., Nebgen, B., Lubbers, N., Isayev, O., Roitberg, A.E., Less is more: Sampling chemical space with active learning. *J. Chem. Phys.*, 148, 241733, 2018.
93. Schütt, K.T., Arbabzadah, F., Chmiela, S., Müller, K.R., Tkatchenko, A., Quantum-chemical insights from deep tensor neural networks. *Nat. Commun.*, 8, 13890, 2017.
94. Schütt, K.T., Sauceda, H.E., Kindermans, P.J., Tkatchenko, A., Müller, K.R., SchNet – A deep learning architecture for molecules and materials. *J. Chem. Phys.*, 148, 241722, 2018.
95. Noé, F., Tkatchenko, A., Müller, K.-R., Clementi, C., Machine Learning for Molecular Simulation. *Annu. Rev. Phys. Chem.*, 71, 361, 2020.
96. Zhang, L., Han, J., Wang, H., Car, R., E, W., Deep potential molecular dynamics: A scalable model with the accuracy of quantum mechanics. *Phys. Rev. Lett.*, 120, 143001, 2018.
97. Zubatyuk, R., Smith, J.S., Leszczynski, J., Isayev, O., Accurate and transferable multitask prediction of chemical properties with an atoms-in-molecules neural network. *Sci. Adv.*, 5, eaav6490, 2019.
98. Senn, H.M. and Thiel, W., QM/MM methods for biomolecular systems. *Angew. Chem. Int. Ed.*, 48, 1198, 2009.
99. Wang, Z., Han, Y., Li, J., He, X., Combining the fragmentation approach and neural network potential energy surfaces of fragments for accurate calculation of protein energy. *J. Phys. Chem. B*, 124, 3027, 2020.
100. Lahey, S.-L.J. and Rowley, C.N., Simulating protein–ligand binding with neural network potentials. *Chem. Sci.*, 11, 2362, 2020.
101. Cover, T. and Hart, P., Nearest neighbor pattern classification. *IEEE Trans. Inf. Theory*, 13, 21, 1967.
102. Yao, X., Evolving artificial neural networks. *Proc. IEEE*, 87, 1423, 1999.
103. Wan, S., Duan, Y., Zou, Q., HPSLPred: An ensemble multi-label classifier for human protein subcellular location prediction with imbalanced source. *Proteomics*, 17, 1700262, 2017.
104. Friedman, N., Geiger, D., Goldszmidt, M., Bayesian network classifiers. *Mach. Learn.*, 29, 131, 1997.
105. Xia, J., Yue, Z., Di, Y., Zhu, X., Zheng, C.-H., Predicting hot spots in protein interfaces based on protrusion index, pseudo hydrophobicity and electron-ion interaction pseudopotential features. *Oncotarget*, 7, 18065, 2016.
106. Ye, L., Kuang, Q., Jiang, L., Luo, J., Jiang, Y., Ding, Z., Li, Y., Li, M., Prediction of hot spots residues in protein–protein interface using network feature and microenvironment feature. *Chemometr. Intell. Lab. Syst.*, 131, 16, 2014.

107. Zhu, X. and Mitchell, J.C., KFC2: A knowledge-based hot spot prediction method based on interface solvation, atomic density, and plasticity features. *Proteins: Struct. Funct. Bioinf.*, 79, 2671, 2011.
108. Hu, S.-S., Chen, P., Wang, B., Li, J., Protein binding hot spots prediction from sequence only by a new ensemble learning method. *Amino Acids*, 49, 1773, 2017.
109. Jiang, J., Wang, N., Chen, P., Zheng, C., Wang, B., Prediction of protein hotspots from whole protein sequences by a random projection ensemble system. *Int. J. Mol. Sci.*, 18, 1543, 2017.
110. Ofran, Y. and Rost, B., Protein–protein interaction hotspots carved into sequences. *PLoS Comput. Biol.*, 3, e119, 2007.
111. Andersen, S.K., Probabilistic reasoning in intelligent systems: Networks of plausible inference. *Artif. Intell.*, 48, 117, 1991.
112. Domingos, P. and Pazzani, M., On the optimality of the simple Bayesian classifier under zero-one loss. *Mach. Learn.*, 29, 103, 1997.
113. Assi, S.A., Tanaka, T., Rabbitts, T.H., Fernandez-Fuentes, N., PCRPi: Presaging critical residues in protein interfaces, a new computational tool to chart hot spots in protein interfaces. *Nucleic Acids Res.*, 38, e86, 2009.
114. Freund, Y. and Schapire, R.E., A decision-theoretic generalization of on-line learning and an application to boosting. *J. Comput. Syst. Sci.*, 55, 119, 1997.
115. Liaw, A. and Wiener, M., Classification and regression by randomForest. *R News*, 2, 18, 2002.
116. Chen, T. and Guestrin, C., XGBoost: A scalable tree boosting system, in: *Proceedings of the 22nd ACM SIGKDD International Conference on Knowledge Discovery and Data Mining*, San Francisco, California, USA, ACM, pp. 785–794, 2016.
117. Friedman, J.H., Greedy function approximation: A gradient boosting machine. *Ann. Stat.*, 29, 1189, 2001.
118. Wang, L., Liu, Z.P., Zhang, X.S., Chen, L., Prediction of hot spots in protein interfaces using a random forest model with hybrid features. *Protein Eng. Des. Sel.*, 25, 119, 2012.
119. Huang, Q. and Zhang, X., An improved ensemble learning method with SMOTE for protein interaction hot spots prediction, in: *IEEE International Conference on Bioinformatics and Biomedicine*, IEEE, p. 1584, 2016.
120. Chawla, N.V., Bowyer, K.W., Hall, L.O., Kegelmeyer, W.P., SMOTE: Synthetic minority over-sampling technique. *J. Artif. Intell. Res.*, 16, 321, 2002.
121. Breiman, L., Bagging predictors. *Mach. Learn.*, 24, 123, 1996.
122. Błaszczyński, J. and Stefanowski, J., Neighbourhood sampling in bagging for imbalanced data. *Neurocomputing*, 150, 529, 2015.
123. Breiman, L., Random forests. *Mach. Learn.*, 45, 5, 2001.
124. Wolpert, D.H., Stacked generalization. *Neural Netw.*, 5, 241, 1992.
125. Liu, Y. and Yao, X., Ensemble learning via negative correlation. *Neural Netw.*, 12, 1399, 1999.

126. Srivastava, N., Hinton, G., Krizhevsky, A., Sutskever, I., Salakhutdinov, R., Dropout: A simple way to prevent neural networks from overfitting. *J. Mach. Learn. Res.*, 15, 1929, 2014.
127. Li, W., Ding, S., Chen, Y., Yang, S., Heterogeneous ensemble for default prediction of peer-to-peer lending in China. *IEEE Access*, 6, 54396, 2018.
128. van der Laan, M.J., Polley, E.C., Hubbard, A.E., Super learner. *Stat. Appl. Genet. Mol. Biol.*, 6, 25, 2007.
129. Zhou, Z.-H. and Tang, W., Clusterer ensemble. *Knowl.-Based Syst.*, 19, 77, 2006.
130. Thomas, P., Semi-supervised learning by Olivier Chapelle, Bernhard Schölkopf, and Alexander Zien (Review). *IEEE Trans. Neural Networks*, 20, 542, 2009.
131. Wang, J., Cao, H., Zhang, J.Z.H., Qi, Y., Computational protein design with deep learning neural networks. *Sci. Rep.*, 8, 6349, 2018.
132. UniProt, C., UniProt: A worldwide hub of protein knowledge. *Nucleic Acids Res.*, 47, D506, 2019.
133. Evans, R., Jumper, J., Kirkpatrick, J., Sifre, L., Green, T., Qin, C., Zidek, A., Nelson, A., Bridgland, A., Penedones, H., *De novo* structure prediction with deeplearning based scoring. *Annu. Rev. Biochem.*, 77, 363, 2018.
134. Kinch, L.N., Shi, S., Cheng, H., Cong, Q., Pei, J., Mariani, V., Schwede, T., Grishin, N.V., CASP9 target classification. *Proteins: Struct. Funct. Bioinf.*, 79, 21, 2011.
135. Cang, Z. and Wei, G.W., Integration of element specific persistent homology and machine learning for protein-ligand binding affinity prediction. *Int. J. Numer. Method. Biomed. Eng.*, 34, e2914, 2018.
136. Unger, E.K., Keller, J.P., Altermatt, M., Liang, R., Matsui, A., Dong, C., Hon, O.J., Yao, Z., Sun, J., Banala, S., Flanigan, M.E., Jaffe, D.A., Hartanto, S., Carlen, J., Mizuno, G.O., Borden, P.M., Shivange, A.V., Cameron, L.P., Sinning, S., Underhill, S.M., Olson, D.E., Amara, S.G., Temple Lang, D., Rudnick, G., Marvin, J.S., Lavis, L.D., Lester, H.A., Alvarez, V.A., Fisher, A.J., Prescher, J.A., Kash, T.L., Yarov-Yarovoy, V., Gradinaru, V., Looger, L.L., Tian, L., Directed evolution of a selective and sensitive serotonin sensor via machine learning. *Cell*, 183, 1986, 2020.
137. Mazurenko, S., Prokop, Z., Damborsky, J., Machine learning in enzyme engineering. *ACS Catal.*, 10, 1210, 2019.
138. Magar, R., Yadav, P., Barati Farimani, A., Potential neutralizing antibodies discovered for novel corona virus using machine learning. *Sci. Rep.*, 11, 5261, 2021.
139. Bao, W., Yuan, C.-A., Zhang, Y., Han, K., Nandi, A.K., Honig, B., Huang, D.-S., Mutli-features prediction of protein translational modification sites. *IEEE/ACM Trans. Comput. Biol. Bioinform.*, 15, 1453, 2018.
140. Cadet, F., Fontaine, N., Li, G., Sanchis, J., Ng Fuk Chong, M., Pandjaitan, R., Vetrivel, I., Offmann, B., Reetz, M.T., A machine learning approach

for reliable prediction of amino acid interactions and its application in the directed evolution of enantioselective enzymes. *Sci. Rep.*, 8, 16757, 2018.

141. King, C., Garza, E.N., Mazor, R., Linehan, J.L., Pastan, I., Pepper, M., Baker, D., Removing T-cell epitopes with computational protein design. *PNAS*, 111, 8577, 2014.
142. Yoshida, K., Kawai, S., Fujitani, M., Koikeda, S., Kato, R., Ema, T., Enhancement of protein thermostability by three consecutive mutations using loop-walking method and machine learning. *Sci. Rep.*, 11, 11883, 2021.
143. Halamka, J., Cerrato, P., Perlman, A., Redesigning COVID-19 care with network medicine and machine learning. *Mayo Clin. Proc.: Innov. Qual. Outcomes*, 4, 725, 2020.
144. Lua, R.C., Marciano, D.C., Katsonis, P., Adikesavan, A.K., Wilkins, A.D., Lichtarge, O., Prediction and redesign of protein–protein interactions. *Prog. Biophys. Mol. Biol.*, 116, 194, 2014.
145. Zhang, W., Liu, J., Shan, H., Yin, F., Zhong, B., Zhang, C., Yu, X., Machine learning-guided evolution of BMP-2 knuckle epitope-derived osteogenic peptides to target BMP receptor II. *J. Drug Targeting*, 28, 802, 2020.
146. Marchetti, F., Moroni, E., Pandini, A., Colombo, G., Machine learning prediction of allosteric drug activity from molecular dynamics. *J. Phys. Chem. Lett.*, 12, 3724, 2021.
147. Navarro, S. and Ventura, S., Computational re-design of protein structures to improve solubility. *Expert Opin. Drug Discovery*, 14, 1077, 2019.
148. Shehu, A., Barbará, D., Molloy, K., A survey of computational methods for protein function prediction, in: *Big Data Analytics in Genomics*, pp. 225–298, Springer International Publishing, Switzerland, 2016.
149. Zhang, C., Freddolino, P.L., Zhang, Y., COFACTOR: Improved protein function prediction by combining structure, sequence and protein–protein interaction information. *Nucleic Acids Res.*, 45, W291, 2017.
150. Yang, M., Fehl, C., Lees, K.V., Lim, E.-K., Offen, W.A., Davies, G.J., Bowles, D.J., Davidson, M.G., Roberts, S.J., Davis, B.G., Functional and informatics analysis enables glycosyltransferase activity prediction. *Nat. Chem. Biol.*, 14, 1109, 2018.
151. Niwa, T., Ying, B.W., Saito, K., Jin, W., Takada, S., Ueda, T., Taguchi, H., Bimodal protein solubility distribution revealed by an aggregation analysis of the entire ensemble of Escherichia coli proteins. *Proc. Natl. Acad. Sci.*, 106, 4201, 2009.
152. Han, X., Wang, X., Zhou, K., Develop machine learning-based regression predictive models for engineering protein solubility. *Bioinformatics*, 35, 4640, 2019.
153. Klesmith, J.R., Bacik, J.-P., Wrenbeck, E.E., Michalczyk, R., Whitehead, T.A., Trade-offs between enzyme fitness and solubility illuminated by deep mutational scanning. *Proc. Natl. Acad. Sci.*, 114, 2265, 2017.

154. Yang, Y., Urolagin, S., Niroula, A., Ding, X., Shen, B., Vihinen, M., PON-tstab: Protein variant stability predictor. Importance of training data quality. *Int. J. Mol. Sci.*, 19, 1009, 2018.
155. Ruiz-Blanco, Y.B., Paz, W., Green, J., Marrero-Ponce, Y., ProtDCal: A program to compute general-purpose-numerical descriptors for sequences and 3D-structures of proteins. *BMC Bioinf.*, 16, 162, 2015.
156. Musil, M., Konegger, H., Hon, J., Bednar, D., Damborsky, J., Computational design of stable and soluble biocatalysts. *ACS Catal.*, 9, 1033, 2018.
157. Li, G., Dong, Y., Reetz, M.T., Can machine learning revolutionize directed evolution of selective enzymes? *Adv. Synth. Catal.*, 361, 2377, 2019.
158. Wu, Z., Kan, S.B.J., Lewis, R.D., Wittmann, B.J., Arnold, F.H., Machine learning-assisted directed protein evolution with combinatorial libraries. *Proc. Natl. Acad. Sci.*, 116, 8852, 2019.

10

Role of Transcriptomics and Artificial Intelligence Approaches for the Selection of Bioactive Compounds

Roshan Zameer[1], Sana Tariq[1], Sana Noreen[2], Muhammad Sadaqat[1] and Farrukh Azeem[1]*

[1]Department of Bioinformatics and Biotechnology, GC University, Faisalabad, Pakistan
[2]Department of Microbiology, GC University, Faisalabad, Pakistan

Abstract
Transcriptomics and artificial intelligence (AI) approaches are used to identify bioactive compounds. Bioactive compounds are classified as flavonoids, isoprenoids, polyketides, and alkaloids, and they are chemically diverse. The demand for bioactive compounds is rapidly increasing due to their use in disease prevention and health improvement through medicines and diet. Moreover, bioactive compounds are intensively used to produce nutraceuticals, functional foods, agrochemicals, and cosmetics. Previously, transcriptome analysis has been applied to various species of plants. In distinct metabolic pathways, transcriptomic analysis identified the functional potential of genes and transcripts associated with the biosynthesis of bioactive substances. The AI study involves whole process and performs intelligent task skillfully with machines. Recently, AI surpassed or neared human-like image recognition and game playing in several tasks. So, with the help of artificial intelligence, the selection of bioactive compounds is easier. It takes less time, and results are valuable. In the future, physicians would become more dependent on AI techniques for clinical practice. In this context, the combination of humans and AI is expected to achieve a maximum potential of effectively selecting bioactive compounds for drug designing.

Keywords: Flavonoids, microarray, RNA-seq, machine learning, deep learning

**Corresponding author*: azeuaf@hotmail.com

Inamuddin, Tariq Altalhi, Jorddy N. Cruz and Moamen Salah El-Deen Refat (eds.) Drug Design Using Machine Learning, (283–318) © 2022 Scrivener Publishing LLC

10.1 Introduction

Secondary metabolites produced by natural bioactive compounds contain an excellent pool of molecules. For living organisms, primary metabolites (i.e., proteins, sugar, amino acids) are essential compared to secondary metabolites [1]. Natural bioactive compounds can be obtained by different extraction or separation methods from several living organisms like plants, fruit, fungi, microbes, and algae [2]. In plants, bioactive compounds are abundant and chemically diverse. These bioactive compounds can be categorized as alkaloids, polyketides, isoprenoids, flavonoids, or phenylpropanoids. These compounds are essential for different mechanisms such as natural defense and stress response mechanisms [3]. In recent years, the demand for bioactive compounds is rapidly increased due to their use in disease prevention and health improvement through diet [4]. To date, natural bioactive compounds produced 60% of approved anticancer drugs and are used in the pharmaceutical industry [5]. Moreover, they are intensively used to produce nutraceuticals, functional food, agrochemicals, and cosmetics [6].

Previously transcriptome research has been applied to various species of plants. Transcriptomic approaches revealed the functional putative genes and transcripts entangled in the biogenesis of bioactive compounds under different metabolic mechanisms [7]. It also elucidates the function of a particular gene. This approach can be made through various methods. In *Physalis angulate*, transcriptome analysis discovers the accumulation pattern of flavonoids under methyl-jasmonate (MeJA) treatment that elucidates the novel gene function for medicinal use [8]. Whereas, artificial intelligence (AI) study the whole process and trained the machines to perform intelligent task skillfully. Recently, AI in several tasks surpassed or neared human-like image recognition and game playing [9]. This method designs the new drug with the desired character through computational approaches. For example, *de novo* designs selected bioactive compounds for future medicinal chemistry [10]. Additionally, it also broadens the application of several computer-assisted discoveries like chemical synthesis planning, identification of the macromolecular target, protein structure prediction, and molecular design [11].

Bioactive compounds show many biological properties such as antimicrobial, anti-inflammatory, anti-plasmodial, anticancer, and antioxidant [12]. So, several attempts have been made through experimental approaches, but their medicinal and pharmacological regulation is made problematic due to variability in chemicals [13]. *In silico* approaches give quick and accurate results by selecting the appropriate bioactive compound for agrochemicals, food additives, and the pharmaceutical industry. This chapter will focus on the types of bioactive compounds, how they are selected through computational approaches and their application.

10.2 Types of Bioactive Compounds

Plants are a rich reservoir of bioactive compounds and promote human health [14]. Plants contain many various varieties of bioactive compounds.

10.2.1 Phenolic Acids

Phenolic (C6-C3) are nonflavonoid compounds and also known for the heterogeneous class of phytochemicals. This dietary compound is divided into two groups: derivatives of hydroxycinnamic acid and derivatives of hydroxybenzoic acid. Hydroxycinnamic acid (i.e., ferulic, caffeic, sinapic, or p-coumaric acid) is hardly present in free form, whereas it is esterified with carbohydrates and tartaric and quinic acid derivatives. It is rarely found in vegetables like eggplant. In esterified form, they are absorbed by the small intestine and digested by the colon. In food, hydroxybenzoic acid is present in a small concentration. The content of ellagic, 4-hydroxybenzoic acid, gallic and protocatechuic acid is probably higher in onion, black/reddish potatoes, and red fruits. Gallic acid is absorbed in both small intestine and stomach [15, 16].

10.2.2 Stilbenes

Stilbenes occur in low quantity in plants, but the presence of resveratrol increases its bioavailability. Resveratrol is present in berries, red wine, pistachios, peanuts, and grapes. Moreover, they are also found in other 72 species of plant and as well in medicinal plants. When resveratrol exposes to light, cis-isomerization occurs. It can be absorbed by passive diffusion and forms complex membrane transporters like integrins. Resveratrol was found in three forms in the bloodstream, i.e., in free form or sulfate and glucuronide derivatives [17].

10.2.3 Ellagitannins

They are bioactive polyphenols rich in nuts (almonds, walnut) or fruits (raspberries, pomegranates, strawberries, and black raspberries). They are not absorbed by the stomach first degraded into ellagic acid (EA), and for digestion, it is converted into urolithins [18].

10.2.4 Flavonoids

Flavonoids are a large group of polyphenols in the diet. To date, 6000 different compounds of flavonoids have been recognized, and new forms are still discovered. They are found in all plants, especially in aromatic and medicinal plants. Based on their structural differences, flavonoids are divided into six classes: flavones, flavanols, flavan-3-ols, flavanones, isoflavones, and anthocyanins. Except for catechins, most flavonoids are present naturally in plants. In the plant kingdom, except mushrooms and algae, flavanols are very common flavonoids. Kaempferol, isorhamnetin, myricetin and quercetin are representative of flavanols. Flavones are present moderately in red pepper, celery, and parsley [19]. The flavone glycosides (apigenin and luteolin) are found in cereals like wheat and millet. Isoflavones are primarily present in legumes, and soybean or by-product are significant sources of the human diet. The content of isoflavones is varied in soybean-derived food. Flavanones are found in citrus fruits like grapefruits, mandarins, lemons, and oranges. Naringenin, eriodictyol, isosakuranetin, and hesperetin are the most frequent flavanones. In the human diet, flavanols are essential flavonoids. They are present in the form of polymers and monomers [20].

In diet, chalcones are poorly found because, during extraction stages, they are transferred to acidic flavanones. Phloretin and its glycoside are the most studied chalcones and present in apples. Anthocyanidins are flavonoids present in cereals, tubers, vegetables, and wine but rich in fruits. They stimulate the ripening of fruits [21].

10.2.5 Proanthocyanidin

Proanthocyanidins are flavonoid derivatives and also called condensed tannins. They do not contain sugar moieties and give food flavor. It is present in fruits (plum, strawberry, apple), chocolate, dried vegetables (hazelnut, common bean), and wine. They combine with salivary proteins to form molecular complexes and are responsible for astringency in some fruits (apples, peaches, grapes, persimmons) or drinks (beer, cider, tea, or wine) and bitterness in chocolates [22].

10.2.6 Vitamins

Vitamins are intricate in the metabolism of carbohydrates, proteins, fats, and the synthesis of numerous compounds required for body function. They are organic compounds and required for the proper functioning of tissues and cells. They are present in an adequate amount in natural food and may or may not be synthesized in the body. The absence and deficiency of vitamins prevent the mileage of different processes and disrupt the body's functions [23].

Vitamins are classified as fat-soluble (vitamins D, K, E, and A) or water-soluble (vitamins C, E, and A), riboflavin, thiamine, niacin, folate, biotin, vitamin B12, vitamin B6, and pantothenate. They show antioxidant properties such as lipid peroxidation inhibition and free radicals scavenging. Due to their antioxidant properties, vitamins reduce diseases like neurological diseases, cancer, cardiovascular and neuropsychiatric disorder.

10.2.7 Bioactive Peptides

In the body, bioactive peptides may be produced in a free state. They are produced by the protein digestion in the gastrointestinal tract or may be delivered through food. Hydrolysis of protein is catalyzed by pepsin in the gastrointestinal tract to produced peptide fragments. There are at least 20 different peptides present on the epithelial cell membrane. They release different types of amino acids and affect peptide bonds. They increase immunity by producing antibodies [24].

The interest of science is growing in bioactive compounds due to their diverse biological properties. Additionally, they prevent and reduce the risk of various chronic diseases. Different transcriptomic and artificial intelligence approaches use different bioactive compounds to reduce the risk of diseases, enhance the availability of food and cosmetics [25].

10.3 Transcriptomics Approaches for the Selection of Bioactive Compounds

Transcriptomics technologies are methods for studying an organism's transcriptome, which is the total number of RNA transcripts. An organism's information content is stored in its genome's DNA and expressed through transcription. Noncoding RNAs perform additional roles, while mRNA serves as a temporary intermediary molecule in the information network [26]. The entire transcripts present in a cell are captured in a transcriptome, which is a snapshot in time. The first attempts to analyze the entire transcriptome were made in the early 1990s, and technical developments have made transcriptomics a widely accepted discipline since the late 1990s. Transcriptomics has been defined by a series of technological breakthroughs that have changed the discipline. Microarrays, which measure a set of preset sequences, and RNA sequencing (RNA-Seq), which employs high sequencing to collect all sequences, are two significant contemporary approaches in the subject. Measuring gene expression in multiple tissues, circumstances, or time periods in an organism yields detailed knowledge about how genes are expressed and exposes detailed characteristics about an organism. It can also be used to predict the roles of genes that have yet to be annotated [27]. Transcriptomic profiling has aided in the knowledge of human disease by allowing researchers to look at how gene expression fluctuates in various organisms. Gene expression analysis in its whole permits for the observation of broad coordinated patterns that are difficult to identify with more customized assays [28].

10.3.1 Hybrid Transcriptome Sequencing

Hybrid sequencing (also known as 'Hybrid-Seq') has emerged as a revolutionary method to combine Third Generation Sequencing (TGS) and second-Generation Sequencing (SGS) data to overcome the restrictions of SGS and TGS data analysis on their own. It can improve the output data's whole execution and performance. In addition, a variety of bioinformatics techniques for Hybrid-Seq transcriptome data have been described, comprising IDP-ASE, IDP, LSC, and IDP-fusion for a more accurate and more sensitive portray model organism at transcript level [29]. In bioinformatics, hybrid sequencing uses various sequencing technologies to assemble a genome from fragmented, sequenced DNA/RNA appearing from shotgun sequencing. Raw sequence analyses are converted to genomic characteristics (i.e., the transcriptome is assembled) using two methods: (1) *de novo* and (2) genome-guided. The transcriptome is reproduced without the requirement of a reference genome in the *de novo* method. It's usually used when the genome is unusual, partial, or heavily reassembled in comparison to the reference genome. [30]. Puglia *et al.*, looked into how partial reconstruction and recognition of isoforms in short inputs constrain transcriptome profiles in nonmodel organisms without annotated genomes. On the other hand, Long-read sequencing approaches have demonstrated that they can build full transcript assembly even without a reference genome. *Cynara cardunculus var. altilis* (DC) is a perennial, resistant crop designed for a harsh climate with numerous manufacturing and nutraceutical purposes owing to the abundance of the secondary metabolism formed primarily on floral heads. The latest release of a draft genome was used to research this species. However, it still doesn't look at the transcriptome pattern throughout capitula production. The report uses a unique RNA-seq hybrid technique that uses both long and short RNA-seq values to analyze the transcriptome of plant and inflorescent cardoon organs. This new approach to hybrid sequence enabled the transcriptome assembly to be improved, over half of the gene annotated/updated and many new genes and as a substitute split isoforms identified. This research adds to our knowledge of an Asteraceae plant's floral cycle, useful plant biology and reproduction asset in Cynara, and an efficient tool for improving genetic annotation [31]. Wu *et al.*, published the next-generation sequence which makes sequence-based molecular pathology and tailored oncology realistic. Before hormone therapy, the primary and metastatic tissue genome and transcriptome of a person reported with conventional, but now aggressive prostate cancer were retrieved and sequenced. The histology and copy number assessments were astonishingly consistent, but the prostate tumor quadrant, which was likely to have the metastatic diaspora, could be suggested. Although the cell type was homogeneous, both luminous and neuroendocrine cell types have been identified by our transcriptome testing. Significantly, the diversity of expressed and unique gene fusions, especially C15orf21:MYC, summed up this biology. We believe that amplification and overexpression of the stem cell gene MSI2 may aid in the maintenance of a steady hybrid cell id. This hybrid lumina-neuroendocrine tumor seems to be a novel and very aggressive kind of prostate cancer with distinct biologic features and a deliberate castrate resistive progression. The significance of intrinsic tumor biology, sequence-based molecular pathology, and customized oncology of linked genome, exome, and transcriptome sequences is highlighted in this study [32].

10.3.2 Microarray

Following genome sequencing, DNA microarray analysis has been the most widely used resource of genome knowledge in the life sciences. Gene expression and other workable genomics are produced in massive quantities by microarray expression research, which assures vital insight into the gene's function and interactions through metabolism. However, the microarray data that have previously been generated are still broadly not accessible to the research community and have standard presentation formats and widely used tools and databases. Many variables work together to keep microarray data out of the hands of the general public. The field is still fresh, but it has reached the maturity level required to detect critical data items. Gene expression data are also more complicated than sequencing data. They are only useful if they are accompanied by a full characterization of the circumstances in that they were formed, such as the status of the underlying biological system and its perturbation. Unlike the genome of an organism, the same number of cell types multiplied by environmental conditions are present [33]. Microarray technology enables the concurrent analysis of thousands of variables in a single trial. Capture microspecies that are mobilized in rows and columns on the solid support and subjected to specimens of the bound molecules. To recognize complicated structures within each microspot, readout methods relying on electrochemistry, fluorescence, mass spectrometry, chemiluminescence, and radioactivity can be employed. Miniaturized parallel obligatory evaluations can be extremely sensitive, and an array-based gene expression study can demonstrate the technique's incredible capability. These systems are exposed to complementary objectives in arrays containing immobilized DNA samples, which measure the degree of hybridization. Latest protein microarray advances include implementations for enzyme-substrate, DNA–protein, and many kinds of protein-protein interactions. External and internal parameters affect the physiological condition of a cell. The microarray technique can be used to track intracellular gene expression and protein expression pathways. At the mRNA level, DNA microarrays are employed for genetic and expression analyses. Protein microarrays are used for protein-level expression and the broad field of interaction analysis [34]. Crucial trends occur in fields ranging as assay diversification, microarrays, genomics, proteomics, and genetic screening as microarray platforms evolve and extend to more research sites, which include universities, research centers, public health laboratories, and diagnostic health centers. The little Arabidopsis thaliana mosquito plant was the initial microarray article, but the technique quickly extended to yeast and animal investigations. The diversification of tests continued at an explosive pace, with more than 100 organisms in the data. Any species in the biosphere can be examined, genomically analyzed, and DNA sequencing information for functional genomic assessment using an unique organism microarray. The microarray platform can also be diversified to include cellular proteins, organic molecules, carbohydrates, peptides, and nanotubes, at a level that expands rapidly beyond DNA. The density of the microarray is also growing steadily over time, as is the number of arrays with tens thousands of elements of the collection, and it allows analyzing the entire genomics on single chips. This population has risen progressively over time as well. The move toward full-genome analysis includes the utilization of 'focused microarrays' which comprise only a few hundred elements. With carefully selected gene subsets, the focused pathway analysis complements the entire genome studies is a highly economical approach [35].

10.3.3 RNA-Seq

To identify and characterize transcripts contained in an RNA extract, RNA-Seq combines a high-throughput sequencing approach with computational tools. The size of the produced nuclear sequences is usually approximately 100 bp; depending on the sequencing process, they can range from 30 bp to 10,000 bp. RNA-Seq uses transcriptome collection of many short transcriptome fragments so that the original RNA transcript can be computerized by aligning reads with one another or with a reference genome (*de novo* assembly). A significant advantage over microarray transcriptomes is the normal dynamic span of 5 levels for RNA-Seq. Input RNA amounts are significantly less than microarrays (microgram quantity) for RNA-Seq (monograph quantity), which allow for more detailed cellular structure analysis to be performed down to one cell level in combination with a linear cDNA amplification [36]. Theoretically, the quantifying limit in the RNA-Seq is not upper, and the background signals in nonrepetitive areas are very low for 100 bp readings. RNA-Seq can be utilized to distinguish genes within a genome or to pinpoint functional genes at a certain phase, and reading counts can be applied to precisely simulate the comparative amount of gene expression. In particular, by developing DNA sequencing technologies for improving throughput, precise reading, and duration, the RNA-seq methods have continuously improved. RNA-Seq has quickly been adopted as the dominant transcriptome technology in 2015 since first descriptions in 2006 and 2008 and overtook microarrays. The search for transcriptome data in each cell led to advances in the preparation methods for RNA-Seq libraries, leading to dramatic sensory advances. Single-cell transcriptomes questioned in fixed tissues using *in situ* RNA-sec are currently fully documented and expanded to encompass transcriptomes of single cells explicitly interrogated in fixed tissues [37]. discovered that Adlay is a tropical plant that has been used in conventional Chinese medicine for centuries and is acclaimed for its nutritious properties. The latest research has manifested that vitamin E compounds are protected from chronic conditions such as cancer and cardiovascular disease in Adlay. Furthermore, the molecular mechanism of Adlay's health advantages is yet unknown. Long-read isoform sequencing (Iso-Seq) and short-read RNA sequencing by *de novo* transfer montage were used to create Adlay gene collections (RNA-Seq). Iso-seq and RNA-seq genes each comprised 31,177 and 57,901 genes, correspondingly. They tested the constructed gene sets for authenticity by looking for prolamine and vitamin E–related proteins in Adlay plant tissues and seedlings. The researchers matched tissue-specific genes from Adlay leaf, root, and young, mature resources to families of neighboring plant species including rice, sorghum, and maize, and scientifically confirmed the differential expression of 12 arbitrarily picked genes. Their research into the Adlay transcriptome will result in useful genetic analyses that will benefit upcoming Adlay breeding efforts [38].

Luo *et al.* reported that Salvia miltiorrhiza is a Chinese plant with considerable pharmacological benefits, thanks to its medicinal tanshinone and phenolic acid components. The production of these compounds has been increased by using methyl jasmone (MeJA) as an effective elixir. The molecular processes of Tanshinone and Salvianolic acid production regulated by MeJA are unknown. The transcribed profiling of S. miltiorrhiza leaves were examined for 12 hours (T12) following MeJA stimulation and sham processed leaves (T0) employing an Illumina deep (RNA-seq) approach for gene expression alterations in reaction to MeJA. Out of approximately 21 million readings, 37,647 single sequences have been obtained, and 25,641 (71,53%) have been recorded based on BLAST public database searches. In a sum of 5287 distinct sequences, substantially every reported gene engaged in Tanzhinone and phenolic acid production in *S. miltiorrhiza* differed between the samples T0 and T12. Many transcriptions (e.g., MYB, bHLH, and WRKY) and genes associated with the production of plant hormones and signal transmission have been conveyed differently in reaction to Meja induction. Crucially, three and four cytochrome P450 (P450s), contenders participating in the biosynthesis of tanshinone and phenol acid, correspondingly, were identified from RNA-seq datasets relying on co pattern investigation with SmCPS1/SmKSL1 or SmRAS, which are key genes accountable for biosynthesis. This extensive research on gene expression profiles induced by MeJA can reveal the molecular processes of MeJA-mediated bioactive chemical production and regulation in *S. miltiorrhiza* [39].

Lateef *et al.*, discovered that the *Solanum trilobatum L.* is an important plant in the Solanaceae family's conventional Indian medicinal scheme. We analyzed the transcriptome of the S. trilobatum leaf with a high-performance RNA sequence. In the *de novo* assembly of 136,220,612, 128,934 nonredundant unigenes with a size of 1347 bp were generated. NCBI nr datasets, Gene Ontology, KEGG, Uniprot, Pfam, and plnTFDB were used to do unique interpretations. Employing the KEGG database,

60,097 unborn persons were assigned to 138 pathways, comprising 48 transcriptional variable families and 14,490 unborn people. The transcripts of key secondary metabolites participating in biosynthesis, such as flavonoids, were discovered using the pathway analysis. In addition, the transcripts were measured using RSEM to detect substantially activated genes in secondary metabolism. The reverse transcript PCR was used to verify the *de novo* constructed unigenes. The expression status of chosen unigenes in the flavonoid biosynthesis route was examined using qRT-PCR. These simple repeat redundancies would perhaps be useful in molecular breeding. This is the initial thorough transcriptome analysis study for *S. trilobatum*,

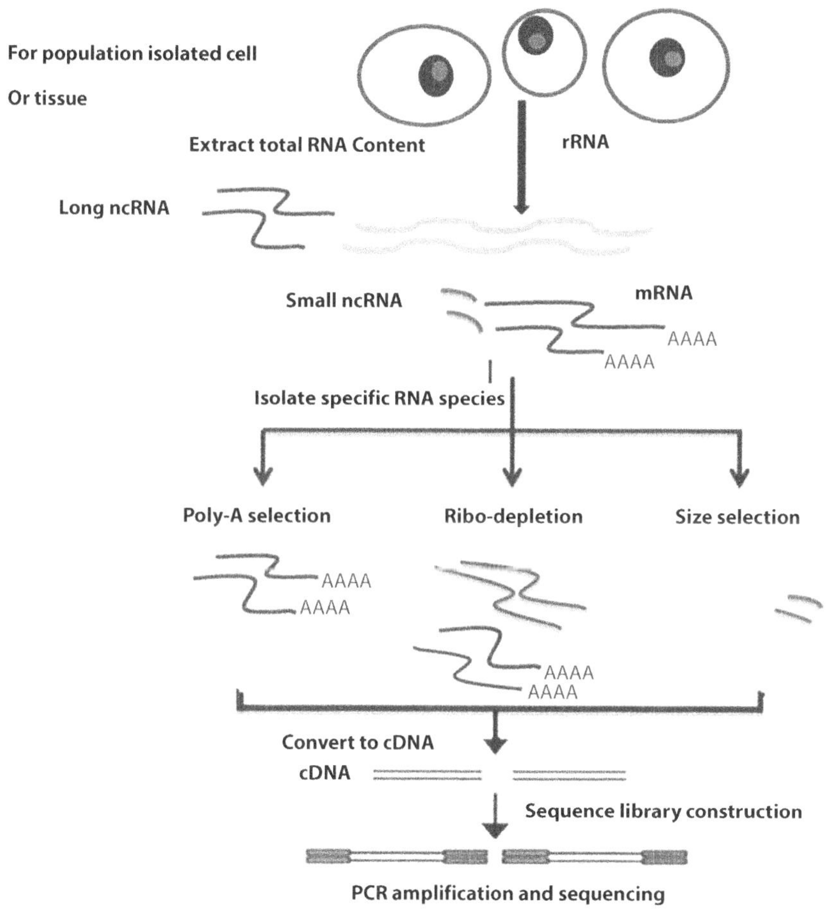

Figure 10.1 Overview of RNA seq. rRNA: ribosomal RNA, mRNA: messenger RNA.

and it will be helpful in future research to comprehend the molecular basis of *S. trilobatum*. [40].

The emergence of high-performance next-generation sequencing (NGS) technology changed transcriptomics. Many of the problems faced by microarrays relying on hybridization and Sanger's gene expression measurement sequencing techniques have been solved by this technical advancement. The separation and transformation of RNA into complementary DNA, the sequencing of the library on an NGS platform, and the sequencing of the library are all part of a typical RNA-Seq experiment (Figure 10.1). Nonetheless, based on a researcher's goals, numerous experimental aspects must be examined before RNA-Seq is performed. These comprise biological and technological duplicates, sequencing depths, and required transcriptome penetration. These trial settings may have a minor influence on the data accuracy in some circumstances. In many circumstances, nevertheless, the researcher should precisely plan the experiment, balancing high outcomes with the time and monetary expenditure [41].

10.4 Artificial Intelligence Approaches for the Selection of Bioactive Compounds

The invention of innovative and effective methods for the focused distribution of multifunctional medicinal substances with the least amount of danger and optimum performance has become a challenge for biological and chemical researchers from the past few decades. Moreover, the time consumption in the production of novel therapeutic agents and development cost was another hindrance in development and drug design. Therefore, scientists worldwide are influenced by computational approaches such as molecular docking and virtual screening (VS) to minimize these hurdles and challenges. Moreover, these methods also force some challenges and hurdles such as inefficiency and inaccuracy. Therefore, there is a surge in implementing novel techniques. The unique methodologies are self-contained, reducing the obstacles that standard computational strategies face. Artificial intelligence (AI) has emerged as a potential option for reducing the challenges and problems encountered during the drug design and development procedure. Machine learning (ML) and deep learning (DL) algorithms are two types of AI algorithms that perform together [42]. Furthermore, the stages involved in medication formulation and development are complicated and time-consuming such as manufacturing practices, clinical and preclinical trials, optimization of lead compounds, screening of therapeutic agents, and target validation and selection. All of these processes present a new problem in determining the most efficient treatment for a condition. Unfortunately, an issue that arises in the minds of pharmaceutical corporations is how to manage the efficiency and expense of the procedure. AI has explained all the answers to these rising questions scientifically, including the process cost and the time consumption. Moreover, in the healthcare sector and the pharmaceutical companies, the increase in data digitization trigger AI implementation to defeat the problems of examining complicated data. AI, often known as machine intelligence, refers to a computer system's capability to understand from previous or input data. AI is defined as the machine that mimics the cognitive behaviors associated with humans' brains during the problem-solving and learning process. Nowadays, AI algorithms are extensively used by chemical and biological scientists in discovering and designing a drug. Computational modeling relied on ML and AI postulates to give a grand parkway for validating and identifying chemical compounds, drug repositioning, drug effectiveness, drug monitoring, evaluation of physicochemical properties and toxicity of the drug, and synthesis of peptide and the identification of targets. Upon the discovery of AI postulates, DL and ML algorithms, VS of bioactive compounds from chemical libraries become time-effective and easy. However, the chemical libraries compromise more than 106 million bioactive compounds. Moreover, AI algorithms eliminate the problems of toxicity, which occur due to the of-target interactions [43].

10.4.1 Machines Learning (ML) Approach for the Selection of Bioactive Compounds

The ML field can be described as applying and studying programs that accomplish prediction and classification challenges through pattern detection. ML has not used any explicitly defined rules. ML has surpassed natural language processing, among other areas. Machine learning has thrived in natural language processing, among several other domains. In the process of drug development, data mining processes (particularly machine learning techniques) are often utilized. For virtual screening duties, they are extremely useful. Highly active chemicals are chosen from huge libraries for virtual screening. Prior to categorization, a classifier learns how to distinguish actives from inactives through a coaching procedure. This is done by giving it a collection of molecules to work with. These compounds are active against a certain target and provide a collection of molecules that have been recognized as inactive. As a result, in numerous scenarios, a predictive framework is required to give class labels to undefined events. There have been several examples of using machine learning approaches in virtual screening [44]. Machine learning approaches for molecular forecasting were investigated in terms of computing technological improvement. To assess ion channel activity, Willet *et al.* applied the Binary Kernel Discrimination (BKD) procedure/approach. Harper reported and analyzed BKD using a fused similar query. The Support Vector Machine was used by Liu *et al.* to create a model. This Support vector machine is used to produce predictors automatically. Lavecchia surveyed the possible opportunities and success(rate) regarding virtual screening in machine learning based on ligand binding. Cross-validation, feature extraction, model training, and parameter selection are all included in this framework. The prediction rate improves by this model [45].

10.4.1.1 Evolution of Machine Learning to Deep Learning

In September 2015, Google's search trend revealed that AI was the most sought phrase following the debut of ML. Some refer to machine learning as the fundamental AI application, while others refer to it as an AI subset. ML is when data are entered into a system and an algorithm such as Hidden Markov models (HMM), Decision Tree (DT), or the Nave Bayes is used to assist the machine learn without being deliberately programmed, but AI is when computer programs can reason and understand like humans. In the future, machines could classify and arrange input data like a human brain with neural networks, which further demonstrate progress in IA. Igor Aizen Berg and his collaborators coined the phrase "deep learning" to describe the artificial neural network (ANN) in the twentieth century. Because DL is a subset of AI's ML, the progression is AI>ML>DL. ML utilizes either supervised learning, in which the input is labeled with the intended output labels, or unsupervised learning, in which the prototype is educated to utilize unlabeled data but looks for input data trends that repeat. Others use a hybrid of supervised and unsupervised learning, which is referred to as semi-supervised learning. Furthermore, self-supervised learning is defined as a special instance that employs a two-step method to create a supervised learning model, with unsupervised learning producing the labels for unlabeled data. One other category is reinforcement learning, which is a type of ML that boosts its algorithm over period via a continuous response loop, and finally, deep learning, which consists of numerous layers of ML algorithms known as brain-inspired algorithms that mimic the human brain but need a lot of computing power to accomplish in training and large amounts of information [46].

10.4.1.2 Virtual Screening

Virtual screening uses a database to estimate the resemblance among the objective (reference structure) and individual molecule. It has origins in chemical information technology, computational chemistry, and structural biology. It is a technique for discovering novel physiologically active compounds. It is the technique of molecularly modeling and docking each chemical agent in a database into the binding region within each macromolecule goal. Docking is the best process in which the macromolecular target is calculated for every medium in the binding region. A study of fast, automated docking techniques has been carried out with Schneider and Bohm, and Feinstein and Brylinski have carried out a detailed study to calculate the optimum molecular docking size for predicted binding pocket sizes [47]. During the period 2008 to 2015, Wang *et al.* examined extensively graphene-based glucose sensors. Huang *et al.* studied on Drosophila, which has the most advanced epigenetic method for Piwi-piRNA site targeting. Their findings shed light on how epigenetic variables enlist the help of their designated locations. Marinov *et al.*, meanwhile, examined Huang *et al.* work and found that their dataset did not support their overall genome outcomes. Lin *et al.*, work verified Marinov *et al.* not discovering a genomic site and reiterating the influence of Piwi on the genome of RNA-polymerase II. Watanabe and Lin have reviewed the piRNA regarding specific biological procedures and found a lot of work has gone into it. The processing sciences of bioactive molecules have evolved in recent years in critical areas, such as lead discovery and compound optimization. Numerous virtual screening procedures and forecasting techniques have been extensively explored in the academia [48].

For example, after paralleling this tactic with multiple linear regression (MLR), master component recovery (PCR), and part-less squares (PLS) (BP), Burden and Winkler established the technique QSAR (quantitative structure-activity relationship) as a treatment to bigger databases and afterward presented back propagation. They practiced QSAR in order to enormous facts from high-performance screening and combinatory chemistry (HTS). QSAR includes a vector representation of molecular structure prophecy of a composite's natal commotion. QSAR is being used successfully for many medicines and agrochemical design issues. Further information on the challenges of QSAR has been outlined in the Burden and Winkler study, and the delinquent of formulating the QSAR and QSPR prototypes was resoled by Rogers and Hopfinger by employing the inherited task estimate method (GFA). Their effort revealed that, rather than using a single method, the GFA's secret lies in creating and using multiple models. In addition, unclear QSARs were established amongst plant-based flavones and their inhibitory effects on aurora B kinases (aurB). Several similitude search methods were suggested in the relevant literature. In the earlier innovation of the leads for a medication sighting venture, Sheridan and Kearsley vindicated the requisite for various organic search techniques. In Bohm and Willett, Shneider and Barnard and Downs, you will find detailed reviews of the search for chemical similitudes and virtual screenings. In order to discover two new 5-HT6R ligands, Smusz *et al.*, adapted their virtual screening, and Me'tivier *et al.* operated the innovation of organizational alerts. Clustering algorithms were utilized in chemistry for the discovery of drugs during recent research. A study compares standard techniques of clustering, namely k-medium, k-mean bisecting and ward grouping. Clustering solicitations comprises QSAR analyses, high-performance screening (HTS), and ADMET prediction for immersion, dissemination, uptake, disposal, and venomousness. In contrast to this, an innovative technique called pkCSM was introduced by Pires *et al.* in order to generate prognostic configurations for minor-compound pharmacokinetics and toxicity employing figure based marks [49].

10.4.1.3 Recent Advances in Machine Learning

Nowadays, machine learning is a well-known field that has been resurgent. This field is defined as the learning and presentation of algorithms which execute estimate or perusing errands by recognizing patterns rather than by specific rules. Such algorithms may also be divided into assemblages like managed and unmanaged learning. The former one discusses to algorithms using and mapping records to classification sets known, and the later stating to algorithms which do not utilize predetermined or identified groups (e.g., "grouping" similarity tasters). For example, algorithms may also be classed into parametric (which assume the data distribution) and nonparametric algorithms (which cannot create distribution assumptions). Machine learning is a rich field in general, and Tarca *et al.* recommended to examine the ML background and concepts further. ML's current rise is mainly due to growing computational resources and large dataset availability. The presentation scalability presented by the capability of the algorithms for their improvement as they acclimatize and acquire from databases is the main inspiration for utilizing Machine learning approaches. These approaches permit their consumers to collect valuable data from enormous, multifaceted datasets on a large scale. In its wide range of applications and approaches, the ML field continues to grow. Media advice, speech recognition/classification, and geographic mapping and navigation included some powerful ML applications. ML is utilized to extract useful evidence from enormous datasets and very complicated data types. These domains, in which ML is used to extract a gesture from multipart data, also encompass natural product biology and chemistry. ML's ability to recognize complex patterns in biology and chemistry can be used to get novel insights into genomic signatures, chemical activity, composite assortment, and beneficial associations [50].

10.4.1.4 Deep Learning

Deep learning is one of the most common machine learning approaches that consists of numerous trainable parameters and sensory inputs for imitating the central human system to develop data patterns with multifarious concepts. Many fields have been considerably studied, for example computer vision, computer games, natural language processing, and automatic automobiles. Biomedical data also profit in large measure from healthcare, medicinal analysis and the assessment of medicines using deep learning technologies [51]. Deep learning means that multiple levels of representation are automatically learned from the basic distribution of the data to be modeled. In other words, the low- and high-level classification features are automatically extracted by a profound learning algorithm. One means a feature which depends hierarchically on others with high-level characteristics. For example, in a computer vision, this implies that a deeper learning algorithm will learn its own low level depictions from the crude picture (e.g., edge detectors, gabor filters, etc.), then develop representations which depend on these low level depictions (e.g., linear or nonlinear combinations), and repeat the same process successively [52]. Automatic representation learning is key to this approach, since the need for a hand-crafted design that takes time is eliminated [53]. Deep learning models for medical diagnostics have reached physician level accuracy and have demon strated great application potential. In order to speed up the identification of compounds with desirable pharmacodynamics and pharmacokinetic characteristics, several techniques to learning machines have been utilized during drug discovery [54]. Various machine learning-based webservers, including as OCHEM, ChemSAR, and LBVS, have been created to accelerate drug development. Machine learning approaches are also frequently employed in target prediction, which is another important aspect of drug development. For drug repositioning and action exploratory mechanisms, machine-based learning target prediction has a lot of promise. Many studies have demonstrated that deep learning algorithms outperform conventional machine learning algorithms in target prediction, ADMET property prediction, virtual screening, and chemical synthesis. These conclusions may be drawn not just from the test results, but also from a data science competition organized by pharmaceutical firms [55]. Another important use of deep learning is *de novo* molecule creation, which uses sequence data to create molecules with desired properties. Deep learning approaches in drug discovery and chemical biology, on the other hand, are restricted owing to a lack of knowledge, data processing, and user-friendly deeper learning tools. As a result, we have created a web server that leverages either public or user-supplied data to assist biologists and chemists in doing virtual screenings of chemical probes or medications for a specific purpose [56].

10.4.1.4.1 Framework of Deep Learning

Figure 10.2 illustrates the context of Deep-Learning Virtual Screening Server DeepScreening. (1) Preparation Dataset: select interest target or upload deep-neural network (DNN) private dataset training. (2) Characteristics: select molecular vectorization characteristics.

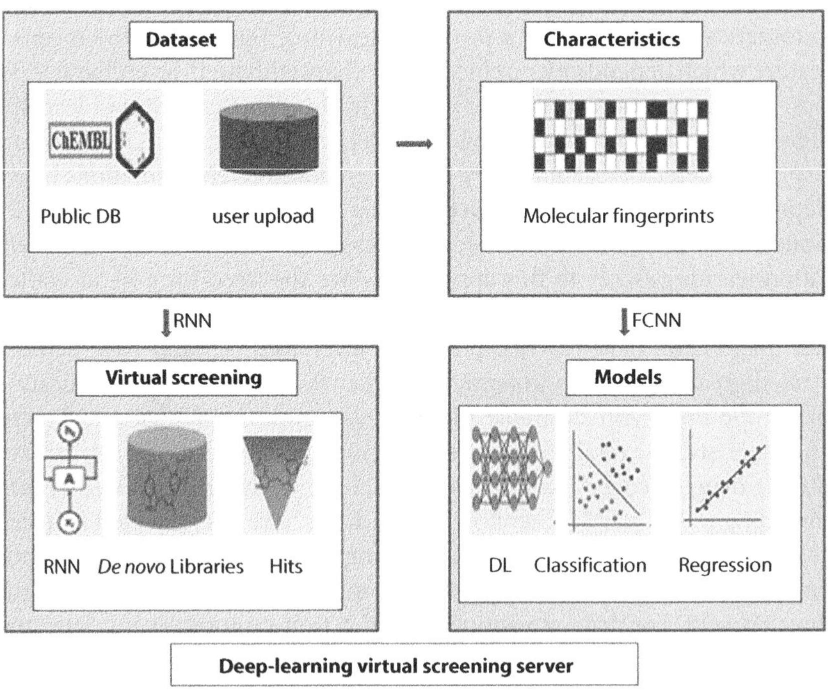

Figure 10.2 The context of deep learning virtual screening server deep screening.

(3) Parameters: choose the training classification model parameters or regression models. (4) Virtual Screening: Virtual screening of chemistry libraries or libraries. DeepScreening is a highly automatic screening server that integrates different data processing, modeling and screening technologies and tools.

10.4.1.4.2 Advances in Deep Learning

DL is an ML subsection that is increasingly important for the biology and chemistry of natural products. DL refers to the ML area, which uses profoundly layered neural networks that function as neuronal networks in the brain of many individuals. Several computational biological procedures, like as sequencing mapping, protein structure estimation, and splicing signal decode, are powered by DL techniques, which are increasing in prominence. For example, high-performance test screening (HTS), QSR, and other studies have all been reported using DL in chemistry. Understanding the variety and chemistry of natural products requires the use of biological and chemical DL. This is particularly obvious in the use of DL natural language processing (NLP) techniques. The bulk of NLP technologies to far have concentrated on comprehending spoken and textual dialects. Nevertheless, researchers are increasingly employing these methods to decipher molecular and genetic codes. Scientists utilize natural language processing (NLP) to describe and characterize genomic components like genes based on their genetic structure, similar to how NLP techniques describe and define words based on their sentence context. Furthermore, NLP methods are being utilized to represent and characterize molecules and fragments as novel mathematical structures, providing new insights and analytical options for understanding chemical agent interactions and activities. These and other DL and NLP techniques disclose fresh information on natural chemical variety, chemical characteristics, and medicinal potential, as well as genome analysis. As DL, NLP, and other ML techniques get enabled, we will continue to discuss these natural products [57].

10.4.1.4.3 Deep Neural Network (DNN)

The deep neural network is a networking architecture of neurons that gains prominence in the learning machine society. DNN comprises a variety of elements and concealed coats. It can learn abstract and advanced structures by using nonlinear alterations for basic types with extraordinary discriminatory authority. This procedure facilitates separating the various explanatory factors from the data from additional theoretical characteristics and high grade demonstration. This distinguishes DNN from the previous algorithms of the learning machine. For example, a standard *in-vitro* trial for the immersion ability of verbally injected medicinal products is the humanoid colorectal carcinoma cell line. Based on Caco-2 test data, *silico* prediction methods can increase the efficiency of a high-performance test for new drug candidates. However, *in-silico* prototypes previously developed which forecast the cell permeability of Caco-2 composites utilize crafted characteristics that can be particular to datasets and cause over-fit issues. It produces higher level functions founded on fundamental characteristics that provide high discrimination and thus an excellent generalized model. Deep Neural Networ based Caco-2 binary penetrability classification is available. Shin *et al.* 2018 have constructed an *in-vitro in vitro* Caco-2 specious data model based on 663 chemical compounds. Two hundred and nine molecular descriptors are used during DNN model production in order to develop high-level attributes [58]. Regularization of dropouts is used to solve the problem of overfitting and nonlinear activation. To minimize the fading gradient problem, the rectified linear unit (ReLU) is accepted. The results show that the high-level DNN features are robust over handcrafted features to predict the structurally diverse

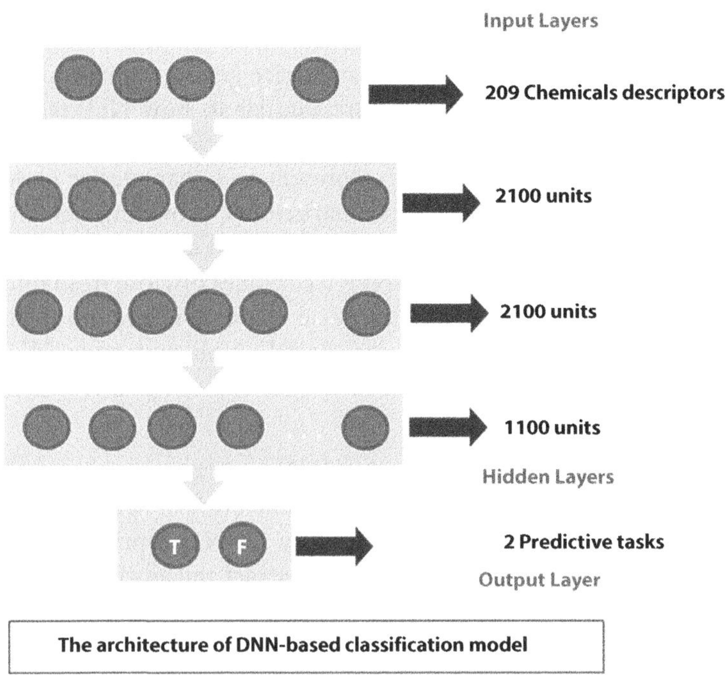

Figure 10.3 The architecture of DNN based classification model.

chemical compound cell permeability of Caco-2 cellular lines. This study included an inner coating (209 molecular descriptors), a SoftMax external sheet (two predictive tasks), and three covered layers of 2,100, 2,100, and 1,100 covering unit (Figure 10.3). The neural network units were fully interconnected, with each link representing a real-life weight. With the activation function, the output of each cached unit in our DNN has been calculated [59].

10.4.2 *De Novo* Synthesis of Bioactive Compounds

The goal of *de novo* design is to create novel compounds that have drug-like characteristics and targeted biological actions. That goal coincides to the core sustainment of early medicine development and encompasses a substantial portion of the work put forward by pharmaceutical companies and academic institutions to create novel remedies for illnesses. *De novo* is analogous to high-performance testing in terms of discovering novel beginning points for drug development. Rather than looking for functional substances in large libraries of physically available screening chemicals, installing chemical pieces from the ground up creates *de novo* design. For candidates for this procedure, computer-assisted *de novo* design methodologies generate hypothetical silicon structures automatically [60].

In contrast, there has also been significant attention to developing computer-aided pharmaceutical products. The numbers published in *de novo* design have evolved steadily from the first computer methods of the late 1980s onward. Most *de-novo* design approaches attempt to emulate a chemical medicine chemist's work: molecules (virtually mounted from fragments) are synthesized and tested for the biological activity of the drugs (calculation-assessed by a scoring function). These procedures vary based on the searching of molecules which are generated, assembled, and marked. For example, the measurement can be done using either the calculation of a certain similitude indeximate of applicant composites and recognized standard ligands (ligand-based approach) (receptor-dependent approach). Regardless of the specific technique, the question of synthesizability has consistently been addressed by automated *de novo* design. One may conclude that this is one of the primary reasons why *de novo* design software is seldom put to the test in the real world. Kutchukian and Shakhnovich have published an article that summarizes successful *de novo* design research. *De novo* drug design has shown to be an effective method for quickly identifying lead structural candidates. Using fragment-based molecular assembly techniques, in particular, automated screening compound invention has been successful. Particle swarm optimization and

Table 10.1 Selected software approaches that use adaptive techniques for compound design and optimization.

Software	Optimization strategy	Required input	References
COLIBREE	PSO	Reference ligand	[77]
ADAPT	EA	Receptor structure	[78]
Chemical Genesis	EA	Receptor structure and Reference ligand	[79]
SYNOPSIS	EA	Receptor structure	[80]
GANDI	EA	Receptor structure and Reference ligand	[81]
LEA	EA	Ligand-based QSAR model	[82]
SME	EA	Neural network QSAR model	[83]

evolutionary algorithms are preferred approaches for iterative virtual synthesis and testing (PSO) [61]. Table 10.1 contains designated software methodologies that utilize adaptive procedures for scheming and improving a compound.

10.4.2.1 Application Examples of De Novo Design

10.4.2.1.1 Design of Histamine H3 Receptor Agonists

The application of Skelgen software to generate new histamine H3 receiver agonists is a further example of an effective *de novo* design project. Like the SPROUT approach, the receptor and ligand information can be used by Skelgen to restrict the design and build new molecular fragments. In order to offer new scaffolds by optimizing fitness, stochastic searching is carried out in the chemical and conformation space. Skelgen has created 100 potential structures of H3 receptor agonists clustered manually in four templates with a familiar but distinct pharmacophore connection. For synthesis, two of these templates have been chosen. Alternative differences led to persuasive and careful H3 receptor nanomolar antagonists [62].

10.4.2.1.2 Receptor-Based Design of Dihydroorotate Dehydrogenase (DHODH) Inhibitors

Gillet *et al.* created the SPROUT program in the early 1990s, which can construct structures from 3D structural realignment using reception data or a pharmacophore modeling. SPROUT consists of two steps: (1) 3D skeleton creation, which fulfills steric restrictions and binds reactive groups, and (2) atom type assignment to skeleton polygons, which satisfies hydrophobic and electrostatic criteria (Gillet *et al.*, 1994). The SPROUT program was recently utilized to efficiently discover DHODH antagonists in the malaria-causing *Plasmodium falciparum* worm. The organizational features of *P. falciparum* DHODH vary from those of human DHODH, as shown in the corresponding X-ray structures. In human and parasite enzymes, Heikkila *et al.* discovered a hydrophobic subpocket with a distinct shape. In this region, the authors have identified two sites of contact with substantially conserved residues. SPROUT created 20 distinct small molecule templates and chose a few for synthesis. The most powerful inhibitor of human DHODH is *P. falciparum* DHODH, which has an IC50 of 43 mM [63].

10.4.2.1.3 Ligand-Based Design of Inverse Agonists of the Cannabinoid-1 Receptor

In the second research, Roche Pharmaceuticals used the *de novo* design program TOPAS to produce novel CB-1 receptor reverse agonists from an original *de novo* created candidates' structure. The identification of benzodioxols as a new CB-1 receptor reverse agonist series was made possible by the refinement of this initial proposition's pharmacophore matching, the application of drug-like criteria, and considerations of chemical tractability. Most importantly, *in vivo* actions in mice were demonstrated; in particular, CP-55940-induced hypothermia was reversed, and fat mass was reduced, indicating pharmacological possibilities for obesity therapy [64].

10.4.3 Applications of Machine Learning and Deep Learning

10.4.3.1 Application of Deep Learning in Compound Activity and Property Prediction

Machine learning approaches, such as artificial neural networks (ANN), have been used in chemical activity estimations for a long time. As a matter of fact, DL techniques are used to solve the challenge of activity projection in the first place. When the same number of molecular descriptors exist substances, the simplest way is to create models with fully connected deep neural networks (DNNs). On the Merck Kaggle DNN challenge dataset, Dahl *et al.* employed a variety of topological 2D descriptors, and DNN outperformed the traditional RF approach in 13 of the 15 overall goals. The following are the study's key takeaways: DNNs can handle thousands of designators without the need to choose a feature; (ii) drop out can mitigate the well-known overfitting dilemma of traditional ANNs; (iii) hyperparameters (layer numbers, number of nodes per layer, activating function, etc.) can be used to improve DNN productivity; (iv) DNN designs with parallel processing outperform single models with singular activities [55].

Another sort of technique is graph convolution models. This approach is similar to UGRNN in that it employs NNs to automatically produce a molecular vector characterization, and training NNs taught us vector values (Morgan, 1965). The neural fingerprint technique was proposed by Duvenaud *et al.* as one of the first attempts to construct a graph convolution model inspired by the Morgan circular fingerprint method. This method's procedure is depicted in Figure 10.3. To begin, each atom's state matrix is read into the 2D molecular structure, which contains information on its atoms and bonds (depending on the bindings connected to the atom) The State matrix will then be transformed to a molecular description with a fixed-length vector using a single-layer NN. The conflating process may be carried out at several stages by taking into account the inputs of neighboring atoms, which are comparable to circular fingerprints at different adjacent levels. SoftMax initially transforms vectors created by multiple conversion processes before summarizing them as the final vector for the molecule, a neural fingerprint storing information at the molecular level. The neural fingerprints are transmitted across a completely connected NN layer to obtain the final result. Training is used to learn and differentiate the neural fingerprint bit values. Better outcomes have been achieved utilizing neural fingerprints than Morgan fingerprints in the three Duvenaud trials [65].

Most notably, in the graph convolution model, the model may be understood with substantial substructures. The graph convergence model benefits from the automated generation of descriptors during training and the absence of predefined molecular descriptors. Such a descriptor is not a broad descriptor but has certain duties and can be distinguished completely.

10.4.3.2 Application of Deep Learning in Biological Imaging Analysis

During the drug development phase, from preclinical research and innovation to clinical trials the biological imaging and image analysis are frequently employed. Imagery permits scholars to observe phototypes and activities of

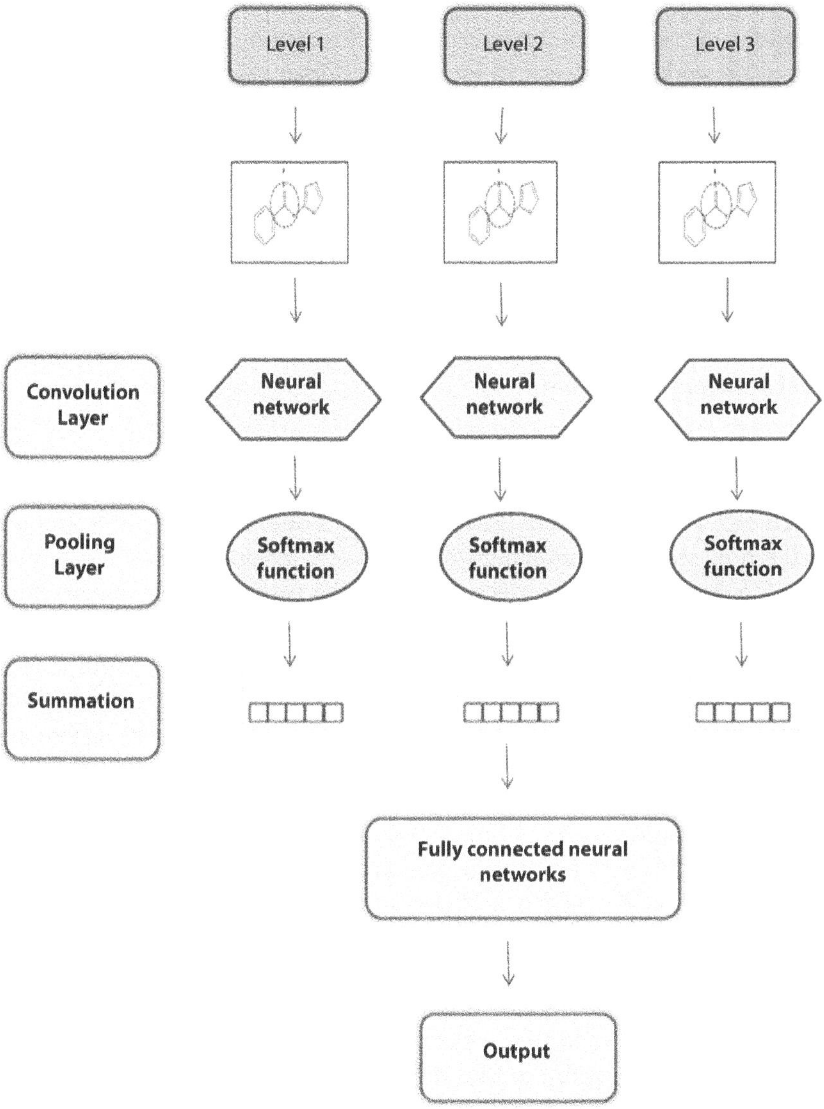

Figure 10.4 Illustration graph of convolutional neural networks (CNNs).

individuals, species, organs, cells, and subcellular components. Digital image analysis reveals underlying biology and disease and the mechanism of the medicine. Fluorescent or nonlabel pictures, CT, MRI, tomography (PET), Imaging of tissue pathology, imagery of mass spectrometry metrology image imaging modalities (MSI). DL has also been successful in biological image processing, with several studies demonstrating that it outperforms traditional pictures. For microscopic pictures, CNNs were utilized for segmenting and subtyping individual fluorescent cells (Figure 10.4), as well as unlabeled images using phase contract microscopy. Illustration graph of convolutional neural networks are shown in Figure 10.4. Other previously tedious activities, such as cell tracking colony counts, might be automated using DL in preclinical settings. Because of the tissue's rich shape, tissue pathology pictures are generally more complicated than fluorescence images. Individual cells were segmented and categorized at the cellular level in breast and colon tissue stained with hematoxylin and eosin (H&E). At the tissue area level, DL detected H&E-stained tumor tissue regions, as well as additional leucocyte and fat tissue categories. DL was previously utilized beyond the primary division of the picture to diagnose histological H&E and stem tissue immunohistochemistry [66–68].

10.4.3.3 Future Development of Deep Learning in Drug Discovery

Machine learning and deep learning methods often require a large amount of learning material; nevertheless, only a few instances allow the human brain to comprehend. As a result, one of the trendiest issues in machine learning is how to learn with very little data. A correspondent network, for example, was presented as a shot learning alternative for exploiting subsidiary data to enhance a model with only a few data points. The findings were enhanced when the supplementary data were provided. Medicinal chemists frequently work toward novel goals with minimal evidence, and approaches like One-Shot Learning are useful in drug development. Altae-Tran *et al.* employed the LSTM approach with chemoinformatic datasets to create models with a simple training framework and showed promising results. In DL, a new form of architecture called neural networks enhanced memory has recently been employed. In the original incarnation, it was a Turing neural machine. This architecture was greatly enhanced with the use of a differentiable neural computer (DNC). DNCs were used to solve a variety of issues, including answering questions and finding the shortest path in graphs. However, until today, these sophisticated designs had not been employed in drug discovery [69–71].

10.5 Applications of Transcriptomic and Artificial Intelligence Techniques for Drug Discovery

In drug development, machine learning models and biosynthetic gene clusters (BGCs) are becoming extremely helpful, particularly for target selection. Conventional specific molecular clinical research is a high-level procedure in which clinical objectives are defined and objectives with a molecule to change a biochemical pathway and for the interest of a therapeutic process are identified and targets with a molecule (for example, a receptor agonist). This procedure's therapeutic effects have been established. This procedure necessitates a great deal of trial and error before the final molecule is deemed a viable, clinically tested therapeutic candidate. Due to their association with illness conditions, BGCs and their natural products might be viewed as beginning factors for selection of treatment goals (e.g. natural recettes), via data analyses (i.e., reverse translation). The analytically determined natural compounds can guide object tracking and can be validated in silicone by quantitative surveillance. The aim to further build alongside this collection of prediction and validation stages may be viewed as a functional BGC screen. A "functional metabolic gene group" is defined in Figure 10.5 to facilitate drug development in the machine learning field. This workflow describes the method by which the biosynthetic gene cluster (BGC) and the consequent natural product is the plumbing compound. The approach begins with identifying the BGCs related with illness disorders in microbiome data sets (blue). The BGC-derived natural product is purified (violet) to determine if the natural product is linked with the disease phenotype (red). Hit the validated molecule can help to build and perform target tests to identify appropriate drug molecules or if the natural product is not a reasonable drug hit When natural product is not a reasonable product (orange). The molecular hits will ultimately turn into (yellow) plumbing compounds for clinical testing. This chart illustrates high-level development pharmaceutical (left) phases and opportunities for machine learning and improvement (right) [72–74].

A new, provocative method to identify the action mechanisms of poorly understood drugs or other bioactive compounds can be helpful through a new approach in a therapeutic objective, and pathway finding called forward pharmacology. The approach incorporates microarrays for the measurement of changes in m RNA by medicines or other bioactive substances to infer from previously unknown activities (Gerhold *et al.*, 2002). Hughes *et al.* have tracked over 6,000 transcripts in 300 experimental settings,

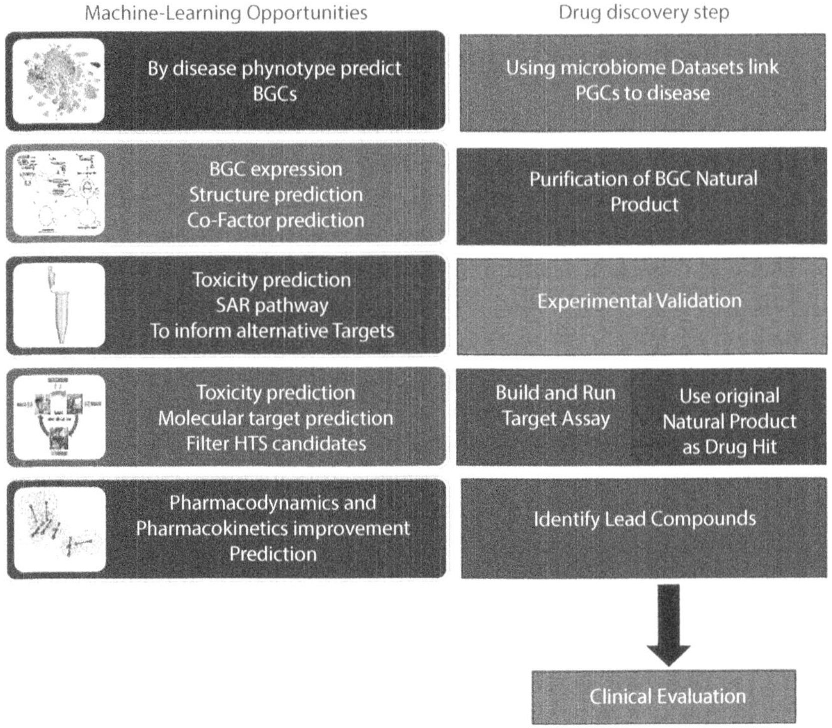

Figure 10.5 Machine learning applications within a "functional biosynthetic gene cluster screen" to facilitate drug discovery.

including 279 gene knockout strains. A reference database was then utilized to assess the impact of many yeast medications on the global profile expressions of those various diseases. Topical dyclonine anesthetic has been used to disrupt the route of the metabolism of ergosterol by using a pattern match. This idea was reinforced by the actions of fenpropimorph and haloperidol on the same route. This example shows the possibility of employing extensive reference databases to identify pharmacological effects, which are generally manifested as direct and indirect changes in mRNA expression (Bataille *et al.*, 2000). The technique of RNA-Seq has been used in drug discovery and development. It is capable of detecting drug-related genes, microRNAs, and fusion proteins. The identification of potentially therapeutic genes is a key issue in drug development. RNA-Seq is a potent method for studying genome-wide changes in drug-induced gene expression. As a result, the technique enables the determination of drug global transcriptions and greatly accelerates the process of drug target identification. Kim *et al.* employed RNA-Seq to investigate the norfloxacin resistance mechanism of the soil bacteria *Acinetobacter oleivorans*. Norfloxacin's effects on the transcriptome of *A. oleivorans* were identified. According to RNA-Seq, 418 genes were differentially expressed by more than twice in norfloxacin-treated cells compared to untreated cells. Norfloxacin was discovered to significantly upregulate genes involved in the SOS response and DNA repair. These pathways may play a role in *A. oleivorans*' norfloxacin resistance [75].

Artificial intelligence in medicine is gaining popularity at the moment. CAD for colonoscopy is the most explored topic in the field of gastrointestinal endoscopy, despite the fact that it is still in the preclinical stage. Colonoscopy is faulty by definition since it is performed by humans. With CAD assistance, the quality of automated polyp detection and characterization (i.e., predicting the pathophysiology of the polyp) is expected to increase. It may aid endoscopists in avoiding missed polyps and providing an accurate visual assessment for those that are discovered. Furthermore, the functions provided by CAD may result in a higher adenoma detection rate and a lower cost of polypectomy for hyperplastic polyps [76].

10.6 Conclusion and Perspectives

RNA-Seq technique has fundamentally transformed how scientists study the transcriptome. It can not only identify the precise expression levels of thousands of genes at the same time, but it can also discover new transcripts, miRNAs, and fusion genes. Other transcriptome approaches, like as expression microarray, can help with drug research, but advancements in this technology will provide important information on drug-target interactions. As sequencing capabilities and bioinformatics analytic tools increase, RNA-Seq will become a critical method in current drug discovery and development. NGS is also a promising tool for studying small RNAs. Using NGS, a general investigation of miRNA in acute myeloid leukemia was done, yielding unique findings of differently indicated miRNAs. Transcriptome sequencing with Illumina and 454 technologies has also shown to be an effective method for detecting new gene fusions in tissues and cancer cell lines.

In cancer diseases, AI approaches, particularly ML and DL, are making significant progress. Several related researchers reported that AI outperformed traditional statistical methods. Despite various limits and roadblocks in AI, such as a lack of well-annotated data and model interpretability, AI will change the diagnosis and prognosis of cancer in the near future, thanks to its efficient processing capacity and learning competency.

AI will arise in a variety of stomach cancer domains due to its processing strength and learning potential. The impact of disease features, psychological, and physiological states of patients and even social communication on the prognosis of stomach cancer patients are being increasingly recognized. Physicians find it challenging to integrate complex data manually. However, because of some ethical and safety concerns, experienced physicians must evaluate and interpret the predictions made by AI. As a result, AI techniques will not wholly replace physicians in clinical practice in the future, and combining humans and AI can achieve the optimum condition of increased efficiency.

References

1. Jimenez-Garcia, S.N., Vazquez-Cruz, M.A., Guevara-Gonzalez, R.G., Torres-Pacheco, I., Cruz-Hernandez, A., Feregrino-Perez, A.A., Current approaches for enhanced expression of secondary metabolites as bioactive compounds in plants for agronomic and human health purposes - A review. *Polish J. Food Nutr. Sci.*, 63, 67, 2013.
2. Gokoglu, N., Novel natural food preservatives and applications in seafood preservation: A review. *J. Sci. Food Agric.*, 99, 2068, 2019.
3. Septembre-Malaterre, A., Remize, F., Poucheret, P., Fruits and vegetables, as a source of nutritional compounds and phytochemicals: Changes in bioactive compounds during lactic fermentation. *Food Res. Int.*, 104, 86, 2018.
4. Winklhofer-Roob, B.M., Faustmann, G., Roob, J.M., Low-density lipoprotein oxidation biomarkers in human health and disease and effects of bioactive compounds. *Free Radic. Biol. Med.*, 111, 38, 2017.
5. Chen, L., Gnanaraj, C., Arulselvan, P., El-Seedi, H., Teng, H., A review on advanced microencapsulation technology to enhance bioavailability of phenolic compounds: Based on its activity in the treatment of Type 2 Diabetes. *Trends Food Sci. Technol.*, 85, 149, 2019.
6. Saucedo-Pompa, S., Torres-Castillo, J.A., Castro-López, C., Rojas, R., Sánchez-Alejo, E.J., Ngangyo-Heya, M., Martínez-Ávila, G.C.G., Moringa plants: Bioactive compounds and promising applications in food products. *Food Res. Int.*, 111, 438, 2018.
7. Issue, I.T., Newsletter of the Mycological Society of America At the grave of William Alphonso Yeast Diversity Studied from the Gut of Australian Passalid Beetles. *Mycologia.*, 63, 277, 2012.
8. Zhan, X., Luo, X., He, J., Zhang, C., Liao, X., Xu, X., Feng, S., Yu, C., Jiang, Z., Meng, Y., Shen, C., Bioactive compounds induced in Physalis angulata L. by methyl-jasmonate: An investigation of compound accumulation patterns and biosynthesis-related candidate genes. *Plant Mol. Biol.*, 103, 341, 2020.

9. Sellwood, M.A., Ahmed, M., Segler, M.H.S., Brown, N., Artificial intelligence in drug discovery. *Future Med. Chem.*, 10, 2025, 2018.
10. Jiménez-Luna, J., Grisoni, F., Schneider, G., Drug discovery with explainable artificial intelligence. *Nat. Mach. Intell.*, 2, 573, 2020.
11. Öztürk, H., Özgür, A., Ozkirimli, E., DeepDTA: Deep drug-target binding affinity prediction. *Bioinformatics*, 34, i821, 2018.
12. Llorent-Martinez, E.J., Ruiz-Riaguas, A., Sinan, K.I., Bene, K., Fernández-de Cordova, M.L., Picot-Allain, C., Mahomoodally, F., Saleem, H., Zengin, G., Exploring chemical profiles and bioactivities of Harungana madagascariensis Lam. ex Poir. leaves and stem bark extracts: A new source of procyanidins. *Anal. Lett.*, 53, 399, 2020.
13. Cornara, L., Biagi, M., Xiao, J., Burlando, B., Therapeutic properties of bioactive compounds from different honeybee products. *Front. Pharmacol.*, 8, 1, 2017.
14. Moldovan, M.L., Carpa, R., Fizeşan, I., Vlase, L., Bogdan, C., Iurian, S.M., Benedec, D., Pop, A., Phytochemical profile and biological activities of tendrils and leaves extracts from a variety of vitis vinifera l. *Antioxidants.*, 9, 1, 2020.
15. Chiorcea-Paquim, A.M., Enache, T.A., De Souza Gil, E., Oliveira-Brett, A.M., Natural phenolic antioxidants electrochemistry: Towards a new food science methodology. *Compr. Rev. Food Sci. Food Saf.*, 19, 1680, 2020.
16. Gutiérrez-Grijalva, E.P., Picos-Salas, M.A., Leyva-López, N., Criollo-Mendoza, M.S., Vazquez-Olivo, G., Heredia, J.B., Flavonoids and phenolic acids from Oregano: Occurrence, biological activity and health benefits. *Plants.*, 7, 1, 2018.
17. Roupe, K., Remsberg, C., Yanez, J., Davies, N., Pharmacometrics of Stilbenes: Seguing Towards the Clinic. *Curr. Clin. Pharmacol.*, 1, 81, 2008.
18. Clifford, M.N., Nature, Anthocyanins -, dietary burden., *J. Sci. Food Agric.*, 80, 1063, 2000.
19. Dhiman, A., Nanda, A., Ahmad, S., A quest for staunch effects of flavonoids: Utopian protection against hepatic ailments. *Arab. J. Chem.*, 9, S1813, 2016.
20. Barreca, D., Gattuso, G., Bellocco, E., Calderaro, A., Trombetta, D., Smeriglio, A., Laganà, G., Daglia, M., Meneghini, S., Nabavi, S.M., Flavanones: Citrus phytochemical with health-promoting properties. *BioFactors.*, 43, 495, 2017.
21. De Pascual-Teresa, S. and Sanchez-Ballesta, M.T., Anthocyanins: From plant to health. *Phytochem. Rev.*, 7, 281, 2008.
22. Hagerman, A.E. and Butler, L.G., The specificity of proanthocyanidin-protein interactions. *J. Biol. Chem.*, 256, 4494, 1981.
23. Burgos, S., Bohorquez, D.V., Burgos, S.A., Vitamin deficiency-induced neurological diseases of poultry. *Int. J. Poult. Sci.*, 5, 804, 2006.
24. Korhonen, H. and Pihlanto, A., Food-derived bioactive peptides-opportunities for designing future foods. *Curr. Pharm. Des.*, 9, 1297, 2003.
25. Udenigwe, C.C. and Aluko, R.E., Food protein-derived bioactive peptides: Production, processing, and potential health benefits. *J. Food Sci.*, 77, R11, 2012.

26. Lowe, R., Shirley, N., Bleackley, M., Dolan, S., Shafee, T., Transcriptomics technologies. *PloS Comput. Biol.*, 13, e1005457, 2017.
27. Shaw, R., Tian, X., Xu, J., Single-cell transcriptome analysis in plants: Advances and challenges. *Mol. Plant*, 14, 115, 2020.
28. Pollina, E.A., *Chromatin and Transcriptional Regulation of Cell Identity and Aging*, Stanford University, 28119887, 2015.
29. Fu, S., Ma, Y., Yao, H., Xu, Z., Chen, S., Song, J., Au, K.F., IDP-denovo: *De novo* transcriptome assembly and isoform annotation by hybrid sequencing. *Bioinformatics.*, 34, 2168, 2018.
30. Grabherr, M.G., Haas, B.J., Yassour, M., Levin, J.Z., Thompson, D.A., Amit, I., Adiconis, X., Fan, L., Raychowdhury, R., Zeng, Q., Chen, Z., Full-length transcriptome assembly from RNA-Seq data without a reference genome. *Nat. Biotechnol.*, 29, 644, 2011.
31. Puglia, G.D., Prjibelski, A.D., Vitale, D., Bushmanova, E., Schmid, K.J., Raccuia, S.A., Hybrid transcriptome sequencing approach improved assembly and gene annotation in Cynara cardunculus (L.). *BMC Genomics*, 21, 1, 2020.
32. Wu, C., Wyatt, A.W., Lapuk, A.V., McPherson, A., McConeghy, B.J., Bell, R.H., Anderson, S., Haegert, A., Brahmbhatt, S., Shukin, R., Mo, F., Integrated genome and transcriptome sequencing identifies a novel form of hybrid and aggressive prostate cancer. *J. Pathol.*, 227, 53, 2012.
33. Brazma, A., Hingamp, P., Quackenbush, J., Sherlock, G., Spellman, P., Stoeckert, C., Aach, J., Ansorge, W., Ball, C.A., Causton, H.C., Gaasterland, T., Minimum information about a microarray experiment (MIAME) - Toward standards for microarray data. *Nat. Genet.*, 29, 365, 2001.
34. Templin, M.F., Stoll, D., Schrenk, M., Traub, P.C., Vöhringer, C.F., Joos, T.O., Protein microarray technology. *Drug Discovery*, 7, 815, 2002.
35. Stears, R. L., Martinsky, T., Schena, M., Trends in microarray analysis. *Nature Med.*, 9, 1, 2003.
36. Conesa, A., Madrigal, P., Tarazona, S., Gomez-Cabrero, D., Cervera, A., McPherson, A., Szcześniak, M.W., Gaffney, D.J., Elo, L.L., Zhang, X., A survey of best practices for RNA-seq data analysis. *Genome Biol.*, 17, 1, 2016.
37. De Wit, P., Pespeni, M.H., Ladner, J.T., Barshis, D.J., Seneca, F., Jaris, H., Therkildsen, N.O., Morikawa, M., Palumbi, S.R., The simple fool's guide to population genomics via RNA-Seq: An introduction to high-throughput sequencing data analysis. *Mol. Ecol. Resour.*, 12, 1058, 2012.
38. Kang, S.H., Lee, J.Y., Lee, T.H., Park, S.Y., Kim, C.K., *De novo* transcriptome assembly of the Chinese pearl barley, adlay, by full-length isoform and short-read RNA sequencing. *PloS One*, 13, 1, 2018.
39. Luo, H., Zhu, Y., Song, J., Xu, L., Sun, C., Zhang, X., Xu, Y., He, L., Sun, W., Xu, H., Wang, B., Transcriptional data mining of Salvia miltiorrhiza in response to methyl jasmonate to examine the mechanism of bioactive compound biosynthesis and regulation. *Physiol. Plant*, 152, 241, 2014.

40. Lateef, A., Prabhudas, S.K., Natarajan, P., RNA sequencing and *de novo* assembly of Solanum trilobatum leaf transcriptome to identify putative transcripts for major metabolic pathways. *Sci. Rep.*, 8, 1, 2018.
41. Kukurba, K.R. and Montgomery, S.B., RNA sequencing and analysis. *Cold Spring Harb. Protoc.*, 11, 951, 2015.
42. Rathi, B.S., Kumar, P.S., Show, P.-L., A review on effective removal of emerging contaminants from aquatic systems: Current trends and scope for further research. *J. Hazard. Mater.*, 409, 124413, 2021.
43. Gupta, R., Srivastava, D., Sahu, M., Tiwari, S., Ambasta, R.K., Kumar, P., Artificial intelligence to deep learning: Machine intelligence approach for drug discovery. *Mol. Divers.*, 25, 3, 2021.
44. Young, K., Reliability and Validity of a Locally Designed Rating Scale: The Case of a Czech Business College, 2021.
45. Hu, Y., Lu, Y., Wang, S., Zhang, M., Qu, X., Niu, B., Application of machine learning approaches for the design and study of anticancer drugs. *Curr. Drug Targets.*, 20, 488, 2019.
46. Zhang, L., Tan, J., Han, D., Zhu, H., From machine learning to deep learning: Progress in machine intelligence for rational drug discovery. *Drug Discovery Today*, 22, 1680, 2017.
47. Feinstein, W.P. and Brylinski, M., Calculating an optimal box size for ligand docking and virtual screening against experimental and predicted binding pockets. *J. Cheminform.*, 7, 1, 2015.
48. Afolabi, L.T., Saeed, F., Hashim, H., Petinrin, O.O., Ensemble learning method for the prediction of new bioactive molecules. *PloS One*, 13, 1, 2018.
49. Vedani, A. and Dobler, M., Multi-dimensional QSAR in drug research. *Prog. Drug Res.*, 105, 135, 2000.
50. Prihoda, D., Maritz, J.M., Klempir, O., Dzamba, D., Woelk, C.H., Hazuda, D.J., Bitton, D.A., Hannigan, G.D., The application potential of machine learning and genomics for understanding natural product diversity, chemistry, and therapeutic translatability. *Nat. Prod. Rep.*, 38, 1100, 2021.
51. Liu, Z., Du, J., Fang, J., Yin, Y., Xu, G., Xie, L., *DeepScreening: A deep learning-based screening web server for accelerating drug discovery*, vol. 1, Database, baz104, 2019.
52. Esteva, A., Robicquet, A., Ramsundar, B., Kuleshov, V., DePristo, M., Chou, K., Cui, C., Corrado, G., Thrun, S., Dean, J., A guide to deep learning in healthcare. *Nat. Med.*, 25, 24, 2019.
53. Arnold, L., Rebecchi, S., Chevallier, S., Paugam-Moisy, H., An introduction to deep learning. *ESANN 2011 - 19th Eur. Symp. Artif. Neural Networks*, vol. 477, 2011.
54. Long, E., Lin, H., Liu, Z., Wu, X., Wang, L., Jiang, J., An, Y., Lin, Z., Li, X., Chen, J., Li, J., An artificial intelligence platform for the multihospital collaborative management of congenital cataracts. *Nat. Biomed. Eng.*, 1, 1, 2017.

55. Ma, J., Sheridan, R.P., Liaw, A., Dahl, G.E., Svetnik, V., Deep neural nets as a method for quantitative structure-activity relationships. *J. Chem. Inf. Model.*, 55, 263, 2015.
56. Jing, Y., Bian, Y., Hu, Z., Wang, L., Xie, X.Q.S., Deep learning for drug design: An artificial intelligence paradigm for drug discovery in the big data era. *AAPS J.*, 20, 3, 2018.
57. Hanrahan, G., *Artificial neural networks in biological and environmental analysis*, CRC Press.
58. Shin, M., Jang, D., Nam, H., Lee, K.H., Lee, D., Predicting the absorption potential of chemical compounds through a deep learning approach. *IEEE/ACM Trans. Comput. Biol. Bioinforma.*, 15, 432, 2018.
59. Chen, Y., Xie, Y., Song, L., Chen, F., Tang, T., A survey of accelerator architectures for deep neural networks. *Engineering*, 6, 264, 2020.
60. Lavecchia, A., Deep learning in drug discovery: opportunities, challenges and future prospects. *Drug Discovery Today*, 24, 2017, 2019.
61. Schneider, G., Hartenfeller, M., Reutlinger, M., Tanrikulu, Y., Proschak, E., Schneider, P., Voyages to the (un) known: adaptive design of bioactive compounds. *Trends Biotechnol.*, 27, 18, 2009.
62. Walter, M. and Stark, H., Histamine receptor subtypes: A century of rational drug design. *Front. Biosci (Schol Ed)*, 4, 461, 2012.
63. Heikkilä, T., Thirumalairajan, S., Davies, M., Parsons, M.R., McConkey, A.G., Fishwick, C.W.G., Johnson, A.P., The first *de novo* designed inhibitors of Plasmodium falciparum dihydroorotate dehydrogenase. *Bioorganic Med. Chem. Lett.*, 16, 88, 2006.
64. Alig, L., Alsenz, J., Andjelkovic, M., Bendels, S., Bénardeau, A., Bleicher, K., Bourson, A., David-Pierson, P., Guba, W., Hildbrand, S., Kube, D., Benzodioxoles : Novel Cannabinoid-1 receptor inverse agonists for the treatment of obesity. *J. Med. Chem.*, 51, 2115, 2008.
65. Duvenaud, D., Maclaurin, D., Aguilera-Iparraguirre, J., Gómez-Bombarelli, R., Hirzel, T., Aspuru-Guzik, A., Adams, R.P., Convolutional networks on graphs for learning molecular fingerprints. *Adv. Neural Inf. Process. Syst.*, 65, 2224, 2015.
66. Cireşan, D.C., Giusti, A., Gambardella, L.M., Schmidhuber, J., Mitosis detection in breast cancer histology images with deep neural networks. Lect. Notes Comput. Sci. (including Subser. *Lect. Notes Artif. Intell. Lect. Notes Bioinformatics)*, 8150 LNCS, 411, 2013.
67. Kraus, O.Z., Ba, J.L., Frey, B.J., Classifying and segmenting microscopy images with deep multiple instance learning. *Bioinformatics*, 32, i52, 2016.
68. Xu, Y., Mo, T., Feng, Q., Zhong, P., Lai, M., Chang, E.I.C., Deep learning of feature representation with multiple instance learning for medical image analysis. *ICASSP, IEEE Int. Conf. Acoust. Speech Signal Process. - Proc*, vol. 1626, 2014.
69. Graves, A., Wayne, G., Reynolds, M., Harley, T., Danihelka, I., Grabska-Barwińska, A., Colmenarejo, S.G., Grefenstette, E., Ramalho, T., Agapiou, J.,

Badia, A.P., Hybrid computing using a neural network with dynamic external memory. *Nature.*, 538, 471, 2016.
70. Bar, Y., Diamant, I., Wolf, L., Greenspan, H., Deep learning with non-medical training used for chest pathology identification. *Med. Imaging 2015 Comput. Diagnosis.*, 9414, 94140V, 2015.
71. Cheng, J.Z., Ni, D., Chou, Y.H., Qin, J., Tiu, C.M., Chang, Y.C., Huang, C.S., Shen, D., Chen, C.M., Computer-aided diagnosis with deep learning architecture: Applications to breast lesions in us images and pulmonary Nodules in CT Scans. *Sci. Rep.*, 6, 1, 2016.
72. Hannigan, G.D., Prihoda, D., Palicka, A., Soukup, J., Klempir, O., Rampula, L., Durcak, J., Wurst, M., Kotowski, J., Chang, D., Wang, R., A deep learning genome-mining strategy for biosynthetic gene cluster prediction. *Nucleic Acids Res.*, 47, e110, 2019.
73. Stokes, J.M., Yang, K., Swanson, K., Jin, W., Cubillos-Ruiz, A., Donghia, N.M., MacNair, C.R., French, S., Carfrae, L.A., Bloom-Ackermann, Z., Tran, V.M., A deep learning approach to antibiotic discovery. *Cell.*, 180, 688, 2020.
74. Du, J., Jia, P., Dai, Y., Tao, C., Zhao, Z., Zhi, D., Gene2vec: Distributed representation of genes based on co-expression. *BMC Genomics*, 20, 1, 2019.
75. Kim, D. and Salzberg, S.L., TopHat-Fusion: An algorithm for discovery of novel fusion transcripts. *Genome Biol.*, 12, 8, 2011.
76. Kudo, S. ei, Mori, Y., Misawa, M., Takeda, K., Kudo, T., Itoh, H., Oda, M., Mori, K., Artificial intelligence and colonoscopy: Current status and future perspectives. *Dig. Endosc.*, 31, 363, 2019.
77. Hartenfeller, M., Proschak, E., Schüller, A., Schneider, G., Concept of combinatorial *de novo* design of drug-like molecules by particle swarm optimization. *Chem. Biol. Drug Des.*, 72, 16, 2008.
78. Pegg, S.C.H., Haresco, J.J., Kuntz, I.D., A genetic algorithm for structure-based *de novo* design. *J. Comput. Aided. Mol. Des.*, 15, 911, 2001.
79. Glen, R.C. and Payne, A.W.R., A genetic algorithm for the automated generation of molecules within constraints. *J. Comput. Aided. Mol. Des.*, 9, 181, 1995.
80. Vinkers, H.M., De Jonge, M.R., Daeyaert, F.F.D., Heeres, J., Koymans, L.M.H., Van Lenthe, J.H., Lewi, P.J., Timmerman, H., Van Aken, K., Janssen, P.A.J., SYNOPSIS: SYNthesize and OPti mize System *in Silico*. *J. Med. Chem.*, 46, 2765, 2003.
81. Dey, F. and Caflisch, A., Fragment-based *de novo* ligand design by multiobjective evolutionary optimization. *Supporting Information. J. Chem. Inf. Model.*, 48, 679, 2008.
82. Douguet, D., Thoreau, E., Grassy, G.A., genetic algorithm for the automated generation of small organic molecules: Drug design using an evolutionary algorithm. *J. Comput. Aided. Mol. Des.*, 14, 449, 2000.
83. Schneider, G., Schrödl, W., Wallukat, G., Müller, J., Nissen, E., Rönspeck, W., Wrede, P., Kunze, R., Peptide design by artificial neural networks and computer-based evolutionary search. *Proc. Natl. Acad. Sci. U. S. A.*, 95, 12179, 1998.

11

Prediction of Drug Toxicity Through Machine Learning

Ariga Gharabeiki, Foad Monemian and Ali Kargari*

Membrane Processes Research Laboratory (MPRL), Department of Chemical Engineering, Amirkabir University of Technology, Tehran, Iran

Abstract
Advances in related technologies and techniques have led to advances in many different fields of science and technology. Machine learning has become an essential tool for planning medication and discovering bit knowledge from massive databases. This chapter provides doable reviews on drug discovery through ml tools and techniques. It's applied at each stage of drug development to expedite the analysis method, cost of clinical trials, and infer risk. Nowadays, software based on machine learning science has provided the possibility of a deeper analysis of data in medicine. Also, by looking at all the stages of drug discovery, it can be concluded how this new method has given purposeful organization to pharmacy science.

***Keywords*:** Machine learning, pharmaceutical, AI technology, drug

11.1 Introduction

Over the past years, improved efficient and advanced systems have purposefully provided the foremost efficient service operators. The most important factors affecting drug discovery are the discussion of cost and time, which minimizes these two parameters by using artificial intelligence and deep learning methods [1]. Researchers worldwide have stirred to process approaches like virtual screening (VS) and molecular binding, conjointly called typical approaches. Be that because it could, these procedures

**Corresponding author*: kargari@aut.ac.ir; Ali_kargari@yahoo.com

Inamuddin, Tariq Altalhi, Jorddy N. Cruz and Moamen Salah El-Deen Refat (eds.) Drug Design Using Machine Learning, (319–338) © 2022 Scrivener Publishing LLC

conjointly impose challenges like quality and wastefulness. Hence, there is a surge in novel techniques independent of killing the impediments practiced in typical process approaches. Due to the advancement of computer science, many methods for providing models for existing data have grown significantly, including machine learning (ML) and deep learning (DL). The purpose of defining data modeling methods is to present computations as a possible solution, which can solve failures and overcome barriers to drug discovery [2].

Drug discovery and planning have various stages which are complex and time-consuming. The steps are target determination, functional screening and optimization of lead composition, fabrication, and clinical trials [3]. During these stages, there are challenges that researchers have overcome in recent years. Early progress was made in 1950 with turning tests. In this first step, computer methods in pharmaceutical discovery science were examined for the first time to optimize data analysis. In this regard, the original AIM NIH Main Workshop demonstrated the importance of computer science in medicine in 1975 [4].

In different words, factory-made neural networks and profound learning calculations need to modernize this region. DP and ML algorithms are enforced in many drug discovery categories containing modeling, pharmacophores, structure and polypharmacology, and little activities amendment the standing of the drug [5]. Additionally, new data management techniques are essential to creating modeling calculations. Computer science and profound knowledge of improvements deliver an excellent chance for drug style and discovery in precis, eventually impacting humanity [6]. Consumption time and costar are the foremost vital considerations associated with drug style and development.

Additionally, factors that inhibit drug delivery and development are unskillfulness, incorrect target delivery, and improper dosing. Computer-aided drug style integrates computer science algorithms with advancements in technology to eliminate ancient drug styles and technology developments [7, 8].

In addition, deep learning, which is one of the sub-branches of a set of machine learning, has been widely applied in the development of medicine [9]. Examples of modeling methods for data classification are drug detection algorithms that include artificial neural networks, deep neural networks, and support vector machines (SVMs). All plans have been used to classify and find appropriate regression of data [10]. Computer technology has gained a foothold in various pharmaceutical fields for improvement, such as amide synthesis to molecular style, digital screening to molecular drug design, quantitative structural correlation with modification of drug function, and removal of the inflexibility of molecular structure in protein cross-pathway. Protein is used in molecular to polypharmacology. Computer science concepts are implemented to classify active and inactive, monitor drug unharness, diagnose and clinical improvement, and primary and second drug screening and biomarkers [11].

Computer science uses engineering to train data by finding connections between data according to machine learning patterns to give researchers valuable results that pave the way for drug discovery. Artificial intelligence (AI) is a data modeling method with various applications, such as finding algorithms to decode and retrieve data. The algorithm also has various capabilities such as pattern recognition, finding applied mathematical relationships, and representing statistical information. Application of multiple strategies such as fuzzy models and neural networks (a process for predicting other data) will be provided. Other advanced applications of this algorithm that can be mentioned are classification, regression, predictions, and data optimization techniques. For any sort of info, machine learning should be modified; for instance, initially, a particular model should be beside the parameters. Therefore, machines will use trained knowledge to master the model with offered parameters [12].

Moreover, the model will predict the knowledge/info for recovering information from data. Recently, there has been a great deal of interest in using machine learning techniques in pharmacy. At each stage, organizing the Mojo data and finding connections can have good therapeutic consequences. With collected data, the appropriate steps that indicate repetition can be avoided, which causes reducing the time and cost of discovery. In the science of drug discovery, each step must be validated to demonstrate the effectiveness of the treatment to discover the possibility of entering the next step. In medical knowledge, these algorithms give the power to extract useful information and are evaluated using several intelligent and accurate automation tools. To deploy any sort of drug within the pharmaceutical trade, machine learning strategies are explored. At this time, if enhancements within the knowledge set seem as size in the course of unlimited storage, varieties will give premises to machine learning. This approach will access Brobdingnagian knowledge from the pharmaceutical trade. Knowledge varieties will have different configurations, like matter knowledge, images, sensing info, biometrics, and high-dimensional omics knowledge. Thus, the sphere of computer science has evolved from theoretical data to real-world knowledge. Information has been widely improved in hardware, such as the GPU, which quickens the process. The deep learning model could be a quite machine learning algorithmic rule. This model develops for more considerable success in daylight challenges. The employment of ML algorithms is widespread in pharmaceutical firms [13].

Within the clinical field, making a drug for determined malady trusted modern medicines. As of late, different medications are ad-libbed to recognize energetic parts from ancient drugs like antibiotics. In chemical laboratories, it contains common substances, very few atoms that facilitate useful drugs determine substances like cells or intaglio organisms named from an old-style medical specialty. As a result of the human ordination has allowed ways to simulate and refine proteins in massive quantities, dynamic screening has become commonplace with many libraries. Screening activity of enormous compounds through biological targets can amend an unwellness referred to as reverse medical specialty [14].

Researchers have used the CADD technique to help organize existing data [15]. Synthetic strategies for molecular properties (i.e., specificity, distribution, adsorption, biological activity, metabolism, aspect effects, and excretion at theoretical levels) are first defined for modeling using this method in drug discovery. Then the lead compounds are defined as Reports ideal properties in silica as the results of the algorithm. Also, the power of these algorithms is the simultaneous communication and review of input data and thus the accuracy of output results. Therefore, several pharmaceutical industries have shown a great desire to participate in technologies, which have made the discovery process shorter and more accurate by using these methods [16]. Finally, this summary proposes AI ways at intervals the sedate revelation vary for that specialize in totally different applications in sedate revelation and advancement by utilizing profound learning procedures. On these lines, the AI field offers anticipated results regarding process intelligence in medicating improvement and discovery. Machine learning algorithms, pharmaceutical development pipelines style are often, for the most part, automatic. These pipelines could guide or accelerate drug discovery, give a higher understanding of diseases and connected biological phenomena, and facilitate preclinical tests during a wet laboratory and even future clinical trials. This automation of the drug development method could also be the key to the low productivity rates that pharmaceutical firms face [17].

Machine learning has influenced many tasks in cheminformatics and modeling, which can be referred to as synthesis designing, toxicity diagnosis, and screening in virtual. Computer science has been extensively employed healthfully in drug design fields. ML needs a set of computer science, and machine learning relies on developing exposure models to academic knowledge. Nowadays, machine learning is often used with numerous knowledge varieties and strategies, like imaging, protein structures, rather than being restricted to antecedently sure knowledge varieties (e.g., protein compounds and sequences). The employment of ML to find medication has attracted the attention of many pharmacists. This algorithmic rule uses pattern recognition, mathematical relationships between experimental observations of tiny molecules, and their extrapolation to predict new compounds' chemical, biological, and physical properties. Achieving results is promising in this method. Machine learning techniques are more employed in massive knowledge sets without processing resources than the physical model [16]. The qualities of AI approaches acceptable for drug development and discovery have been considered.

11.2 Drug Discovery

Drug discovery could be a method that aims at distinctive a compound therapeutically valuable for curing and treating unwellness. This method is selected following a synthetic molecule or a biomolecule as a potential drug candidate for comprehensive analysis. The most crucial issue in pharmaceutical business management is to avoid the risks associated with drug discovery and development. In addition, limited-time should be taken for patents and their general replacement so that the profits and successive growth of the pharmaceutical business are not harmed. Given these conditions, a method to reduce investment and innovative analysis was considered by researchers. The concern of replacing the old drug discovery methods is to minimize the adverse environmental effects of prescription drugs and to provide clear guidelines by government pharmaceutical organizations to ensure that the necessary measures are taken and reduce the side effects of this strategy [18]. The new drug development method should continue through many stages to create a safe, effective drug and has approved all restrictive needs. One overall concern is that the process is sufficiently long, complex, and expensive. Several biological targets should be considered for every modern drug eventually supported for clinical use, and alternative fact-finding tools could also be needed to explore every new target. In general, the modern drug discovery method includes distinctive the unwellness for treatment and unmet medical wants, choosing a variable molecular target and confirmatory it, developing a laboratory technique for high-throughput screening of hybrid versus target libraries to spot strokes, and optimization for the assembly of lead compounds that exhibit spare efficiency and property for biological functions *in vitro* and unwellness animal models. Consequently, lead compounds are more optimized to enhance their effectiveness and materia medica before drug

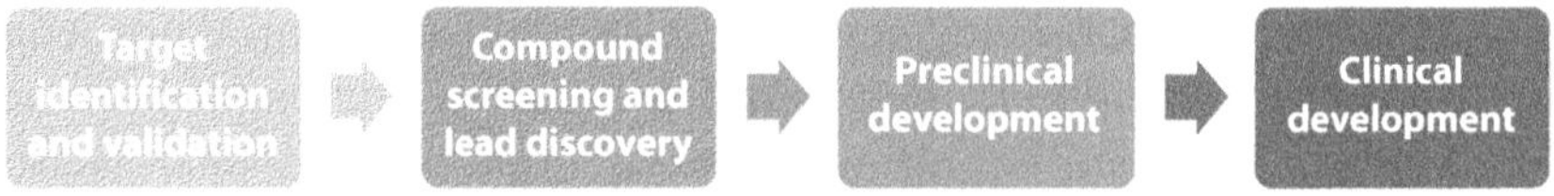
Target identification and validation
Compound screening and lead discovery
Preclinical development
Clinical development

Figure 11.1 Steps of drug discovery.

development. The drug development method is often divided into diagnosing and clinical development stages [19].

In addition, studies are being conducted on the efficient processes required to produce a new drug and present its best formulation. It is assumed that the new drug is sufficiently effective and safe in the preclinical analysis phase. In this case, drug-limiting organizations can initiate clinical development to evaluate the new drug's effectiveness by pilot and pilot studies [20]. From initial discovery to the generation of an attractive drug could also be a long and challenging trip. One million molecules are screened on average. However, only one is explored in late-stage clinical trials and is finally offered for patients. This text provides a quick layout of recent drug revelation and improvement processes. Drug discovery could be a diverse method involving distinctive a drug chemical therapeutically valuable for treating and managing unwellness. Typically, researchers realize new medication through new visions into an unwellness method that allows the investigator to style drugs to prevent or contrary the consequences of the unwellness. Drug discovery and development are expensive because of the high allow analysis and development and clinical trials. It takes close to tens of years to develop a replacement drug molecule, from the time it's discovered to once it's offered on the market to treat patients [21]. The steps to find a drug are shown in Figure 11.1, which describe in the following.

11.2.1 Target Identification

Identifying the goal is the first step in this process. Even medicine is not mentioned, realizing the objectives is more reliable in this step. The target contains misfolded proteins, DNA mutations, and potential disease biomarkers include the target. Despite identifying targets and working on drug development as possible, drug development is more complex than them. For most medications, this process takes about two-plus years [22].

11.2.2 Lead Discovery: Preclinical

One of the significant steps in the cycle is lead discovery. In this preparation, thousands of compounds that can be effective in improving the disease are screened. Through this method, the activity of potential compounds affecting the target is limited. The cycle takes 1 to 2 years in general [23].

11.2.3 Medicinal Chemistry: Preclinical

Employing the restricted combinations in analyzing the intelligence with the targets that caused the infection is the main task of this stage. Using three-dimensional (3D) arrangements of materials and associating their intelligence with illness targets is used in some examinations. Outputs are from the research and advanced optimization towards the targets. The duration of this cycle is from 1-2 years [24].

11.2.4 *In Vitro* Studies

Compounds are filtered and tested in the cellular system for the preclinical stage. By taking place petri dish studies, laboratory researches are started. A drug's success is tested by examining a compound that affects the goal [25].

11.2.5 *In Vivo* Studies

On animal studies, research has been done as follows: compounds moving through the vitreous stage are taken and these compounds examine animals such as rabbits or mice. *In vivo* studies on animals are more outstanding than *in vitro* two-dimensional (2D) cell structure models. However, the failure in this stage is also more remarkable because of the architectural differences in animal models. So, the difference between the laboratory results and *Vivo* results is occurred [25].

11.2.6 Clinical Trials

A combination that demonstrates some reliable specifications is then subjected to clinical trials. For this purpose, human volunteers are chosen and tests performed on them [26].

11.2.7 Food and Drug Administration Approval

Submitting for the FDA approval is the last phase of this cycle. Available for public use in the market with FDA approval. Approved drugs lasted an average of 6.5 years in clinical development from 2005 to 2006, while it was an average of 9.1 years from 2008 to 2012 [3].

After the clinical trial, the drug failure may have happened. Drug failure and a time-consuming process can be frustrating because it takes long periods and huge costs, especially when our successful paths have not been successful enough. Learning from the former experiences and data and helping to unknown parameters omission and reducing bad human effort, cost, and time are some ML benefits in this field [27].

11.3 Drug Design Through New Techniques

Due to their essential role in the planning and discovery of drugs, Computational strategies have caused a change in the whole drug design [18]. However, many issues such as time, computing, and reliability are still less prominent in some situations than in traditional computing methods. Artificial intelligence can overcome all the bottlenecks in the design of computational drugs and lead to the development of drugs by computational methods [28]. In 2019, Schott *et al.* developed a DL science-based algorithm called SchNOrb, which can accurately predict the molecular orbit of organic molecules and wave functions. The properties of molecules are determined by employing these inputs [29]. Therefore, SchNOrb can be an effective aid to researchers in designing new drugs. In addition, molecular dynamics (MD) simulation can analyze the behavior and interaction of molecules at the atomic level.

One of the ways for protein-ligand interaction rating and binding stability is employing the MD simulations in drug discovery, but it is complex and time-consuming, which requires sufficient knowledge and accuracy to work with this method. Artificial intelligence can speed up the MD simulation process. Researchers have found that neural networks are calculated using data with almost similar accuracy and used in MD simulations [30]. MD simulation can be accelerated by ML techniques. However, some training data is required to achieve this purpose. In addition, the design of new drugs in recent years to take advantage of artificial intelligence can design 3D drugs in the form of 3D proteins. One of these methods is

MolAICal. It designs the ability of 3D drugs with two components: (i) the first component is used by the DL algorithm and trained genetics to design new drugs, (ii) the second component is the molecular binding combined and trained by the DL model [31]. Generating new combinations and predicting compound properties are the benefits of a model application. In addition, artificial intelligence has recently been used to improve drug production planning. A DT-based program has been developed to plan a new synthesis method for target molecules [32]. Another way for this purpose is using the ICSYNTH, in which the complex and fast chemical guidelines associated with ML models are occurred in this method [33].

In addition, numerous statistics-driven tools can assist diagnose conventional drugs. Any other technique known as NLP can be used as it should be for brand new analytical insights. NLP is a department of artificial intelligence that lets computer systems system and analyze through artificial intelligence-based algorithms [34]. This approach uses these strategies based on synthetic intelligence. The ability to appropriately examine facts in addition, DisGeNET is an outcomes-primarily based database consisting of a wealth of information about gene-sickness relationships and ailment kinds. Analyzing numerous biological strategies (e.g., harmful drug reactions, pathways of the molecule affect in sickness and the effect of medication on objectives) can be happened by DisGeNET method.

Further, STRING is another database that could provide many statistics about protein interactions by extracting statistics from the statistics [35]. In addition, the stitch is any other textual content-based extraction database that incorporates statistics about the interplay between proteins and chemicals. The STITCH (Search Tool for Interactions of Chemicals) database can also be used to determine drug affinity and the connection among drugs and genes across genomes and their interactions contained in the STRING database. Synthetic intelligence has appeared as a viable solution to the chemical environment of the pharmaceutical enterprise or the classical chemistry matters [36]. Synthetic intelligence algorithms, including ML to DL in software program design (CADD), have expanded with generation and improved high-performance computer systems [37]. However, the primary intention of scientists today is to improve the drug discovery methods and the reliability of classical chemistry activities through ML algorithms methods. It encourages chemists to discover the capacity of artificial intelligence techniques to respond to two vital factors of medicinal chemistry. But, advances have been made in CADD, which has been prioritized as a tool for locating new therapies [37].

11.4 Machine Learning as a Science

Machine learning has brought about fundamental changes by creating changes and improvements in how data is collected, used, and stored in various fields, including engineering and medicine. Different variables are numerical, batch, or related.

These new models can be divided into four categories: regression, classification, correlation, and clustering. According to recent approaches and new applications of machine learning, biological materials such as metals, polymers, and ceramics are examined by ML to predict their properties instant. Prominent candidates in this method can be mentioned: cognitive immutability of data, learning mechanism, innate ability to obtain results, skills, and abstract concepts. One of the exciting developments in this field is that appropriate models are generated in this method, using systems with specific computational science [38].

One of the main goals of machine learning is to discover alternative learning mechanisms, including finding various induction algorithms. In the first step, a set of initial information is required for the learner to provide data through inadequate information training and develop work areas by building workable techniques. Deep learning methods exhibit the relevant results in knowledge and skills gaining. However, it cannot be considered as the only possible way in this regard. Most theoretical work in machine learning focuses on creating, describing, and analyzing existing

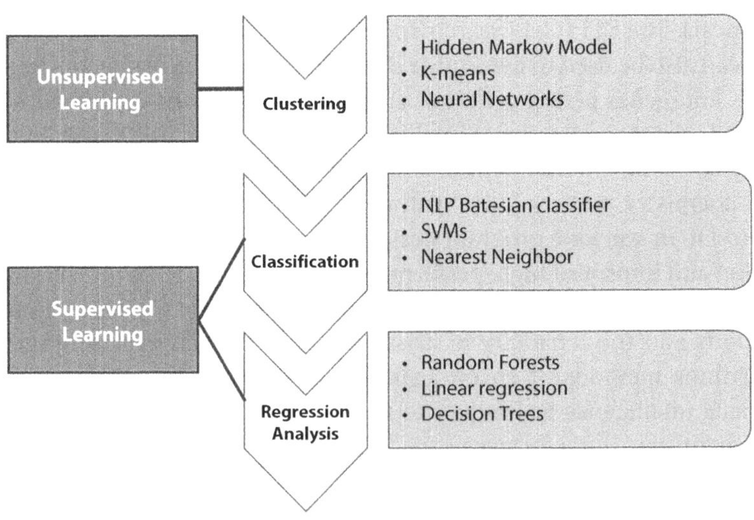

Figure 11.2 Machine learning category.

learning methods and emphasizes generalities. While theoretical analysis provides a means of exploring space for possible learning methods, it still has a task-oriented approach to testing and improving system performance. By creating and testing applied learning systems, algorithms can be obtained with good accuracy to conclude the input data process. In this method, according to the input data in the space of learning systems, it has the potential to explore, creating a centralized space for a better understanding of the relationship between the data [38, 39]. There are three categories of machine learning (Figure 11.2)

11.4.1 Supervised Machine Learning

Supervised machine learning: Supervised machine learning refers to using labeled datasets to achieve algorithms to classify data or accurately predict results. When input enters the model, it adjusts the weights using the reinforcement learning process to perfectly fit it. Many kinds of real-world problems are solved by this method. Classification and regression are two essential issues in supervised learning:

- → **Classification:** categorizing and separating data into appropriate categories by employing an algorithm in the classification section. These data are formed in a given dataset and labeled by classification.
- → **Regression:** Regression has been used to figure out the dependent and independent variables' relationship. Typical algorithms for supervised learning are SVM, KNN[1], random forest, decision trees, linear regression, Naive Bayesian classifier, and polynomial and logistical regression [40].

11.4.2 Unsupervised Machine Learning

Unsupervised machine learning: In Unsupervised learning, the input variable is accessible, without corresponding output variables. Its primary purpose is to learn more information by realizing distribution grouped in relation and clustering [41]. Clustering and association are two methods in unsupervised machine learning. In the first one, data are grouped depending on a particular pattern of behavior for a clustering problem. In the last one, rules are discovered to describe a large part of data for communication.

---

[1]K-nearest neighbor

11.5 Reinforcement Machine Learning

In a given task, the model concludes what to do without the date while the educational data is the answer key in supervised learning. In reinforcement learning, the model learns from its experience in the absence of educational data. Positive and negative are two types of reinforcement learning. An increment in the strength and frequency of a particular behavior is an event that occurs as positive reinforcement learning. Maximizing the performance and keeping the changes for longer are its advantages.

Stopping a harmful condition to strengthen the behavior is applied by another type of reinforcement called negative reinforcement learning. Its benefit is increasing model behavior.

The first step in learning a machine is to prepare an educational data set. The training data set is retained from the collection of the data on which the model is run. On some occasions, information is labeled with attributes and classifications, and sometimes without labels, where the model is forced to, it extracts those attributes and performs the category lonely. In either case, preparation of the training dataset is necessary. Choosing an algorithm to start the dataset is known as the next step of the machine learning implementation. A set of statistical measures makes up an algorithm. Depending on labeled or unlabeled data, various algorithms are formed. For labeled data, there are some algorithms that include decision trees, regression, and sample-based algorithms. For instance, there are some algorithms such as communication algorithms, clustering algorithms, and neural networks for unlabeled data. Comparison between the generated outputs with the actual results, and variables running repetition, are known as the next step is to train the algorithm by adjusting the weights. By this procedure, the correct results are achieved in typical [42].

11.6 AI Application in Drug Design

This section examines several programs based on the artificial intelligence used in the drug discovery procedure. Activity is a protein structure that is considered as an application in drug design. The cause of protein dysfunction can be side effects in the collision of the drug in the human body. Structure-based drug design strategies to create a distinctive structure of small protein molecules are used to achieve a goal by overcoming a specific patient. The protein structure is three-dimensional, predicts a new structure, and needs time and knowledge to organize the collected data.

However, for example, more accurate new predictions in 3D design are complex. The use of deep learning tools has improved the process of predicting the secondary structure of the protein. Information on the relationship between protein structures can be obtained by studying existing data on similar structures. The next goal is to predict the structure of three-dimensional proteins using deep learning techniques to increase accuracy. Many researchers have paid attention to research on the PPI interface to recovery information from the pharmacological plan of the protein-protein computer structure. Artificial intelligence has been employed to forecast drug-protein interactions, detect drug effects, and ensure the safety of biomarkers [16].

11.7 Machine Learning Methods Used in Drug Discovery

ML approaches have a priority due to the power of accurate analysis in the input data. Deep learning methods automatically extract various features very quickly from existing raw data because, in this method, all data is categorized in different layers. Each layer, according to the existing algorithm, checks its accuracy with the top layer. This method is performed simultaneously. Deep learning methods have a small number of generalized errors that lead to more accurate results. RNN, CNN, Auto Encoder, RBN, and DNN are considered different DL algorithms. Several popular models such as random forest (RF), SVM, DP, and multilayer perception (MLP) are employed in drug discovery practical application [29, 43].

11.7.1 Support Vector Machines

A support vector machines (SVM) model is a supervised learning algorithm that predicts class-labeled data, like binary data. The various cores of SVM are widely assisted in drug discovery. This method was used for the quantification of anti-cancer drugs by the characteristics of cancer cells. The SVM version is supervised, gaining knowledge of a set of rules used to predict information. For instance, the SVM approach was utilized to quantify anti-most cancers drugs based totally on the traits of most cancer cells. Twenty-four tablets were examined on most cancers cell traces to find the connection between most cancers' cellular properties and drug resistance. In treating this disease, the SVM-RBF (radial basis function) technique has been used to discover therapeutic compounds from an intensive set of trendy databases. RBF is a prominent center feature used in diverse gaining knowledge of algorithms. The SVM approach works higher than other techniques. As the objective protein is identified, one can detect the proper combination for it. This method is mainly used for the prediction of the outcome of targeted drugs.

Unlike other ANNs, SVM verified the capability to test the similarity prediction of drugs in many compounds. Based on the reports of descriptors, the SVM model can predict enzyme inhibitory quality better for conventional QSAR [40, 44].

11.7.2 Random Forest

As the name of the random forest algorithm says: "This method does not use all the data for analysis". The random forest algorithm has the advantage of the more suitable for regression and classification problems. In regression and classification methods, the need for input data is not excessive [45].

11.7.3 Multilayer Perception (MLP)

MLP model is also known as a leading neural network. The MLP provides a result based on the set of input data. The backpropagation method is used to teach information data. This model is similar to a guide diagram for finding a suitable algorithm because the nature of multiple layers as input and output nodes is related to weights. After processing the data, it can determine the weight for analyzing any data connected to the network and reports the degree of compliance. In this way, the actual output errors can be compared with the expected result. In general, MLP can be used very easily and quickly [46].

11.8 Deep Learning (DL)

One section of ML is deep learning (DL), by which more levels of features can be extracted using multiple layers of input data. Generally, deep learning is similar to the neural network architecture consisting of different layers, and data can be deformed through them. Another structure in neural networks is the integration layer. By the integration of layers, the spatial size of the display can be reduced, and consequently, the system boundary calculations and measurements and work independently on each feature (channel) map would be reduced. The final goal for maximizing the number of combined layers in different networks is that the features after testing an input structure would be effectively detected in this situation and over-fitting would be prevented.

The DNN architecture follows the results in a mathematical model that can find up to a linear or nonlinear matching relation. In DNN, each mathematical model is considered as a layer. The network was therefore labeled "deep." In QSAR modeling, DL models are automatically represented to recovery chemical characters [44, 47].

11.9 Drug Design Applications

They are classified according to the function of ML in medicine, and their applications such as target identification, impact detection, and lead optimization techniques and effect are discussed. Drug design methods are based on databases from various ML algorithms. In most drug design processes, ML methods decrease time consumption and increase accuracy [48, 49].

Before prescribing a drug in the human body, it is essential to identify a metabolic site for any new chemical or drug organism. Therefore, preclinical studies to predict drug metabolism can be performed using animal models. There are several modules for predicting metabolism. One of them is ADMET predictor, a simulation tool that relies on artificial intelligence algorithms. This tool was used to calculate the dose, toxicity, and other side effects [50].

One of the primary bases for evaluating the safety parameters of drugs with new combinations is predicting skin sensitivity. For this purpose, artificial intelligence models, such as MACCS (RF_MACCS) based on forest and SVM algorithms (SVM_PaDEL) based on machine learning have approximately 1400 ligands related to the sensory information of trained nodes [38].

11.10 Drug Discovery Problems

Several experts should review all methods and algorithms in developing and discovering drugs in invalidation, computational pathology, and identification, of biomarkers [23].

According to the available data, once the causative agent has been searched for that purpose, it can be side the target identification. However, trying to validate goals for successful projects must be considered.

Conditions include metabolic, transcriptomic, proteomic profiles present in the patient's clinical material. The use of clinical databases makes it possible to reuse data through public databases, initial identification, and target validation [22, 25].

Identifying the correlation between disease and purpose is the first step in starting drug design. Using ML approaches, predictions can be determined based on the characteristics, causes, and goals that motivate the goals. Therefore, several critical parameters in the data learning model, namely finding a path for cellular design, are metabolic pathways. John *et al.* have improved the SVM classification model with genomic details to classify proteins relative to non-pharmacological and pharmacological sites in ovarian and breast cancer [4, 51].

11.10.1 Prognostic Biomarkers

The discovery of biomarkers with drug differentiation and learning about drug mechanisms for patients by ML procedure improves the performance of clinical trials and reduces drug design costs. In clinical trials, it is necessary to use the predicted models in the initial steps and after validating the model, the designed drug should be proposed. Various factors such as model reconstruction, design, data access, and software are essentially identified. The main issue was that ML approaches evaluate community efforts to develop regression and classification models. ML methods in detecting biomarkers have been successful, and still, several issues need to be corrected [52].

11.10.2 Digital Pathology

ML methods combined with immunopathology research help create high-potency medicinal properties to provide thousands of cells related to spatial tissue. This algorithm enables the ability to overcome defective points in nonpathological stages. DL methods have also been reported to show a more real improvement in the diagnosis of tissues and cells in cancerous environments. It provides helpful information to pathologists by giving the algorithm to the input data. The issue of transparency is another challenge of digital pathology. A well-known method is mentioned in the black box in deep learning strategies [53, 54].

11.11 Conclusion

In the pharmaceutical industry, AI technology uses ML science and deep learning techniques. New strategies have been developed to improve drug discovery. ML models can provide information to predict protein structure. Furthermore, DL models could offer chemical structures and QSAR models, which have helpful information such as protein success in clinical trials and compliance with input conditions. Artificial intelligence technology is a decisive step toward improving the organization of input data and extracting information that provides the ability to interpret the relationship between data. The main challenge in this regard is implementing correct deep learning strategies that directly affect the accuracy of information extraction.

This model is used by theoretical and practical frameworks and many parameters during the neural network training course to optimize these models. Innovation in computer science, computing, and pharmaceutical design science has improved the power of predictive decision-making and deep learning algorithms for designing biomolecules and determining treatment side effects and therapeutic benefits. In the design phase of clinical trials, the presence of these models has been successful. Also, by using machine learning in organizing data, more accurate analysis has caused a positive change in medicine. It has significantly reduced the operating cost and time of drug discovery. Hence the motivation pharmaceutical companies in the use of these methods. In the future, drug discovery and development are eagerly awaiting the coverage of all aspects by artificial intelligence technology.

References

1. Yang, S.Y., Pharmacophore modeling and applications in drug discovery: Challenges and recent advances. *Drug Discovery Today*, 15, 444, 2010.
2. Jing, Y., Bian, Y., Hu, Z., Wang, L., Xie, X.Q.S., Deep learning for drug design: An artificial intelligence paradigm for drug discovery in the big data era. *AAPS J.*, 20, 1, 2018.
3. Hughes, J.P., Rees, S., Kalindjian, S.B., Philpott, K.L., Principles of early drug discovery. *Br. J. Pharmacol.*, 162, 1239, 2011.
4. Gershell, L.J. and Atkins, J.H., Brief history of novel drug discovery technologies. *Nat. Rev. Drug Discovery*, 2, 321, 2003.

5. Butler, K.T., Davies, D.W., Cartwright, H., Isayev, O., Walsh, A., Machine learning for molecular and materials science. *Nat.*, 559, 547, 2018.
6. Ramesh, A.N., Kambhampati, C., Monson, J.R., Drew, P.J., Ann., R., Artificial intelligence in medicine. *Coll. Surg. Engl.*, 86, 334, 2004.
7. Kuntz, I.D., Structure-based strategies for drug design and discovery. *Science*, 257, 1078, 1992.
8. Hessler, G. and Baringhaus, K.H., Artificial intelligence in drug design. *Mol.*, 23, 2520, 2018.
9. Moustafa, H., Youssef, A.M., Darwish, N.A., Abou-Kandil, A., II, Eco-friendly polymer composites for green packaging: Future vision and challenges. *Compos. Part B Eng.*, 172, 16, 2019.
10. Negoescu, D.M., Frazier, P., II, Powell, W.B., The knowledge-gradient algorithm for sequencing experiments in drug discovery. *INFORMS J. Comput.*, 23, 346, 2010.
11. Ishibashi, M., Ota, H., Akutsu, N., Umeda, S., Tajika, M., Izumi, J., Kageyama, Y., Technology for removing carbon dioxide from power plant flue gas by the physical adsorption method. *Energy Convers. Manage.*, 37, 929, 1996.
12. Moran, M.S., Heilman, P., Peters, D.P., Holifield Collins, C., Agroecosystem research with big data and a modified scientific method using machine learning concepts. *Ecosphere*, 7, 01493, 2016.
13. Gawehn, E., Hiss, J.A., Brown, J.B., Schneider, G., Advancing drug discovery via GPU-based deep learning. *Expert Opin. Drug Discovery*, 13, 579, 2018.
14. Xu, X., New concepts and approaches for drug discovery based on traditional Chinese medicine. *Drug Discovery Today Technol.*, 3, 247, 2006.
15. Hopfinger, A.J., Computer-assisted drug design. *J. Med. Chem.*, 28, 1133, 2002.
16. Sellwood, M.A., Ahmed, M., Segler, M.H., Brown, N., Artificial intelligence in drug discovery. *Future Med. Chem.*, 10, 17, 102018, 2025.
17. Nassar, A.F., Wisnewski, A.V., Raddassi, K., Progress in automation of mass cytometry barcoding for drug development. *Bioanalysis*, 8, 14, 1429, 2016.
18. Ou-Yang, S.S., Lu, J.Y., Kong, X.Q., Liang, Z.J., Luo, C., Jiang, H., Computational drug discovery. *Acta Pharmacol. Sin.*, 33, 1131, 2012.
19. Schneider, G., Automating drug discovery. *Nat. Rev. Drug Discovery*, 17, 97, 2017.
20. Dickson, M. and Gagnon, J.P., The cost of new drug discovery and development. *Discovery Med.*, 4, 172, 2009.
21. Rao, V.S. and Srinivas, K., Modern drug discovery process: An *in silico* approach. *J. Bioinforma. Seq. Anal.*, 3, 89, 2011.
22. Gibbs, J.B., Mechanism-based target identification and drug discovery in cancer research. *Science*, 287, 1969, 2000.
23. Blundell, T.L., Jhoti, H., Abell, C., High-throughput crystallography for lead discovery in drug design. *Nat. Rev. Drug Discovery*, 1, 45, 2002.
24. Ooms, F., Molecular modeling and computer aided drug design. Examples of their applications in medicinal chemistry. *Curr. Med. Chem.*, 7, 2, 141, 2000.

25. Csermely, P., Agoston, V., Pongor, S., The efficiency of multi-target drugs: The network approach might help drug design. *Trends Pharmacol. Sci.*, 26, 178, 2005.
26. Traxler, P., Bold, G., Buchdunger, E., Caravatti, G., Furet, P., Manley, P., Zimmermann, J., Tyrosine kinase inhibitors: From rational design to clinical trials. *Med. Res. Rev.*, 21, 499, 2001.
27. Johnson, J.R. and Temple, R., Food and Drug Administration requirements for approval of new anticancer drugs. *Cancer Treat. Rep.*, 69, 1155, 1985.
28. Greer, J., Erickson, J.W., Baldwin, J.J., Varney, M.D., Application of the three-dimensional structures of protein target molecules in structure-based drug design. *J. Med. Chem.*, 37, 1035, 1994.
29. Schütt, K.T., Gastegger, M., Tkatchenko, A., Müller, K.R., Maurer, R.J., Unifying machine learning and quantum chemistry with a deep neural network for molecular wavefunctions. *Nat. Commun.*, 10, 1, 2019.
30. Boggara, M.B. and Krishnamoorti, R., Partitioning of nonsteroidal antiinflammatory drugs in lipid membranes: A molecular dynamics simulation study. *Biophys. J.*, 98, 586, 2010.
31. Bai, Q., Tan, S., Xu, T., Liu, H., Huang, J., Yao, X., MolAICal: A soft tool for 3D drug design of protein targets by artificial intelligence and classical algorithm. *Brief. Bioinform.*, 22, 3, 161, 2021.
32. Shen, W., Hu, T., Yin, Y., He, J., Tao, F., Nee, A.Y.C., Digital twin based virtual commissioning for computerized numerical control machine tools, in: *Digital Twin Driven Smart Design*, pp. 289–307, Academic Press, Massachusetts, United States, 2020.
33. Bøgevig, A., Federsel, H.J., Huerta, F., Hutchings, M.G., Kraut, H., Langer, T., Saller, H., Route design in the 21st century: The IC SYNTH software tool as an idea generator for synthesis prediction. *Org. Process Res. Dev.*, 19, 357, 2015.
34. Chowdhury, G.G., Natural language processing. *Annu. Rev. Inf. Sci. Technol.*, 37, 51, 2003.
35. Piñero, J., Queralt-Rosinach, N., Bravo, A., Deu-Pons, J., Bauer-Mehren, A., Baron, M., Furlong, L., II, DisGeNET: A discovery platform for the dynamical exploration of human diseases and their genes. *Database*, 2015, 28, 2015.
36. Kuhn, M., von Mering, C., Campillos, M., Jensen, L.J., Bork, P., STITCH: Interaction networks of chemicals and proteins. *Nucleic Acids Res.*, 36, 684, 2007.
37. Wasser, S.K., Houston, C.S., Koehler, G.M., Cadd, G.G., Fain, S.R., Techniques for application of faecal DNA methods to field studies of Ursids. *Mol. Ecol.*, 6, 1091, 1997.
38. Jordan, M., II and Mitchell, T.M., Machine learning: Trends, perspectives, and prospects. *Science*, 349, 255, 2015.
39. Mahmoudi, A., Asghari, M., Zargar, V., CO2/CH4 separation through a novel commercializable three-phase PEBA/PEG/NaX nanocomposite membrane. *J. Ind. Eng. Chem.*, 23, 238, 2015.

40. Kim, J., II, Kim, B.S., Savarese, S., Comparing image classification methods: K-nearest-neighbor and support-vector-machines, in: *Proceedings of the 6th WSEAS International Conference on Computer Engineering and Applications, and Proceedings of the 2012 American Conference on Applied Mathematics*, vol. 1001, p. 48109, 2012.
41. Gentleman, R. and Carey, V.J., *Unsupervised machine learning. in: Bioconductor Case Studies*, pp. 137–157, Springer, New York, 2008.
42. Kaelbling, L.P., Littman, M.L., Moore, A.W., Reinforcement learning: A survey. *J. Artif. Intell. Res.*, 4, 237, 1996.
43. Stephenson, N., Shane, E., Chase, J., Rowland, J., Ries, D., Justice, N., Cao, R., Survey of machine learning techniques in drug discovery. *Curr. Drug Metab.*, 20, 185, 2019.
44. Gozalbes, R., Doucet, J.P., Derouin, F., Application of topological descriptors in QSAR and drug design: history and new trends. *Curr. Drug Targets - Infect. Disord.*, 2, 93, 2002.
45. Shi, T. and Horvath, S., Unsupervised learning with random forest predictors. *J. Comput. Graph. Stat.*, 15, 118, 2006.
46. Porta, R., Sabbah, M., Di Pierro, P., Biopolymers as food packaging materials. *Int. J. Mol. Sci.*, 21, 4942, 2020.
47. Deng, L., Deep learning: methods and applications. *Found. Trends Signal Process.*, 7, 197, 2014.
48. Verma, J., Khedkar, V.M., Coutinho, E.C., 3D-QSAR in drug design–A review. *Curr. Top. Med. Chem.*, 10, 95, 2010.
49. Piano, S.L., Ethical principles in machine learning and artificial intelligence: cases from the field and possible ways forward. *Humanit. Soc Sci. Commun.*, 7, 1, 2020.
50. Zamora, I., Afzelius, L., Cruciani, G., Predicting drug metabolism: A site of metabolism prediction tool applied to the cytochrome P450 2C9. *J. Med. Chem.*, 46, 2313, 2003.
51. Hussain, M., Wajid, S.K., Elzaart, A., Berbar, M., A comparison of SVM kernel functions for breast cancer detection, in: *2011 Eighth International Conference Computer Graphics, Imaging and Visualization*, pp. 145–150, 2011.
52. Dhanasekaran, S.M., Barrette, T.R., Ghosh, D., Shah, R., Varambally, S., Kurachi, K., Chinnaiyan, A.M., Delineation of prognostic biomarkers in prostate cancer. *Nat.*, 412, 822, 2001.
53. Yao, L.C., Aryee, K.E., Cheng, M., Kaur, P., Keck, J.G., Brehm, M.A., Creation of PDX-bearing humanized mice to study immuno-oncology, in: *Target Identification and Validation in Drug Discovery*, pp. 241–252, Humana Press, New York, NY, 2019.
54. Lavecchia, A., Deep learning in drug discovery: Opportunities, challenges and future prospects. *Drug Discov. Today*, 24, 2017, 2019.

12

Artificial Intelligence for Assessing Side Effects

Aarati Panchbhai

Sharad Pawar Dental College & Hospital, Datta Meghe Institute of Medical Sciences (Deemed to be University), Sawangi-Meghe, Wardha (Maharastra), India

Abstract

Artificial intelligence is the simulation of human intelligence processes by machines; it aims to mimic human cognitive functions. The combination of artificial intelligence and healthcare is bringing wonders to healthcare delivery system. The abundant healthcare data and speedy analytics techniques have made the greater progress in the healthcare field. There can be many applications of artificial intelligence healthcare and biomedical research. Artificial intelligence techniques that can be widely applied to medicine are machine learning, machine vision, and modern deep learning methods. Cardiology, neurology, and oncology could be the domains where artificial intelligence tools can effectively handle the structured or unstructured data. The potential application of artificial intelligence in the field of pharmacology and toxicology to assess the side effects is greatly being researched these days. Anticipating that artificial intelligence may be able to predict side effects of different drug combinations in patients, it will open many avenues for healthcare professionals to prescribe various treatments or enable them to make informed decisions in regard to drug combinations to be prescribed for patients with multiple or complex ailments.

***Keywords*:** Artificial intelligence, side effects, drug, adverse effect

12.1 Introduction

Artificial intelligence leverages computers and machines to mimic the problem-solving and decision-making capabilities of the human mind.

Email: artipanch@gmail.com

Inamuddin, Tariq Altalhi, Jorddy N. Cruz and Moamen Salah El-Deen Refat (eds.) Drug Design Using Machine Learning, (339–350) © 2022 Scrivener Publishing LLC

It is the imitation of human intelligence processes by machines, especially computer systems. Artificial intelligence systems can handle enormous data and analyze it for various applications in terms of its programming embracing three cognitive fields, such as learning, reasoning, and self-correction. Artificial intelligence tools often complete task with few errors and speedily, at times, it can make predictions more accurately than human. Artificial neural networks and deep learning artificial intelligence technologies are quickly evolving. Considering that enormous data are collected in medical colleges routinely, the input of this data can turn into actions to be performed. Strong artificial intelligence is capable of imitating the cognitive abilities of the human brain using fuzzy logic to have various applications. The various categories of artificial intelligence initiated with the system of intelligence has now reached to the system with self-awareness and consciousness. The technologies of machine learning and machine vision can have wide applications in health care filed [1–3].

12.2 Background

The role of artificial intelligence is identified first in early as the 1950s; with the idea that computer-aided programs can be used to perk up the diagnosis. Drug reactions that are adversely affecting the body is the area which is largely being focused upon. Artificial intelligence using a range of tools and networks may act as the imitator for human intelligence; it can be applied to various types of healthcare data with extended scope for human functions to be performed by this approach [1–9]. The availability of enormous amount of digital data made is mandatory to use the machine for assistance. Artificial intelligence that imitate human acts, such as adaptation, thought, understanding, engagement, and deep learning. It utilizes software and computational technologies to interpret input data to make decisions. The advancement in artificial intelligence has revealed its potential applications towards healthcare fields. It may be anticipated that some of the activities performed by healthcare professionals may be left to the tools used for artificial intelligence [10–12]. The combination of healthcare and artificial intelligence may open up possibilities for improved, efficient, economic, and accessible healthcare. Artificial intelligence necessitates the knowledge and skills to handle, manage, and interpret the given data. The research work is being done to explore the possible role of artificial intelligence in healthcare. The various domains of healthcare where it can have applications would be patient data and diagnostics, health services management, clinical decision making and diagnosis. Additionally, it may have a role in predictive medicine customizing treatment paths and predicting the spread of diseases [1, 2].

12.3 Traditional Approach to Pharmacovigilance and Its Limitations

Conventional approaches to estimate the toxicity profiles were based on human effort, manpower and were time-consuming, the implementation of computational technology speed up the work. The time-consuming labor intensive ways have halted the progress. Besides, the diversity among the patients and polypharmacy has put forth the challenges in regard to safety of a drug. The artificial intelligence with computational alternatives envisaged to fasten the work [14, 16, 17]. Initially, the targets were sought through receptors in relation to their ligands; however, nowadays, the means have become more systematic and sophisticated using the methods of relating targets by their ligands. Artificial intelligence techniques that can be widely applied to pharmacology are machine learning, machine vision, and modern deep learning methods [18].

12.4 Role of Artificial Intelligence in Pharmacological Profiling for Safety Assessment

When a new drug or drug combinations need to be introduced, it is essential that pharmacological profiling be done which necessitates the evaluation of the functional effects of new drug on various body systems, which will help in its selection and safety assessment. Pharmacovigilance is the science to study the drug monitoring, and its side effects or adverse drug reactions. The pharmacodynamic safety of a newly introduced molecule is the prime concern [7, 17]. The goal should be the introduction of data collection using more sophisticated and refined technologies, evaluation of new therapeutic targets with uncertain toxicities, and utilization of transgenic animal models to explore novel targets of toxicity. Pharmacological toxicity may be defined as pharmacological activity of a new agent or drug that would be undesirable as well as that is both unintended. The range of toxicities disclosed includes a multiplicity of or physiological or functional effects that are usually reversible; rarely may they be life-threatening. The safety profile and pharmacological toxicity of newly introduced drug can be determined by drug dose, types of reactions, nature of the effects, therapeutic margin of safety and risk-to-benefit ratio. It is essential to do the pharmacological profiling of drug as it facilitates the selection of new drug with reduced toxic potential, the design and conduct of preclinical toxicology studies, the investigation of preclinical and clinical safety issues, and the identification and monitoring of potential functional effects of the drug. Lately, there has been a rise in data digitalization in the pharmaceutical sector [7, 11, 17, 19–26].

12.5 Artificial Intelligence for Assessing Side Effects

The application of artificial intelligence to pharmacology is the emerging science especially to the field of toxicology to assess the side effects. The drugs given to the patient can result in detrimental side effects and thus requires careful monitoring once inserted into the body. Drug safety is a matter of grave concern due to the lack of systematic and reproducible method of assessment. It is hypothesized that artificial Intelligence may predict side effects of drug combinations. It enables the healthcare professional to make informed decisions before prescribing combinations of drugs to patients, for the treatment of complex or multiple diseases. Huge numbers of people around the world take two or more medications daily. The concern behind this is that a single drug taken by the patient may have many side effects and the combination of drugs may have side effects in multiple combinations or patterns, which are very difficult to assess based on investigation. So here the computational interventions based on artificial intelligence will come into play [7, 9, 13, 19, 20].

The various tools of artificial intelligence are identified to have specificity and sensitivity in prediction of drug toxicity. The identified network should encompass the biological organization of a patient from gene to mRNA to protein and the components involved in determining drug toxicity. The advances in artificial intelligence tools and models may render the development of integrated systems pharmacology-based prediction of drug safety [2, 11, 16]. Rao *et al.* configured the new computer aided approach to predict off-Target Interactions for small Molecules. The side effect or adverse effects are result of these off-target interactions in which the drug molecules interact at target that are not predicted or assumed. Early recognition of such off-target interactions novel computational approach may decrease the safety-related attrition. Under polypharmacology, the interaction of the drug with protein molecules or a drug molecule with multiple receptors producing off-target adverse effects can be assessed [7, 9, 13, 15, 17, 23]. Off-Target Safety Assessment involves the computational process to foresee pharmacological activities for an assortment of 857 drugs. Nowadays, new drug leads are revealed characterizing the targets determining their function and structure thus relating targets by their ligands. This suggested the bases for their side effects and molecular targets underlying phenotypic screens [18]. Target identification for bioactive molecules may facilitate the understanding of drug repurposing, mode of action of drugs and their side effects. By screening a compound against a protein database, it is possible to identify potential target candidates that fit with this specific compound. Notably, the ligand based target prediction methods have marked by substantial progress in the given sector [14]. The unintended off targets are widely associated with adverse drug reactions; here the recognized side effects and ligand chemistry are utilized to organize drugs into networks by similarities among the profiles [2, 11, 16, 27–30].

Tools, Models and Networks for Assessing Side Effects [9–11, 16–20, 31–39].

- human Ether-à-go-go-Related Gene (hERG) and Pred-hERG
- chemTox, Deepchem
- ProTox, DeepTox
- Tox21 Data Challenge 2014
- LimTox, pkCSM, admetSAR, and Toxtree
- TOPKAT (Toxicity Prediction by Komputer Assisted Technology,
- *e*ToxPred, hitdexto
- TargeTox and PrOCTOR
- Deep neuralnet, QSAR, organic, potentianet, deltavinna, neural graph fingerprint, AlphaFold, Chemputer
- Deep neural networks, elastic nets
- Random forests, support vector machines

The available tools, models, and networks for artificial intelligence (Tables 12.1 and 12.2) have various modes of handling and operating healthcare data provided as an input which would be processed to give desired output. Artificial intelligence involves several domains, such as machine learning and deep learning linked to artificial neural networks consisting of set of interconnected computing elements to act similar to human brain that converts input to output using various algorithms. It is cumbersome to discover the relevant therapeutic targets or unintended off-targets for drug-like molecules, to estimate adverse drug reactions by means of experiment or researches, hence it is highly recommended to have computational approach to perform the work of detecting potential targets of drug

Table 12.1 Tools, models and networks for artificial intelligence.

	Modes for artificial intelligence
Tools	chemTox, Deepchem ProTox, DeepTox LimTox, pkCSM, admetSAR, Toxtree *e*ToxPred, hitdexto TargeTox, PrOCTOR QSAR, organic, deltavinna,
Models	TOPKAT (Toxicity Prediction by Komputer Assisted Technology, Tox21 Data Challenge 2014 Random for Neural graph fingerprint, AlphaFold, Chemputer nests, support vector machines

Table 12.2 Networks for artificial intelligence.

Sn	**Networks**
1	Deep neural networks (DNN)
2	Elastic nets, potentianet
3	Remote neural networks
4	gene regulatory networks (GRNs)
5	Counter-propagation networks
6	Deep Belief Network (DBN)
7	Deep convolutional neural networks (CNNs)
8	Time Series Network Identification (TSNI)
9	and Dose-Time Network Identification (DTNI)

interaction quickly. TarPred, is considered as newly launched computational model which can detect the targets of interaction more precisely, it is based on a reference library containing 533 individual targets with 179,807 active ligands. TarPred is known to receive interactive graphical input or input in the chemical file format [23].

Several web-based tools, such as pkCSM, LimTox, Toxtree, admetSAR, etc, are available. The Tox21 Data Challenge was arranged with a purpose to appraise the computational techniques using DeepTox to forecast the toxicity of various drug, as well as the available compounds in nature. Models in DeepTox are combined to determine the toxicity of novel drug or compounds. *e*ToxPred prepared through machine learning method uses molecular fingerprints of chemical compounds to estimate toxicity with accuracy of around 72%. It is said to be useful handling heterogeneous datasets. The TargeTox and PrOCTOR are beneficial tools to predict toxicity by generating protein network data. Harboring random forests models PrOCTOR deals with molecular characteristics, drug-likeliness properties, target-based features, and protein targets. The toxicity prediction is the vital arm of modern computer-assisted drug delivery system. For example, a group of drugs can induce lethal cardiac arrhythmia due to blockage of the human Ether-à-go-go-Related Gene (hERG) potassium ion channels, hence detection of putative hERG blockers should be done to predict cardiotoxicity, the Pred-hERG has characteristics that guides the quantitatively structured alternative relationship models of the blockage of hERG [11, 16, 17, 19, 22].

The chemTox use parameters, such as lethality and mutagenicity, to determine toxicity using molecular descriptors to make quantitative-structure property relationships models as similar to ProTox. ProTox also evaluates possible targets linked to toxicity mechanisms and adverse drug reactions based on protein-ligand pharmacophores. It is known to perform better than the TOPKAT, the toxicity prediction computer assisted technology. It appeared that ET-based classifier employing molecular fingerprints would forecast even specific toxicities as carcinogenicity potency, acute oral toxicity, cardiotoxicity and endocrine disruption [11, 16, 17, 22].

Decagon, a novel artificial intelligence system to foresee side effects of diverse drug combinations, enables physicians to prescribe various treatments. When more than 2 drugs are taken, there can be possibility of unknown sequences. It is known that the side effects occur due to the drug actions various proteins in the body, consequently, the way the varied drugs affect the body proteins and how the many proteins in the body interact are being explored. Using model of deep learning of artificial intelligence complex data is derived establishing the patterns. Decagon, the innovative system, is still under exploration so as to be precise and user-friendly. Nonetheless, Decagon may prove to be more efficient predicting the patterns of drug interactions and side effects [13].

The broad-spectrum profiling of drug safety can be done using various complex network. The advanced machine learning model for safety assessment uses the multilayer drug-gene-adverse drug reaction interaction network. Network biology along with bioinformatics handles the available biological and chemical data. It can be used at several levels of complexity and provides improved knowledge of a drug's safety profile. Utilization of network biology in drug discovery may render a novel way to augment drug efficacy and lessen adverse drug effects through molecule and protein's function collectively. The network-based computational methods provides to explore the drug action across multiple scales of complexity in relation to human body to have improved perspective towards effect of chemicals in human health.[16] Various network explorers are MLP, ADALINE, RNNs, gene regulatory networks (GRNs), CNNs, Kohonen, RBF, LVQ, counterpropagation networks, and Deep Belief Network (DBN) etc. [9, 11, 12, 17]. Deep convolutional neural networks (CNNs) are a class of DL networks that learn representations of raw images from pixel information as a hierarchy of images from which features can be extracted and used to classify complex patterns [17]. The Deep Belief Network (DBN) is a probabilistic model provides platform for the visible layer for the subsequent sub-network. Because the gene regulatory networks are known to evolve over a time, the repeated measurement of expression of gene at several points will offer valuable data in regards to the adverse effects of compounds. Time Series Network Identification (TSNI) and Dose-Time Network Identification (DTNI) are the additional tools to serve the desired purposes towards assessment of side effects. It is observed that Dose-Time Network Identification functions better than Time Series Network Identification in inferring toxicant-induced gene regulatory networks. it is also revealed that Dose-Time Network Identification provides in detail information about the action of compounds, such as potential molecular initiating events and various unfamiliar interactions which otherwise need to have to be confirmed [9, 11, 12, 17].

It is revealed that use of KinomeX, an artificial intelligence-based medium using Deep neural networks for the detection of polypharmacology of kinases can be beneficial. Thus, it has potential to explore drug selectivity toward the kinase family and subfamilies. It provides the accurate guesses for primary targets and off-targets. The cyclica's cloud-based proteome-screening artificial intelligence platform can interact at molecular level to generate off-target interactions to facilitate acquaintance to the probable adverse drug effects [11, 35–37].

Several factors add to the failure of novel pharmaceuticals, one of the most important being its adverse effects or side effects. Early identification of off-target compound activity in advanced will help to curtail safety-related attrition. In vitro profiling of drug against targets has profound role in selection of compound; it aids to screen Roche small molecules produced across a diverse range of therapeutic targets. A Roche panel basically helps in external screening; it provides a commercial screening panel for assessing many safety-relevant targets along with indiscriminate compound mixtures [38, 39].

12.6 Conclusion

Although artificial intelligence is considered as an emerging field, the speedy progress in automation can be anticipated to alter working in pharmaceutical industry. Practicing artificial intelligence necessitates the skills and awareness for data-intensive analysis and knowledge-based management. Artificial intelligence applications can deal with the vast amount of data produced in healthcare sector and find new information that would otherwise remain unattended, thus, it is gradually changing medical practice. Although, definite challenges remain to be addressed; nonetheless, artificial intelligence will become very useful tool in the pharmaceutical industry shortly. The brighter and smarter future can be envisaged using artificial intelligence guided new scientific accomplishments in the field of pharmacovigilence.

References

1. Mrinmoy, R. and Jamwal, M., An overview of artificial intelligence (AI) intervention in Indian healthcare system. *Int. J. Sci. Res.*, 1217, 9, 2016.
2. Secinaro, Davide, C., Aurelio, S., Vivek, M., Paolo, B., The role of artificial intelligence in healthcare: A structured literature review. *BMC Med. Inform. Decis. Mak.*, 125, 21, 2021.
3. Gomez-Gonzalez E, Gomez E, Marquez-Rivas *et al.*, Artificial intelligence in medicine and healthcare: A review and classification of current and near-future applications and their ethical and social impact, arXiv:2001.09778, 2020, https://doi.org/10.48550/arXiv.2001.09778.
4. Murali, N. and Sivakumaran, N., Artificial intelligence in health care. *Int. J. Modern Comput., Informat. Commun. Technol.*, 1, 103, 2018.
5. Rong B., Mendez A., Assi E. B., Zhao., B., Sawan., M., Artificial intelligence in healthcare: Review and prediction case studies. *Engineering.*, 291, 6, 2020.
6. Jiang, F., Jiang, Y., Zhi, H., Dong, Y., Li, H., Ma, S. *et al.*, Artificial intelligence in healthcare: Past, present and future. *BMJ*, Stroke Vascular Neurology 2017, 0:e000101, 1-12. http://dx.doi.org/10.1136/svn-2017-000101.
7. Bass, A.S., Hombo, T., Kasai, C., Kinter, L.B., Valentin, J.P., Bass, A.S., A historical view and vision into the future of the field of safety pharmacology. *Handb. Exp. Pharmacol.*, 45, 229, 2015.

8. Hassanzadehetal, P., Atyabi, F., Dinarvand, R., Significance of artificial intelligence in drug delivery. *Adv. Drug Delivery Rev.*, 2019, 151-152, 169-190. doi: 10.1016/j.addr.2019.05.001.
9. Rao, M.S., Gupta, R., Liguori, M.J., Hu, M., Huang, X., Mantena, S.R., Mittelstadt, S.W., Blomme, E.A.G., Van Vleet, T.R., Novel computational approach to predict off-target interactions for small molecules. *Front. Big Data*, 17, 25, 2019.
10. Feng, Q. and Padme, A deep learning-based framework for drug–target interaction prediction. *Computer Sci.*, arXiv. 2018. arXiv: 1807.09741, 1-29. https://doi.org/10.48550/arXiv.1807.09741.
11. Paul, D., Sanap, G., Shenoy., S., Kalyane, D., Kalia, K., Tekade., R., Artificial intelligence in drug discovery and development. *Drug Discovery Today*, 26, 80, 2021.
12. Karimi, M., Deep Affinity: Interpretable deep learning of compound–protein affinity through unified recurrent and convolutional neural networks. *Bioinformatics*, 3329, 35, 2019.
13. Farooq, I., Leskovec, J., Marinka, Z., A.I., Monica, Artificial intelligence may predict side effects of drug combinations. *Eur. Pharm. Rev.*, 17, 7, 2018.
14. Yang, X., Concepts of artificial intelligence for computer-assisted drug discovery. *Chem. Rev.*, 1052, 119, 2019.
15. Muthas, D. and Boyer, S., Exploiting Pharmacological Similarity to Identify Safety Concerns - Listen to What the Data Tells You. *Mol. Inform.*, 32, 37, 2013.
16. Pu, L., eToxPred: A machine learning-based approach to estimate the toxicity of drug candidates. *BMC Pharmacol. Toxicol.*, 20, 2, 2019.
17. Basile, A.O., Yahi, A., Tatonetti, N.P., Artificial intelligence for drug toxicity and safety. *Trends Pharmacol. Sci.*, 2019, HYPERLINK "https://www.ncbi.nlm.nih.gov/entrez/eutils/elink.fcgi?dbfrom=pubmed&retmode=ref&cmd=prlinks&id=31383376" \t "_blank", 40, 9, 624–635.
18. Keiser, M., Irwin, J., Schoichet, K., Chemical basis of pharmacology. *Biochem.*, 49, 48, 2010.
19. Hamon, J., Whitebread, S., Techer-Etienne, V., Le Coq, H., Azzaoui, K., Urban, L., *In vitro* safety pharmacology profiling: What else beyond hERG? *Future Med. Chem.*, 645, 1, 2009.
20. Williams, P., The role of pharmacological profiling in safety assessment. *Regul. Toxicol. Pharmacol.*, 12, 238, 1990.
21. Valentin, J.P., Bass, A.S., Atrakchi, A., Olejniczak, K., Kannosuke, F., Challenges and lessons learned since implementation of the safety pharmacology guidance ICH S7A. *J. Pharmacol. Toxicol. Methods*, 52, 22, 2005.
22. Pugsley, M.K., Curtis, M.J., Pugsley, M.K. *et al.*, Safety pharmacology in focus: New methods developed in the light of the ICH S7B guidance document. *Pharmacol. Toxicol. Methods*, 54, 94, 2006.

23. Gao, K., Interpretable drug target prediction using deep neural representation. in: *Proceedings of the Twenty-Seventh International Joint Conference on Artificial Intelligence (IJCAI)*, Lang Jérôme (ed.), pp. 3371-77, 2018.
24. Yu, H., A systematic prediction of multiple drug–target interactions from chemical, genomic, and pharmacological data. *PloS One*, e37608, 7, 2012.
25. Lusci, A., Deep architectures and deep learning in chemo informatics: The prediction of aqueous solubility for drug-like molecules. *J. Chem. Inf. Model.*, 1563, 53, 2013.
26. Lysenko, A., An integrative machine learning approach for prediction of toxicity-related drug safety. *Life Sci. Alliance.*, 1, 5, 2018.
27. Singh, S., Preclinical pharmacokinetics: an approach towards safer and efficacious drugs. *Curr. Drug Metab.*, 165, 7, 2006.
28. Lounkine, E., Large-scale prediction and testing of drug activity on side-effect targets. *Nature*, 486, 361, 2012.
29. Thafar, M., Comparison study of computational prediction tools for drug–target binding affinities. *Front. Chem.*, 7, 1-19, 2019.
30. Mahmud, S., iDTi-CSsmoteB: identification of drug–target interaction based on drug chemical structure and protein sequence using XGBoost with over-sampling technique SMOTE. *IEEE Access*, 48699, 7, 2019.
31. Mayr, A., eepTox: toxicity prediction using deep learning. *Front. Environ. Sci.*, 3, 80, 2016.
32. Zeng, J., Deep learning with feature embedding for compound–protein interaction prediction. bioRxiv 2016, 16, 6, 1-20, doi: https://doi.org/10.1101/086033.
33. Koromina, M., Rethinking drug repositioning and development with artificial intelligence, machine learning, and omics. *Omics*, 539, 23, 2019.
34. Wang, F., Computational screening for active compounds targeting protein sequences: Methodology and experimental validation. *J. Chem. Inf. Model.*, 282, 51, 2011.
35. Li, Z., KinomeX: A web application for predicting kinome-wide polypharmacology effect of small molecules. *Bioinformatics*, 5354, 35, 2019.
36. Cyclica., C., Cyclica launches ligand Express™, a disruptive cloud–based platform to revolutionize drug discovery, Cyclica 2017, https://www.cyclicarx.com/press-releases, 20171130005015.
37. Xiao, X., iDrug-Target: predicting the interactions between drug compounds and target proteins in cellular networking via benchmark dataset optimization approach. *J. Biomol. Struct. Dyn.*, 2221, 33, 2015.
38. Peters, J.U., Schnider, P., Mattei, P., Kansy, M., Pharmacological promiscuity: Dependence on compound properties and target specificity in a set of recent Roche compounds. *Chem. Med. Chem.*, 680, 4, 2009.
39. Bendels, K., Caterina, B., Bernhard, F., Grégori, G., Wolfgang, G., Kansy, M. *et al.*, Safety screening in early drug discovery: An optimized assay panel. *Pharmacol. Toxicol. Methods*, 106609, 99, 2019.

Index

Printed and bound by CPI Group (UK) Ltd, Croydon, CR0 4YY

17/09/2026

14964276-0004